MW00461055

PUBLISHING

DR. SIEGFRIED MERYN
DR. MARKUS METKA
GEORG KINDEL

MEN'S HEALTH

& THE HORMONE REVOLUTION

NDE Publishing
2000

Men's Health and the Hormone Revolution

By **Dr. Siegfried Meryn, Dr. Markus Metka and Georg Kindel**

Translator: **Warner Patels**

Editor: **Earl Warhus**

Illustrator: **Eduard Gurevich**

Desktop Publishing and Typesetting:
Natalie Romashkin and Aidyn Ismailov

Original title: **DER MANN 2000**
Copyright © 1999 by Verlag Carl Ueberreuter, Vienna, Austria
Copyright © 2000 NDE Canada Corp. for North American English Language Edition
Paperback Edition

Vladimir Mazour, President and Publisher
NDE Publishing*, 15-30 Wertheim Court, Richmond Hill, Ontario
Canada   L4B 1B9   tel (905) 731-1288 fax (905) 731-5744
www.ndepublishing.com

Canadian Cataloguing-in-Publication Data

Meryn, Siegfried
      Men's health & the hormone revolution

    1. Middle aged men–Health and hygiene. 2. Aging–Endocrine aspects. 3. Climacteric, Male. I. Metka, Markus II. Kindel, Georg III. Title. IV. Title: Men's health. V. Title: Men's health and the hormone revolution.
RM288.M47 2000   613'.04234   C00-900710-5
ISBN 1-55321-103-0

Printed in Canada

* *NDE Canada Corp., a member of NDE Group of Companies*

Contents

Contents

Contents

The Right Nutrition 121

The First Step Toward a Healthy Lifestyle

Fit for Life 140

More Power for the Male Body

Contents

Mental Fitness   153
How To Use Your Brain Power

How To Beat Stress   171
Strategies Against the Epidemic of the Third Millennium

Contents

Contents

Foreword

Growing old is a triumph, a victory of human willpower and endurance, and a tribute to technological progress. Today, on the cusp of the third millennium, the challenge of prolonging the human life span is spawning all sorts of developments.

How can we apply new and existing technologies to filling that ever-increasing span of human life with more quality? A rapidly expanding, and aging, world population is essentially a new development in human history. Due to greater life expectancy and a drastically declining fertility rate, the proportion of people over the age of 65 is expected to climb by an estimated 82% in the next 25 years, while the birthrate may increase by only 3%. By the year 2050, according to the United Nations, the number of people over 60 years of age will exceed the number of people under 15 for the first time ever. What is more, according to this forecast, 13 countries will have over 10% of the world's people over 80 years of age.

The next 25 years will see the number of older people rise by 82%

The last century marked great progress in the lengthening of the human life span. We had the satisfaction of seeing our life expectancy increase by more than 50% over 100 years. The development of antibiotics and inoculations, better drinking water, and improved sanitation and hygiene have greatly extended our lives to the point where acute illnesses are no longer the primary cause of death. Today, people die more from chronic and degenerative diseases, metastasizing cancer, weakened immune systems, and other conditions with extended periods of incapacitation, immobility and dependency. To die from one of these causes is a long, drawn out, painful and expensive process.

This past century has been marked by a huge increase the human life span

Despite enormous medical progress in the past decades, we spend about 25% of our life after the age of 65 suffering from physical ailments. The last years of our life are often characterized by one impairment after another. "Health expectancy" needs as much attention from researchers as does life expectancy. Health authorities should be encouraged to publish data on both health and life expectancy. Otherwise, frailty, disability and dependency will create an intolerable burden on the welfare and health care systems of the future.

Health expectancy will have to improve along with life expectancy

With the high cost of these services, the health and welfare infrastructure, as well as the political infrastructure, will be strained to the limit. This will be true not only of second- and third world countries, but also of the industrialized world. Not having to depend on others for help and being free of any disabilities lends dignity to the aging process. Preventing or drastically reducing the incidence of disease and disability, and promoting healthy living in older people must play a central role in health and welfare policies in the new century. These measures will also go a long way toward reducing the overall cost of health care.

The goal has got to be aging with dignity and without disabilities

Key to this strategy will be our attitudes toward aging. Effectively implemented, promoting healthy living and preventive maintenance could significantly reduce welfare and health care costs. Pain and suffering would be significantly reduced, and the quality of life for older people would rise, enabling them to remain productive and contributing members of society.

Men experience a gradual decline in their hormone levels

In past years, discussions have largely revolved around the health and social position of women, and deservedly so. However, health issues specific to men have generally been ignored. Men still have a higher rate of disease and mortality than women, and their life expectancy remains significantly lower in many parts of the world. The effects of disease and society's attitudes toward them indicate a gender bias. As a result, diseases are often treated differently in men and women, and their access to preventive care is managed in quite different ways.

Health issues specific to men have so far been neglected

As they grow older, women experience a rapid decrease in the production of sexual hormones and they stop menstruating. With men, the decline in the number of hormones produced by the body is slow and gradual, but their ability to reproduce does not fade as they advance in years.

As men grow older, hormonal changes and the slowing of endocrine functions in the body result in the production of fewer hormones by the peripheral endocrine glands and lead to changes in the "central control system" of hormone production.

In the course of aging, the levels of testosterone, DHEA (dehydroepiandrosterone), the growth hormone, IGF-1, and melatonin gradually decrease. Moreover, the SHBG (sex hormone-binding globulin) level rises, which further reduces the concentration of free, biologically active androgens. However, since the Leydig cells in the testicles remain functional throughout the aging process, there is no "andropause" in the strict sense of the word. Still, a growing number of books and scientific articles support the view that most men experience a real decrease in gonadal and adrenal androgens as well as a diminished production of the growth hormone when they reach about 50 years of age, and this leads to partial hormonal deficits.

The "partial endocrine deficiency syndrome" in the aging male (PEDAM), or andropause, has come to be associated with a wide range of symptoms: a decline in general well-being; a loss of body hair, libido and cognitive functions; a decreased cell volume in erythrocytes; diminished muscular strength; the occurrence of osteoporosis; a weakened immune system; an increase in the fat mass, accompanied by changes in the content and distribution of body fat; and a rise in cardiovascular disease. In the aging male, the secretion of melatonin is also diminished, and its circadian regularity (the continuity of the day-night rhythmic cycles, with the hormone being produced mostly at night) appears to be impaired. Older men experience a shallow sleep characterized by frequent interruptions. These changes primarily affect the production of growth hormones, which happens during deep-sleep phases. It has been shown that the decline in the production of melatonin and changes in the circadian rhythmic cycles in older men are accompanied by mood swings, reduced cognitive skills and an increase in sleeping disorders. Therefore, treatments such as hormone-replacement therapy or the use of anti-oxidant drugs may, in fact, bring relief for some of the symptoms in the aging male.

During male menopause, well-being, libido, the immune system and cognitive skills are weakened

The changes especially affect the production of growth hormones

The discovery of andropause, the "male menopause," sheds new light on the typical "male problems." For many years, the idea of a male menopause was rejected. Today, we have proof that it is not a figment of our imagination, but a reality.

Today we have proof that andropause is real, and not a figment of our imagination

Unlike the menopause in women, andropause is not easy to diagnose. It is a slow process characterized by a decrease in hormone production. For a long time, symptoms such as a diminished libido or erectility, as well as exhaustion, irritability, depression, osteoporosis and myalgia, were not seen as classic symptoms of andropause. Knowing the influence that hormones have on the male body opens up new therapeutic possibilities. Carefully balanced hormone-replacement therapies can help replenish the hormones in the body. With preventive measures and a change in lifestyle, it becomes possible to raise the hormone levels in a sixty-year-old man, giving him new strength and an improved quality of life.

Hormone-replacement therapies can replenish hormone levels

Preventive care for men will have to undergo major changes in the new millennium. Medicine will no longer focus on healing alone as much of the

Help Wanted: andrologist!

attention shifts to prevention. Men should have their own doctor or andrologist, and andrology should be established as a new medical specialty dedicated to men's quality of life, vitality and virility.

The "International Society for the Study of the Aging Male" (ISSAM) has created a special program to prepare future doctors for this new challenge. It offers courses and seminars around the world, and doctors and hospital staff are trained to provide patients and the general public with the best possible care and with protection from improper treatment by unqualified people. Growing old with the dignity afforded by good health should be a legal right, not a privilege.

This book summarizes the latest developments in the study of aging

This thought-provoking and, at times, controversial book, is a compilation of the latest scientific findings and other developments on the subject of men, their nature and the factors that control them. The book provides a detailed analysis of the influence that hormones have on the male body, and of the different conditions that can be caused by a hormone deficit. It also deals with effective ways of controlling the symptoms related to hormonal imbalances. But it is more than just a book on hormones. It describes men in their totality—everything from treatment and prevention of physical disorders to mental fitness.

It conveys to the reader what it means to get old

Provocative though this book may be, it will raise the reader's awareness of the factors affecting the aging of the human body. It shows how crucial it is for men to have preventive strategies throughout their lives. And it makes a good case for selective treatments such as hormone-replacement therapy or the active use of vitamins, anti-oxidants, proper nutrition and physical exercise. The goal here is to enable men to exercise some control over the conditions and the symptoms of illness and aging, and in doing so put off the inevitable for as long as possible.

Prof. Dr. Bruno Lunenfeld, *FRCOG, FACOG*
President of the "International Society for the Study of the Aging Male"

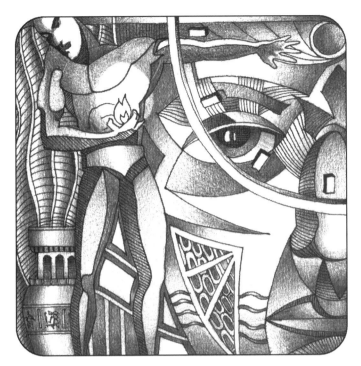

The Man of the Future

The Man in 2050

A Glimpse of Our Future

His mission lasted only nine days. But the insights into the aging process, gained from his stay in a weightless environment, will have a lasting effect on medical research and development here on earth. The oldest astronaut ever to go into space, John Glenn circled the earth 144 times aboard the space shuttle "Discovery" in October 1998. When the 77-year-old returned from orbit, the US had a new "old" national hero. In 1962, Glenn made his historic space flight in the tiny space capsule "Freedom 7," in which he circled the earth three times and almost burned up upon re-entry into the atmosphere. Thirty-six years later, the agile space veteran proved that humans are not really limited by age in what they can do during their time in space. Glenn conducted 10 different experiments that were intended to shed light on the aging process in conditions of zero gravity. His brainwaves were monitored, as were his sleep rhythms, blood readings, cardiovascular system and vestibular sense.

John Glenn, aged 77, circled the earth 144 times

The American Academy of Anti-Aging Medicine, an association of 6000 doctors and scientists from 44 countries, took advantage of Glenn's enormous popularity as a pioneer in retarding the aging process. In December 1998, they adopted him as a model of the new higher consciousness at their sixth world congress in Las Vegas. In return, he promised: "I'll make it to 100."

We All Die Much Too Soon

In 2050, people will settle on Mars

John Glenn will no longer be here when people settle on Mars round about 2050. By that time, most of us will live to be 120. Surprisingly enough, we die much too soon, and are far from reaching our biological limit. For thousands of years, people did not live beyond 30 or 40 years of age. They were felled by infections, epidemics, cancer and the "diseases of civilization."

Even at the end of the 19th century, average life expectancy was only 47 years. It was only after the turn of the century that people gradually began to live longer. So, today we have a greater life span than any generation that came before us.

Our genetic life span ends at 120 years

Nevertheless, it is a known fact that our genetically encoded age, the maximum life span of the human organism, is approximately 120 years, which is equivalent to the life expectancy of other mammals. This is based on the so-called "7-rule," which states that the life expectancy of a living being is seven times longer than the time its skeleton requires to become fully grown. But man is the only being whose life expectancy today—the human skeleton takes between 18 and 20 years to grow—is significantly lower than would be warranted by this rule. So, why do we die prematurely? What causes the human body to age so quickly? And what can we do to slow this aging process?

In the last few years, medicine has identified a number of cultural causes of premature aging, such as poor nutrition, excessive use of alcohol, nicotine and drugs, and lack of exercise. Fortunately, it has also given us a new understanding of the aging process.

Hormones Are the Key

Sex hormones control the aging process

The key to a longer life is in the hormones. Aging is a complex, hormone-controlled process. In this process, the endocrine system—the human hormone system and, more particularly here, the sex hormones, which are among the essential "clocks" of the aging process—plays a decisive role. It functions as a fundamental Zeitgeber, or "regulator" of the biological clock that governs the aging process in both sexes and determines the life span of each person.

Hormones are chemical substances produced by the various glands and transported through the blood to targeted organs and other parts of the body. They are responsible for regulating metabolism. As an example, melatonin is a hormone that reduces the efficiency of various organs so as to increase their life span, while the super hormone DHEA (dehydroepiandrosterone) lowers stress levels.

Melatonin reduces the efficiency of organs

For many decades, scientists and doctors suspected that hormone levels in people were decreasing because of the aging process. Modern medical science has established that the causal connection is just the reverse. People grow older because hormone production falls off and because the human body produces fewer and fewer hormones. The effects of this drop in hormone levels can be dramatic, especially in men. They may experience loss of energy, excess weight gains, imbalances in the immune system, increased risk of cardiovascular and autoimmune diseases, reduced libido, and depression.

People age because of diminishing hormone levels

Male Menopause

The facts about menopause in women are well documented. This book, for the first time, sets forth scientific data and recent research findings that prove that men, too, are controlled by their hormones to a much wider extent than previously assumed. Over the last decades, science has dealt with hormone levels in women, especially with the effects and the consequences of menopause. We can accept as a given that men experience the same problems.

Medical science has established, quite incredibly, that menopause is not an exclusively feminine problem, that men also go through menopause. Men experience a climacteric that normally sets in around the age of 55, and sometimes even earlier. The resulting hormone deficiency makes a man's life more complicated.

Men experience "menopause" at about age 55

In order to fend off disease, increase life span, raise the biological age, and massively enhance quality of life, men may be given extra hormones to compensate for lower production levels. Today it is possible to raise the hormone levels of a 60-year-old to those of a 35-year-old man producing all the accompanying effects: less body fat, more muscle mass, more energy, increased libido and a better memory. Although this branch of medicine is still in its

60-year-olds can be given the hormone levels of 35-year-olds

infancy, medical research in the coming millennium will focus very much on retarding the aging process rather than on fighting infectious diseases and the scourge of cancer, the great challenges of the late 20th century.

Taking 20 Years Off

Pioneer: David Rudman treated war veterans with HGH

David Rudman, an endocrinologist, was among the first to deal with the ways and means of slowing down the aging process in men. He attracted worldwide attention when the renowned New England Journal of Medicine published the results of his study in 1990. At the Medical College of Wisconsin, he had treated twelve war veterans between the ages of 61 and 81 with the human growth hormone HCH for six months, with amazing results. The men lost up to 14% of their body fat while gaining between 9% and 12% muscle mass, the thickness of their skin increased, they felt more energized, and their sex drive was restored. In other words, their bodies were like those of people 10 to 20 years younger.

They lost 14% of their body fat and felt energized

Dr. Edmund Chein, a doctor and lawyer born in Hong Kong, took Rudman's results and built upon them. Rudman could not exclude the possibility that the accelerated cell growth induced by the hormone supplement might also accelerate the growth of cancer cells. Chein's findings supported the notion that other hormones prevent that from happening. If there is a hormone accelerating the growth of cancer, then there must also be an anti-hormone. The key is to balance the hormone level. For example, in supplementing sex hormones, he cautioned against adding only one of the seven (eight in women) known sex hormones.

Each cancer-accelerating hormone has a counterpart

Chein founded the Life Extension Institute in Palm Springs in 1994. Since then, he has treated more than 3,500 patients, adjusting their hormone levels to match those of 20-year-olds. Chein's is the only institution for anti-aging hormone therapy in the world that is allowed to advertise treatment using the human growth hormone (HGH).

The Four Stages of Life

According to Prof. Bruno Lunenfeld, the "high priest" of andropause medicine, the life of a man has four essential stages:

1. Growing Stage
The male body continues to grow up to the age of 20. At that point, it reaches

its maximum functional capacity, and its DNA, the human genetic code, starts to lose 1% of its reproducibility per year. It would follow from there that the DNA death, and thus the death of the person, should occur around the age of 120. The fact that people die much younger than 120 has many causes.

From the age of 20, DNA loses 1% of its reproducibility each year

2. Primary Prevention Stage

From the age of 20 on, special attention must go toward keeping up a healthy lifestyle. Plenty of sports and proper nutrition, among other measures, are needed in order to maintain the functional capacity of the body. It is interesting to note that, only 20 years ago, children and young adults had about 20% more bone mass than they do today. Modern lifestyles have led to deterioration in the physical condition of children and young men. Instead of milk, many kids today prefer to drink Coke; instead of playing football, they choose to spend hours in front of the computer or the TV. The explosion of technology is gradually wreaking havoc on the human body. "The empire strikes back."

Only 20 years ago, children had more bone mass

3. Preventive Strategies Stage

From the age of 40, massive countermeasures against aging must be taken. These preventive measures must become very active, involving departures from established habits. Apart from extending life expectancy, the next century will also be about enhancing men's health expectancy. The primary goal will be to maintain good health for as long as possible and to postpone the aging process as best one can.

The motto for 2000: Stay healthy and postpone aging for years

4. Aging Stage

The goal of the future will be to maintain and improve quality of life. The role of medicine will be to make it possible for people to live longer and better. However, this will bring on other social and sociological problems. For each newborn today, there are 10 men turning 65. According to estimates by the World Health Organization (WHO), that ratio will be 15:1 in 2020. In 2050, it might even be 25:1.

In 2050, there will be 25 65-year-olds for each newborn

On the other hand, the fertility rate among men is declining. "It is actually lower than the rate necessary to keep the population constant," says Prof. Lunenfeld. This means that an ever smaller group of people will have to work to pay for an ever larger population of older people. The drastic effects on social security and pension funds and thus on society at large are not yet fully known.

We Will Live to Be 120

"Healing" medicine becomes prophylactic medicine

In 2050, living to be over 100 will be taken for granted, and many will actually be around for their 120th birthday. In order to achieve this, it will be necessary to take certain preventive action. Future medical science will have moved away from "healing" and become a prophylactic discipline.

Men have been somewhat neglected in research done on aging, prolonging life span, and improving quality of life. The focus has been more on the female sex. Knowing as we do now that the male body reacts not so differently from the female body when it comes to hormones, we can take many of the medical findings connected with women and apply them to men. The effect of hormones on the lives of men is massive, and more complex than originally assumed. The man of the 21st century is controlled by his hormones not only in his sex life, but also on the job and in just about every other routine that makes up his day. And modern man is at the threshold of actually applying this knowledge.

The fascination with the female breast is evolutionary

Evolution has taught us that life is focused on reproduction. If a man is fascinated by a woman's hips, it is due to evolution. A well-formed pelvis indicates a fertile and prolific female and stimulates a man's reproductive drive. Men's fascination with big breasts comes from an instinct to provide food for their offspring.

For a long time now, we have been removing ourselves from the constraints of evolution. Much of this process will have been completed by the turn of the next millennium. Even now, reproduction has been decoupled from evolutionary precepts by means of in-vitro fertilization or more complex methods such as micro-manipulated sperm injections. But the future promises to be even more spectacular.

The Man of the Future

The revolution in the male body is already underway. Join us on a provocative but realistic journey into the future of medicine. For practical purposes, set aside moral and ethical, as well as sociopolitical and philosophical concerns. What sounds like science fiction today may very well be reality 50 years from now.

Personal Anti-Aging Strategies

By 2050, as mentioned already, every man in the Western world will have his own personal "anti-aging strategies." As he turns 40 and his testosterone level falls to 70%, he will start hormone-replacement therapy. His hormones will be adjusted so that he can enjoy the second half of his life almost as much as he did the first. By the time he is 60, that is, when his testosterone level has dropped to 55% of the original level if left untreated, his endocrinologist will already have adjusted his hormone level to match that of a 35-year-old. Every man will maximize his quality of life by regularly taking in antioxidants, vitamins and trace elements.

From the age of 40, every man will undergo hormone-replacement therapy

Reproduction Without Sex

Sexuality in 2050 will be completely separate from reproduction. Only those who actively wish to reproduce will do so. A man will be able to have his sperm frozen at the most favorable time genetically, around the age of 20, so that he can put off having children until later in life. If he decides when he is 80 to become a father, he can put the frozen sperm, which will have been kept in germ-free conditions at the sperm bank, to work for him.

At 20, men will have their sperm frozen

The same will be true for women. Egg cells, while they are still "fresh," will be frozen and saved for some day in the future when her home and work life are more suited to pregnancy.

Sterilization for Men and Women

It will be quite normal for both boys and girls to undergo sterilization upon reaching puberty. The sole purpose of sex will be to satisfy, not to reproduce. If a person wishes to procreate, sperm can be taken from the epididymis for in-vitro fertilization, or frozen sperm could be used. The world will be free of the fear of unwanted pregnancies. It will be a place without anti-baby pills, blood clots and the public debate over abortion.

The purpose of sex will be to satisfy

The quality of a man's sperm will not affect his ability to reproduce, and any woman who wishes to have children will be able to do so.

Every woman can have a baby

Birth by Cesarean Only

In the highly industrialized countries, children will be born almost exclusively by Cesarean. Evolution has shown that human females are not "designed" for birth the way quadrupeds are.

People will find it hard to believe that, in former times, women would suffer a ruptured pelvic floor to have a natural birth, and that 50% of women would have tremendous incontinence problems after the age of 50. They will find it incredible that, not too long ago, babies were exposed to the immense strain of natural childbirth. Over the course of evolution, the increase in brain mass and thus in the size of the human head has brought about these birth complications. As people become more intelligent, our head gets bigger, and vaginal birth becomes ever more difficult. The incidence of birth complications is much higher among humans than it is among animals, with those few minutes during birth being the most dangerous in a person's life. The mortality rate, which was very high up until our century, will no longer be an issue by 2050.

The human head will be too big for vaginal birth

Defeating Cancer

Manipulation of the genetic structure may help prevent cancer

The struggle against cancer will largely be won. Based on findings stemming from the decoding of human genes, long-term prophylactic measures will be devised or the genetic structure manipulated.

Prevention Over Healing

"Growing old in good health should be a legal right, not a privilege."

Prof. Bruno Lunenfeld

Medicine will move away from healing and toward prevention. In the past, the treatment of women in the decades following menopause was not a regular practice, for they died before they were able to experience the consequences of hormone deficiency.

Osteoporosis will be a new problem for men

Since men's life expectancy has long been six to seven years shorter than that of women, the later consequences of aging such as osteoporosis or arteriosclerosis are still not primary issues. However, hormone deficiency will undoubtedly matter much more 20 to 30 years from now, when a rapidly increasing life expectancy will lead most men to suffer from those conditions. Professor Lunenfeld expects that by 2010, osteoporosis in men could be as frequent as in women. Even today, 30% of all hip fractures occur in men, and the mortality rate of men is higher than that of women.

Andrologists and Andropause Institutes

By 2010, women will continue to see their gynecologists, and men will seek out their andrologists. Urologists will primarily perform surgery, but andrologists will go far beyond that, providing medical-prophylactic services to lower the mortality rate associated with many diseases and as a result raise the life expectancy for men.

Men all across the Western hemisphere will have their favorite clinic, or andropause institute. Using regular screening and lab tests, male problems will be detected in the incipient stage and endocrine deficits—a drop in hormone levels—will be brought back up to norms.

Help Wanted:
Andrologist

A New Lifestyle

In order to make it to 100 years of age while living their life in style, people in the West will adapt themselves more and more to Asian values. The Asian cultures, with several thousand years of experience, long ago developed a lifestyle based on meditation, good nutrition and healthy living. Asian countries have fewer cases of modern "civilization diseases" such as heart attacks and hypertension than does the West. Increasingly, advances in Western medical science will merge with the behavioral standards and the standards for living that Asians have practiced for thousands of years.

The West will
adopt Asian values

Anti-Aging Hormones

Manipulating hormones effectively will become a routine medical practice. Hormone-replacement therapies will raise men's life expectancy significantly, and old age ailments will be avoided.

Only 15 years ago, a hormone analysis was a highly complex and expensive process. It required a specialized laboratory, and the test person's urine had to be collected several times over a period of 24 hours. This analysis was therefore only performed in very severe cases of hormonal imbalance such as goiter. This has resulted in a shortage of empirical data on the workings of hormones in men. It has long been known that hormones exert an influence over men, but not to what extent.

Fifteen years ago,
urine was used to
analyze hormones

With the development of radioactive immunoassays, a new era of hormone diagnostics was born. For the first time, it was possible to perform routine radioactive hormone tests on blood. These tests were very expensive, so they could only be undertaken in select cases. Today it is possible to analyze a man's hormones by a simple and inexpensive process using a blood sample. A comprehensive screening for hormonal deficiency is now possible where only 15 years ago it was seen as pure science fiction. One lab workstation can now analyze 5000 hormones a day, fully automated. Back then, it would have required an entire institute and 20 lab workers.

The new era began
with radioactive
immunoassays

A hormonal
analysis costs only
$100

Some of the findings of modern endocrinology gleaned from technological advances in the measurement and analysis of hormones have far-reaching implications for the man of the future:

- Men, too, are strongly dependent on sex hormones. Their entire work life as well as their sex life is controlled by them.

The decline in hormone levels in men is gradual

- The climacteric is not a female phenomenon. Men also experience menopause, during which levels of hormones such testosterone and estrogen drastically decrease. But men do not experience as rapid a drop in those levels as women do. It is a more gradual process.

- Osteoporosis, so far seen primarily as a female problem, also occurs in men. Measuring bone density will clearly reveal the effects of changes in hormonal balance. Men's bones are actually quite dependent on sex hormones, especially estrogen.

- Hair loss in men is also tied to estrogen levels.

- Medical explanations for these hormonal phenomena, which had been suspected but never proven, have become public knowledge thanks to new and better testing methods.

- For the first time, selective intervention in the hormone system of men could be a decisive factor in the battle against disease. Hormone therapy will experience a major boom in the 21st century.

Hormones could be the key to living well past a hundred. In fact, a life span of 120 years will be well within the realm of possibility in the not too distant future if we take clear and decisive action to consistently improve our health standards. What was seen as science fiction only recently is now beginning to take shape even for scientists.

The Delphi Report predicts medical breakthroughs

The Delphi Report of 1998 is a study of the future conducted by the German Fraunhofer Institute for Systems Engineering and Innovation Research in Karlsruhe. Carried out by 2,453 experts from numerous fields, the report predicts a series of revolutionary discoveries and fundamental changes in medicine to take place as early as the first 15 years of the new millennium:

2005: AIDS is cured

2005: A treatment for AIDS that can stop the disease in its initial phase is used in clinics. An insulin preparation that can be administered orally comes on the market.

2006: Causes of Alzheimer's is discovered

2006: Genetic analyses help determine an individual's risk of contracting diseases such as cancer or hypertension. The cause and the pattern of development of Alzheimer's have been determined.

2008: The underlying genetic and molecular causes of diseases such as diabetes and hypertension have been discovered.

2010: Microcomputers move through our bloodstream

2010: Vaccines against AIDS are used for the first time. The neurochemical workings of alcoholism and its genetic components have been revealed. Microcomputers that can propel themselves through the human bloodstream are employed to diagnose blood and treat thrombosis.

2011: A treatment for Alzheimer's has been developed. The cause of Parkinson's has been determined. A treatment for the shakes, and for vestibular and orientation problems is expected for 2018.

Decoding the Genome

In 1953, Francis Harry Compton Crick, a molecular biologist, together with his colleague James D. Watson decoded the double-helix structure of the DNA molecule, which contains all the genetic information relevant to life. In so doing, Crock and Watson made one of the most important discoveries of the 20th century. "We have discovered the secret of life," said Crick, when he received the Nobel Prize for his research. Without the work of Crick and Watson, modern medicine as we know it would not have been possible.

Francis Crick decoded the DNA double helix in 1953

In the decades since, researchers and scientists around the world have been working on the Human Genome Project, decoding the entire genetic code of humans. Scientists agree that within the next five years the code will be unraveled. This will open up tremendous possibilities for medicine to detect disease-specific mutations in the genetic material and to develop new kinds of treatment. Many diseases that are fatal today may suddenly become treatable.

At American laboratories in particular, such as the National Institute of Aging (NIA), scientists are working feverishly to identify the genes that could help prolong life. The cells of tissues begin to deteriorate at a specific point in time, which triggers the aging process. If the genes responsible for that deterioration can be identified, another mystery of human mortality will be solved.

In microscopic worms such as nematodes (roundworms), American scientists have successfully isolated a type of "longevity gene" that puts nematode larvae into absolute stasis if there is an insufficient supply of food. In this state, which may last up to 60 days, the larvae do not take in any food, and this extends their life span by up to 100%. Michal Jazwinski of the Louisiana State University School of Medicine in New Orleans says, "It is the goal of our research to allow people to die at a very old age, while still being young. The genes that trigger the aging process in people are to be manipulated one day in such a manner that they suppress the diseases they would normally cause so that people can remain healthy, even in old age."

By 2004, the full genetic code will be revealed

Nematodes have a "longevity gene"

Are We Trying to Deceive Nature?

What do manipulation of the genetic structure and tinkering with the human hormone system really mean? Are we trying to deceive nature and alter its course? Are we about to eliminate the mechanisms of natural selection? Up to the ages of 40 or 50, i.e., as long as we are able to procreate, we are useful to the process of evolution. Nature guarantees that we produce a sufficient number of sex hormones to experience libido, to maintain our attractiveness and to guarantee the survival of our species. But as our usefulness to this evolutionary process wanes, nature cruelly begins to deprive us of the essential substances of life, the sex hormones. In the future, however, mankind will have ways of adjusting these natural developments.

Humans deceive
evolution

In fact, with current developments in the replenishing of hormones, we are already exerting an influence on evolution. Many old cultures before us, such as the Chinese, had an intuitive understanding of this. They have long replenished their hormone levels from plants such as ginseng. Modern man, however, has discovered subtler, more scientific ways of outsmarting evolution.

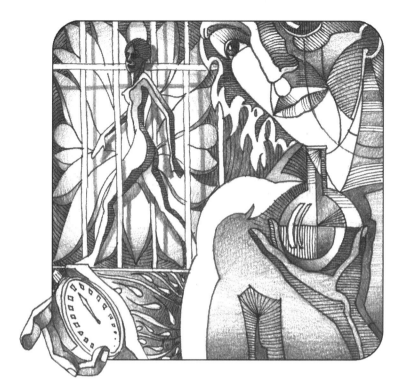

The Climacteric of Men

Factors in Aging

Living means aging from the time we are born. This is part of life, and the real meaning of fate. In the great evolutionary scheme of things, the aging process in humans is unique, for Homo sapiens lives much longer than just about any other mammal on the planet.

But the reason that cells, organs and organisms lose their functionality over the course of their life span and finally die off remains, in large part, a mystery for scientists. It is thought that hormones play a key role. If hormone production in the body falls off, we age.

The reason cells die is still a mystery

This raises an important question. Can aging be postponed simply by replacing missing hormones? Could it be possible to remain forever young?

Telomerase: Making Human Cells Immortal

Is one enzyme the key to immortality?

Humanity has long sought the causes of aging. With the discovery of the enzyme "telomerase," it appeared for the first time as if the mystery might be solved. In 1998, scientists found that telomerase plays an important role in the division of human cells. Each cell division consumes some quantity of telomerase. After 75 divisions, the supply of telomerase is exhausted and the cell dies.

Telomerase prevents cell death

After many years of research on the subject, scientists from Texas discovered that cell death can be prevented by adding telomerase. They started human cell cultures in a telomerase bath in order to make them especially resistant to disease. "Even after 300 divisions, there were no signs of wear and tear," reported Carmen P. Morales of the University of Texas Southwestern Medical Center, writing on the "Methuselah effect" of telomerase in an article in the journal Nature Medicine.

"This is the beginning of the end of the aging process"

The effect of telomerase begins with a constant buildup of so-called "telomeres" at the chromosome ends of the DNA, the repository of our genetic information that doubles with each cell division. It is the task of the telomeres to keep the chromosomes apart and to ensure that their structure remains stable. However, some of the telomeres are lost with each cell division. They need to be replenished by the enzyme telomerase. The lower the level of telomerase, the more advanced is the aging process.

In laboratory tests, Morales succeeded in preventing cell death by adding telomerase. American scientific journals called it the beginning of the end of the aging process.

The Modern Picture of Dorian Gray

He is about 20 years old, innocent, but very elegant and full of masculine beauty. He is tempted into recklessly pursuing his innermost desires. They are so strong that he searches desperately for the secret to eternal youth so that he can enjoy life's pleasures forever. To be forever young as in the portrait on the wall: "For this, I would give my soul." Oscar Wilde's character Dorian Gray symbolizes, like no other, the human desire for eternal youth, and this obsession can be traced back to the ancient Greeks.

Even in the Bible, eternal youth is a powerful motive. According to the first book of Moses, Genesis 5:27, Methuselah died at the age of 969. Abraham, who was in very good health, died at 170 (Genesis 25:8), and his son Isaac lived to 180. Moses' life ended early at 120. According to the 90th Psalm, "The days of our years are threescore and ten; and by reason of strength they be fourscore years."

Eternal youth: Methuselah died at the age of 969

The longest a person could live, according to the ancient Egyptians, was about 110. Buddha set the maximum at 100 years. It is no surprise that ages mentioned in the Bible are corrected downward the closer the events were to the time of their being recorded in writing.

The list of important old men reads like a Who's Who of human history. Plato and Sophocles, for example, lived to be 90 years old. Cato the Elder, Cicero and Seneca reached, surprisingly for their time, the ripe old age of 80. Michelangelo and Titian, who both died at approximately 90 years of age, depicted the Almighty, the Creator, with gray hair and beard, while giving him the taut and highly conditioned body of an athlete in the prime of his life. They saw God as a symbol of wisdom, physical strength and long life in perpetual good health.

The list of admirable "young old men" goes on indefinitely. They can be found in literature and in the fine arts, in Shakespeare's "King Lear" and in Lessing's "Nathan the Wise." Voltaire, who wrote his masterpieces when he was over 50; Giuseppe Verdi, who completed his opera "Falstaff" at 80; and Pablo Picasso, who continued painting until he died at 91, are all impressive role models.

Verdi completed his opera "Falstaff" at 80

The Secret of Aging

What is aging? One thing is known for sure. Aging cannot be traced back to a single cause. In all probability, a series of simultaneous processes are responsible. From there, two main theories of cell aging diverge.

The Wear-and-Tear Theory

This theory is based on the assumption that the cell ages from chemical wear caused by free oxygen radicals. These aggressive substances, which are responsible for causing cancer, are a by-product of everyday metabolism.

Cells age because of free oxygen radicals

Scientists have discovered that free radicals can be partially deactivated or neutralized by the body's own defenses (i.e., antioxidants), but obviously not to an extent sufficient to completely protect vital proteins and the genes.

Antioxidants neutralize free radicals

The Program Theory

According to this theory, the aging of cells is controlled by an internal life clock. If the telomeres, the chromosome ends, lose their protective layers, the chromosomes themselves become unstable and disintegrate. With each cell division, a small amount of this layer is lost. In other words, the telomeres break down. Once a critical point is exceeded, the cell dies. There are only two types of cells that can resist this natural cell death. They are, so to speak, immortal, and can be divided infinitely without ever aging at all. These cells are:

Egg, sperm and tumor cells are the only cells that divide without aging

● egg and sperm cells
● tumor cells

Recent research, outlined in detail for the first time in this book, provides proof of another cause, a third theory, of cell aging and supplies one more missing link in the puzzle of why cells die.

The Hormone Theory

People age because of a hormonal imbalance

Molecular changes in the body are triggered by an increase in hormonal miscommunication, deterioration in the interaction of hormones. From the age of 30 onward, the body of a man produces fewer and fewer hormones. If this highly complex hormonal system gets out of balance, communication within the body and its organs will be disturbed. And this decline in hormone levels suddenly becomes one of the fundamental causes of aging.

Men's Weakness in Old Age

The aging process of organs, indeed of each tiny cell and each molecule, would defeat even Michelangelo's David in his quest to be young forever. The skin becomes thin and wrinkled, the muscle mass shrinks, and the subcutaneous fatty tissue moves to the stomach and hip areas. The body of a man decreases in size by an average of five to six centimeters between the ages of 35 and 80. And there are other accompanying symptoms of advancing age.

● Bad Joints

From the age of 30, we start losing our body water

The most striking change in the body's composition concerns the ratio of fat to body water. From the ages of 30 to 70, total body water decreases by about 10%. The bones become more brittle and lose their stability. At about 40, the bone tissue slowly starts to disintegrate. The spinal column, hips and legs are affected the most (see the section on Osteoporosis). This deterioration is accelerated by a lack of physical exercise. With increasing age, the fluids in the joints become more watery and lose some of their effect as "lubricants." The result is a breakdown of the protective joint cartilage. The action of the joints is not smooth anymore, and the joint wears out and may even become inflamed.

• Wrinkles

Wrinkles first appear as a result of a loss of elastic and collagenous sustentacular fiber in the skin. The tanning craze, which has been around for years, has helped accelerate this process through excessive UV exposure of the skin. The sebaceous glands in the skin produce less and less sebum with advancing age, causing the skin to dry out. Because of inconsistent and declining production of the pigment melanin, men (and women) develop brown spots or "age spots" on the skin. A controversial but interesting hypothesis from the US states that shaving almost daily "rejuvenates" the facial skin of men, along the lines of the "peeling" procedures performed on women by cosmetic studios. Peeling keeps the skin elastic for a longer period of time and makes it appear younger than the skin of other women of the same age.

Lack of melanin causes age spots

• Gray Hair

Hair turns gray because of the increasing buildup of air deposits in the keratin and also, though less intensively, in the hair-root cells. In many men, hair also becomes thinner, and hormonal shifts in the sex hormones may result in baldness.

Air in keratin turns hair gray

• Hearing Problems

The older you get, the worse your hearing. For some unknown reason, more men than women are affected by significant hearing impairment, the so-called senile deafness. This may be linked to higher noise levels in typical male professions, or to a greater frequency of circulatory disturbances.

In the process of aging, three biological communication systems deserve special attention: the nervous system, the hormonal system and the immune system. These will be discussed in detail later in the book. The immune system breaks down mainly because the body's defense cells (T-lymphocytes) become less effective in old age and do not respond well to outside attacks. For that reason, infections usually have more a dramatic effect on older people than on the young. Chronic bronchitis and pneumonia are the leading causes of death among men aged 65 and older. The severity and frequency of these attacks depends on the age and sex of the person affected. With advancing age, the lungs usually lose breathing capacity, and the pulmonary alveoli become less elastic and expand,

After 65, chronic bronchitis often ends in death

especially in smokers. The walls of the lungs become thicker, which makes the exchange of gas more difficult, all while the blood supply is deteriorating. The respiratory muscles also weaken, which renders the thorax less flexible.

● Poor Eyesight

After 45, presbyopia often sets in

The eyes start losing their ability to focus after the age of 45. Doctors call this presbyopia. The fibers of the lens change their structure considerably, become discolored and allow less light to pass through. As a result, the lens becomes clouded and vision is generally impaired.

● Degeneration of Organs

Spleen, liver and kidneys degenerate

In the course of aging, some organs degenerate, especially the spleen, liver, pancreatic gland, kidneys and muscles. The blood supply to the liver of a 65-year-old male may be only half that of a 25-year-old.

The brain, too, loses volume, primarily the white brain matter and its nerve fibers. The nerve cells of the crucial, and often talked about, gray cerebral cortex remain largely unchanged, apart from senile pigmentation.

The Day Hussein Shadli Died

The oldest man who ever lived reached 148

Hussein Shadli, from the village of Mussaifira in Syria, was a wise old man. He could remember when his home was part of the Ottoman Empire, and he would tell horror stories about the young Sultan Abdul Hamid II, born in 1876, whom he met while in his early teenage years. And he could recall October 1918, when World War I was still on and when an alliance of the British, the French and the Arabs expelled the Turks from Syria. Shadli would also vividly recall April 15, 1946, the day the last soldier of the French occupying forces left the country. When Shadli died in April 1999, he was no less than 148 years old and the oldest person ever recorded. The newspaper Es Saura reported that Shadli, born in 1851, had a remarkable memory, was able to read without glasses and had around one hundred grandchildren and great-grandchildren. The official title of the oldest person alive was passed on after Shadli's death to Sarah Knauss Clark, an American, who at 118, is much younger than he was.

Why Women Live Longer

Provided his date of birth was correct, Hussein Shadli was an exception in the sexes' competition for longevity. All the studies done in the industrialized countries, especially in Austria, Germany and the US, have reached the same conclusion. Men's average life expectancy is six to eight years lower than that for women, and men usually suffer from more afflictions and diseases in old age.

THE TEN MOST FREQUENT REASONS FOR IN-PATIENT TREATMENT OF MEN IN AUSTRIA

Main diagnosis	Patients	% of all patients
Cardiovascular disease	147,259	16.3
Injuries or poisoning	133,040	14.7
Cancer	99,659	11.0
Digestive-tract diseases	90,984	10.1
Diseases involving the skeleton, muscles and connective tissue	76,876	8.5
Diseases of respiratory organs	76,765	8.5
Diseases of nervous system and sensory organs	59,093	6.5
Diseases of the urogenital tract	49,038	5.3
Psychiatric conditions	43,901	4.9
Symptoms and insufficiently defined affections (e.g., senility)	30,912	3.4
Total number of male in-patients	903,023	

Source: STAT(Austrian Central Statistical Office) 1998

Why does the male body age faster than the female? The two most common causes of death among men in Western countries, heart attack and stroke, can be traced back to one cause—arteriosclerosis, i.e., the hardening, narrowing and blocking of arteries by fatty and calciferous deposits in the vessels.

Arteriosclerosis causes strokes and heart attacks

The main risk factors in this context leading to arteriosclerosis are: being male, family medical history, smoking, hypertension, excess weight, high cholesterol levels and little exercise.

Based on a direct statistical comparison of men and women, all these risk factors appear to apply primarily to men. Analysis of the risk factors points to three possible causes:
1. the male genetic material
2. the hormones
3. typical male social behavior

These and other factors are responsible for the fact that women outlive men:

During childhood and adolescence, more boys die as a result of accidents

• The mortality rate among men before the age of 25 is far higher than that of women. In the neonatal phase and in early childhood, boys are more prone to health problems. Boys suffer more deformities, injuries and other pathological conditions in the course of labor and birth than girls. During childhood and adolescence and in early adulthood, the primary causes of death among men are accidents.

By the age of 70, the difference in average life expectancy between men and women is down to 2.5 years. This means that the considerable difference in the life spans of men and women is due to events early on in life.

Men are reluctant to see their doctors

• Men are known to be careless when it comes to their bodies. They go to see their doctor less often than women. Only half of all men, compared to women, undergo preventive cancer tests. The fact that they may be diagnosed with an illness scares most men. "They deal with illness in a way," says Professor Anita Schmeiser-Rieder of the Institute for Social Medicine at the University of Vienna, "that must comply with the male status and the social role of males. Signs of weakness, especially with respect to health matters, do not fit that image. Quite frequently, men postpone appointments to see their doctor, or they go to their doctor only if there is a problem. They only speak about symptoms that are compatible with their idea of what it means to be a man."

• The typical man's diet is much more unhealthy than that of women. Seventy percent of men between the ages of 30 and 50 are overweight. Men are also more likely to develop hypertension (high blood pressure) and high cholesterol levels.

Men seek risks

• Men seek out danger and engage in extreme sports. However, they are less consistent than women when it comes to regular exercise and general fitness. According to Professor Schmeiser-Rieder, "They frequently exhibit compensatory, aggressive and risky behavior, which makes them prone to disease, injury and even death. They often see themselves as invulnerable." In addition, accidents caused by the influence of alcohol occur ten times as often among men as among women.

• Men also have more emotional and social problems as well as less support than women in the same age group. Says Professor Schmeiser-Rieder: "They must play different roles—they are fathers and providers for their families—and these roles correlate to their state of health." It is also interesting to note that statistics show an increase in the mortality rate of men following the end of a marriage (twice as high as for women).

● Men do not have an "andrologist" to go to—someone who, as gynecologists do for women—regularly examines and treats them right from adolescence all the way to old age.

The Chromosomes Are to Blame

One of the fundamental reasons that men do not live as long as women, however, is not their fault—it is the fault of their genes.

The chromosomes of a man consist of 22 pairs, and the sex chromosomes X and Y. Women have an XX combination. According to genetics expert Professor Christine Mannhalter of the Institute for Medical and Chemical Laboratory Diagnostics at the University of Vienna, the "masters of creation" are disadvantaged by their genetic material despite their larger average body size and stronger muscles.

Men have only one X-chromosome, and that makes them prone to disease.

While women have two X-chromosomes in each cell, men have only one X-chromosome and a Y-chromosome. This causes instability. Genetic research has shown that the X-chromosome contains the genetic information for essential bodily functions. If this sole X-chromosome becomes damaged, it will invariably have negative consequences for the man. For a woman, one damaged X-chromosome is not so bad because the second one can usually compensate.

Many male diseases are based on the defective X-chromosome

A whole range of diseases that affect only men are based on defects in the X-chromosome. These include, for example, hemophilia (many kings suffered from this condition) and "male dementia," a very serious condition affecting one in a thousand men. According to Professor Wolfgang Schnedl, director of the Advisory Center for Human Genetics at Wilhelminenspital, a Vienna hospital, these psychological illnesses affect men three times as often as women. Other conditions related to the single male X-chromosome, such as albinism of the eyes, narrowing of the visual field, hypergamma globulinemia and spastic paralysis of the arms and legs, are rare, but affect only men. Birth statistics also show that more boys are born than girls, but more of them die at birth. Most cancer statistics show men in the lead. This is especially true of lip cancer, mouth cancer, laryngeal cancer, lung cancer and cancer of the genitals. And even sleep apnea, a severe sleep disorder that has received increased

Men lead the list in almost all cancer statistics

attention over the past few years, affects men almost exclusively. It leads to phases of asphyxiation and morning fatigue and significantly reduces life expectancy.

It is also a fact that more men than women have trouble coping with life. According to the Central Statistical Office in Vienna, almost three times as many men have committed suicide in the last few years as women.

Many researchers believe that men have to change their ways if they want to live longer. They have to stop thinking of themselves as invulnerable. Men have to learn to listen to their body's signals as women do, and they have to treat their body better.

Chasing After the Fountain of Eternal Youth

The quest for the immortal human cell, the fountain of eternal youth and the causes of the aging process is fully underway. The discovery of telomerase has given us valuable new insights. Adding telomerase compensates for wear-and-tear on the protective layers (telomeres) at the chromosome ends. Telomerase gives the basic substance of life, the DNA, a new lease on life. This discovery goes a long way in the quest to slow the biological clock.

Can telomerase turn healthy cells into tumors? However, it has yet to be proven that the addition of telomerase would not turn healthy cells into tumors. In preliminary experiments done at the University of Texas and at Geron, a genetics and pharmaceutical company, human cells have divided 300 times without any sign of cancerous growth. But what they would look like after 500 or 600 divisions?

It should be kept in mind that a single gene cannot stop the aging process. A lot of research is still to be done before there is any chance of decisively prolonging the life span of humans. But with the latest findings on hormones, the revolution in human health and longevity is already well underway. Hormones control life and death, and knowing their properties and how they work opens the door to a fascinating new world.

The Climacteric of Men
The Debunking of a Myth

For decades, medical science denied the existence of a male menopause. Male menopause? Impossible. A climacteric in men? There is no proof and therefore it is not a serious scientific subject.

Only a few years ago, most doctors not only doubted the existence of a male climacteric, but they vehemently denied it, ignored its symptoms, or simply shrugged the symptoms off as "part of growing old."

The existence of andropause was denied for a long time

Men affected by it were not keen on discussing the symptoms such as loss of muscular strength, energy, vitality and potency. Men try to pass themselves off as confident and in control, and they cannot admit to such weaknesses. Their self-image is chauvinistic. They are fixated on their social roles and cannot admit to others that they are losing their strength and their potency. Being perceived as tough and durable is more important to men than improving their personal well-being. Anyone who doubts a man's virility is seen as the enemy.

A few years ago, medical science, and particularly endocrinology, began classifying andropause as a disease with its own symptoms, possible diagnoses and treatments. Today, we have scientific proof of the existence of the male climacteric.

Andropause has been a topic for only a few years

Andropause May Set in at 30

The term "andropause" derives from the Greek words "andro" (man) and "pausis" (end) and is analogous to the word "menopause" ("menses" signifies 'periods'), which was coined by French scientists in 1874.

Andropause = climacterium virile = male menopause

Since discovering the male climacteric, scientists have been mulling over the correct term. "Andropause," "climacterium virile" and "male menopause" are a few examples. In the end, the term "andropause" has come to be accepted in the everyday vernacular.

Andropause is a crisis affecting both masculinity and vitality. But it is important to stress that this male menopause is not an end to masculinity, but only a decline. The first signs of andropause may set in at the age of 30, but in 70% of cases, the typical symptoms appear between the ages of 50 and 55. The characteristic signs are:

It usually sets in between the ages of 50 and 55

● decrease in libido
● decrease in or loss of erectility
● exhaustion
● irritability

- lethargy
- depression
- nervousness
- osteoporosis
- muscular and articular pains

When going through andropause, a strong, enthusiastic and positive man may become pessimistic, negative and possibly depressed, and very difficult for those around him to deal with. A vicious circle is started.

The Climacteric—A Vicious Circle

The first signs of the male climacteric tend to show up in bed. More than 80% of men experience a gradual decline in their sex drive. Their sex life becomes more and more of a problem, which, if left unattended, may end in disaster. Not only the frequency with which men have sex, but also the frequency with which they fantasize about sex declines.

80% of men lose their sex drive

This puts a lot of mental stress on men, and problems with their partner as well as sleep disorders frequently result. Quite often, the partner suspects an affair with another woman to be responsible for the loss of libido.

Erectile dysfunction, even complete impotence, may accompany the lack of libido. Among men going through andropause, 75% to 80% experience this type of problem. They cannot have an erection or cannot maintain it, so they find themselves unable to have sexual intercourse. This takes its toll on the man's self-esteem, his sense of himself as a "real man." Erectile dysfunctions can be the biggest problem men face during the climacteric.

Erectile dysfunctions and impotence on the rise

Erections in the morning will occur less frequently as well. This symptom is an important one in diagnosing the male climacteric, for it corresponds directly to a drop in the level of the hormone testosterone, especially of free and active testosterone. Erectility may be seriously affected by the ingestion of small quantities of alcohol, or by stress, but the beginning of the end of the morning erection is often the clearest signal of the onset of the male climacteric.

Morning erections getting rare

How a man deals with it depends largely on his partner. If the woman massages the penis, performs oral sex or employs other techniques to help him achieve an erection, then erectile dysfunction does not have to escalate into a dramatic personal crisis.

A British study has shown that, with the reduction in testosterone levels and sexual activity, the PC muscle—the muscle around the urethra and the bladder—no longer contracts as well. A reduction in the size of the penis when erected also results from a lack of testosterone, further aggravating problems in the relationship. Particularly if sexual partners have been together for years, a shortened penis size may reduce the intensity of stimulation in certain areas of the vagina, resulting in dissatisfaction for both partners.

The PC muscle of the man becomes less contractible

The Feeling of Permanent Exhaustion

The man will lack energy at work. Approximately 80% of men experience a prolonged state of exhaustion during the climacteric.

Four out of five men going through andropause have a constant feeling of exhaustion

To counter this, he increases his consumption of coffee for its stimulating effect, and he may even resort to alcohol. But that will in turn increase his nervousness. He will find it increasingly difficult to concentrate or to remember things, and he will lose some of his self-confidence. During andropause, creative work becomes very strenuous, and it can be a problem for the man to convince others of his ideas.

Often, these personal and professional problems lead to depression, which occurs to varying degrees in about 70% of all men during andropause. His social life changes overnight. His partner, family, friends and colleagues begin to suffer under the darkness that surrounds him.
He isolates himself. At home, he prefers to sit around quietly, staring at the TV screen or the computer for hours at a time, and more and more often he avoids social contact with friends.

Depression and sleeplessness occur

He may treat his sleeplessness with pills that only serve to reinforce the feeling of fatigue during the day. Professionally, his positive energy is gradually replaced by an insidious pessimistic outlook on life.

Men experiencing andropause are irritable and may overreact to trivial matters. At the office, he might scream at colleagues and see conspiracies everywhere. At home, he feels misunderstood. Sometimes but not always he may experience circulatory problems, such as cold hands and feet.

Another problem may be osteoporosis. It has traditionally been regarded as a female condition, but 13% of men already suffer from this decline in bone density, and this number will drastically rise in the next decades.

There are also external symptoms of andropause, such as thinning hair and dry skin.

All of these warning signs—too much stress, not enough sleep, showing his age, and so forth—are often ignored or attributed to personal lifestyle.

Andropause Is Not a Midlife Crisis

We could shrug these symptoms off as just a midlife crisis the man is experiencing, but that assumption would be false.

There are clear distinctions between andropause and a midlife crisis.

• A midlife crisis is based on emotional problems

The word crisis comes from the Greek "krisis" meaning "decision." It implies change, or a turning point in life. During andropause, a man is often too exhausted, lethargic or depressed to even consider big changes in his life.

The midlife crisis is based on emotional problems—the children move out, parents die, friends have heart attacks, unbearable stress, and so forth.

Andropause, however, is a hormonal state, one that has emotional effects, but is not caused by them.

• Andropause usually sets in later

The midlife crisis tends to set in between the ages of 35 and 45. Andropause, however, occurs between 50 and 55.

• Social factors

One's parental home, upbringing, and even professional success, no matter how paradoxical this may seem, can be contributing factors to the occurrence of a midlife crisis. Often it has a single, direct trigger such as the death of a loved one. The midlife crisis often occurs immediately after a period of success.

• Increased libido

During the midlife crisis, men may experience a heightened sex drive. For them, sex is just a vehicle for running away from problems. During andropause, however, both the libido and erectility are often reduced.

The Discovery of Andropause 200 Years Ago

It was toward the end of the 18th century that a Dr. Hooper in London first wrote about andropause in his Medical Dictionary. Back then, he called it "decline." He referred to the male climacteric as an "illness," and said that a man will recover from it "as soon as a new woman enters his life."

Andropause was discovered and classified as a disease in the 18th century

Modern scientists take a more empirical approach, analyzing the male hormones and looking into the biological causes of the climacteric.

Testosterone was first isolated and synthesized in 1935. As early as the 1940s, doctors described the symptoms of the male menopause as being "comparable to those of women."

The first breakthrough came in 1944, when the Journal of the American Medical Association published the results of a study that caused an uproar among scientists. Men who exhibited the symptoms typical of andropause were injected with testosterone, which led to a rapid improvemen in their condition. A second test group, who received placebos, did not show the same results. Reader's Digest jumped on the topic and, virtually overnight, andropause became a household term.

Reader's Digest focuses on the male menopause

At the end of World War II, the interest suddenly faded. In any discussions or papers on the subject of hormones, the focus was exclusively on the influences and the effects of these hormones on women. It was not until the mid-1990s that hormones were once again put in a male context.

This has resulted in a number of positive developments. To name one, testosterone has been proven an essential hormone in the prevention of cardiovascular disease. American studies have shown that men with low testosterone levels and relatively high estrogen levels developed heart disease more frequently than men with normal levels.

The Sex Hormones' Bad Image

For a long time, sex hormones such as testosterone had a very negative image. Artificial supplements, according to popular myth, would simply bring out the "beast inside the man." This was not helped by the fact that a special breed of hormone, anabolic steroids, have been misused for performance enhancement

It was believed that hormones would bring out the "beast in men"

in extreme sports such as bodybuilding with some disastrous results, including complete impotence, severe liver damage and, in the most serious cases, death by cardiac arrest.

Many hormones, such as testosterone, have been known to us for over 60 years, and have been tested in clinical studies. Next to the male menopause, the most important discovery of modern endocrinology is that its symptoms can be treated, using a selective hormone-replacement therapy that replenishes the hormones depleted in the male body.

Hormone revolution worldwide

This is a key to the future of preventive medicine. This century will see a hormone revolution worldwide. Social economists predict that supplementing essential hormones during the second half of a man's life will prolong his vitality, and this will have important social and political consequences.

So how does the male hormone system work? What does a man have to do, by way of treatment or changing his lifestyle, to actively manipulate his hormones? Which sex hormones control his life? And what can he do to maintain his vitality and virility?

Before he reads about the "The Hormone Revolution" in the next chapter, our male readers may want to take a few minutes out for a self-test to find out whether they are already showing the first symptoms of andropause or whether they have already entered the andropause phase of their lives. Here is the "andropause checklist" for men.

The Andropause Self Test

Am I Already Going Through the Climacteric?

The symptoms usually creep up on you, and they are hard to interpret. Exhaustion, depression, irritability and a reduced libido may be the first signs of the male climacteric, which usually sets in between the ages of 50 and 55.

By taking the following test, you can find out, quite reliably, whether andropause has already started for you or whether you are already in the middle of it.

MIDLIFE CRISIS: YOUR PERSONAL CHECKLIST

	never	seldom	sometimes	often	very often
1. I am exhausted, I lack energy.	☐	☐	☐	☐	☐
2. I am fearful or nervous.	☐	☐	☐	☐	☐
3. I am depressed, I am often in a bad mood.	☐	☐	☐	☐	☐
4. I am very irritable or angry.	☐	☐	☐	☐	☐
5. My concentration and memory are worse.	☐	☐	☐	☐	☐
6. I have relationship problems with my partner.	☐	☐	☐	☐	☐
7. My libido and sexual drive are down.	☐	☐	☐	☐	☐
8. I have problems having an erection or problems with potency.	☐	☐	☐	☐	☐
9. My skin, especially on my face and hands, is dry.	☐	☐	☐	☐	☐
10. I have back pains, or aching joints.	☐	☐	☐	☐	☐
11. I sweat a lot (during the day or night).	☐	☐	☐	☐	☐
12. I drink excessively.	☐	☐	☐	☐	☐
13. I constantly feel stressed.	☐	☐	☐	☐	☐
14. I am not physically fit.	☐	☐	☐	☐	☐

	30s	40s	50s	60s	70s
15. How old do you feel?	☐	☐	☐	☐	☐

	never	seldom	sometimes	often	very often
TOTAL number of boxes checked per column:	.....	.....	.....	......	.....
Multiply the number of boxes checked per column by the following numbers:	0	1	2	3	4
PRELIMINARY score:	.....	.....	......	......	.....

Add the preliminary score of all columns. If you had any of the following diseases, please add 4 points for each disease to the total score:

● prostatitis or prostate surgery
● mumps
● testicular disease
● chronic infections of the urinary tract

YOUR PERSONAL ANDROPAUSE SCORE:

ASSESSMENT

0-10 points

Be happy. It is highly unlikely that you have already entered the male climacteric.

11-20 points

It is possible that andropause has already set in for you.

21-30 points

You are probably going through the climacteric.

31-40 points

You are in the middle of the male climacteric. Consult your doctor.

Above 41 points

You are in the advanced stages of the climacteric.

If you want to be absolutely sure, see a doctor experienced in the field of endocrinology for a complete check-up and a hormonal analysis.

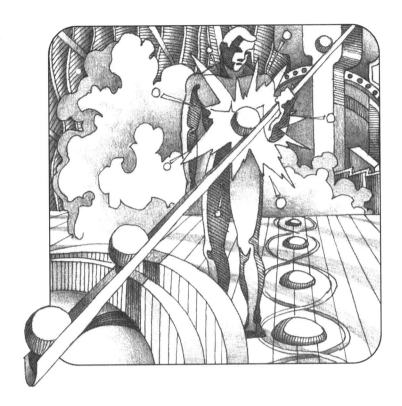

The Hormone Revolution

The Hormone Story

Hormones Fully Control Our Lives

"The most difficult of tasks is the one that ought to be the easiest: to see what lies ahead of us."

Johann Wolfgang von Goethe

It was well worth the try, even though his assistants at the Physiological Testing Institute in the Vienna Prater, also known as the "Vivarium," had voiced their concerns. Eugen Steinach's idea of performing "sex-change operations" on rats sounded just a little too outlandish.

It was the year 1912 when the energetic professor with a trimmed white beard, a sharp mind and a passion for horses, set out to feminize males and masculinize females. The 51-year-old professor removed the testicles of male rats and transplanted them to female rats. The results of his experiments, which also included pseudo-hermaphrodite rats suffering from an impaired hormone function surprised even Steinach himself. After surgery, the female rats suddenly showed male behavioral patterns, and vice versa.

Steinach transplanted testicles of "normal men" to homosexuals

Driven by those results, Steinach went one step further. Six years later, together with the urologist Robert Lichtenstern, he transplanted the testicles of "normal" men to homosexuals, thinking that the causes of "abnormal sexual behavior" were to be found in the "inner secretion." Steinach assumed that the testicles of homosexual men produced female hormones. One of his few failures, the project failed to confirm his hypothesis.

Pioneering Hormonal Research

Binding of the spermatic duct gives men new strength

Another discovery of Eugen Steinach's shortly thereafter gave an entire generation hope for prolonged youth. By performing vasoligatures (i.e., binding the spermatic duct) on old lab rats, Steinach noticed, the cell tissue between the spermatic canals, which he called the "puberty gland," was rejuvenated. On November 1, 1918, Lichtenstern and Steinach performed the first vasoligature on a human patient. The effects were spectacular and were promulgated around the world as the "Steinach operation." The patients were invigorated and revitalized. As a result, thousands of well-to-do men of the time underwent the surgery in the hope of regaining their potency and general vitality. Over a hundred doctors, many of them university professors, even had the operation done, including Steinach's friend, Sigmund Freud, and the famous orthopedist, Adolf Lorenz. Lorenz, who was 72 years old, reopened his practice and, with his new strength, treated patients for years to come. The world media reported euphorically the "Steinach era." But Steinach also had some vicious critics. Some called him a criminal who violated the laws of nature.

Steinach performed the first vasoligature in 1918

Sigmund Freud also had a vasoligature

The professor decide to turn his attention to isolating the sex hormones, following up on another notion he had of synthesizing them. He believed that hormone substitution could have a positive effect on a person's hair and skin, on their mental faculties, and could even lead to outright rejuvenation. Steinach was among the first scientists to establish a connection between hormones and a person's mental state.

Eugen Steinach, who died in Montreux in 1944 at the age of 83, is seen as one of the pioneers of modern hormone research. He not only tackled sexual taboos, but he also laid the groundwork for the scientific analysis of hormones. As a Jew in World War II Austria, he was obliged to discontinue his work and emigrate to Switzerland.

His student and assistant, Walter Hohlweg, who would later establish the field of neuro-endocrinology, went to Berlin and continued Steinach's studies. Hohlweg, according to some a bona fide genius, was the first to produce progesterone. Meanwhile, Adolf Friedrich Johann Butenandt, a chemist from Gdansk, isolated the first androsterone in a pure and crystalline form from 1500 liters of male urine at the Kaiser-Wilhelm Institute in Berlin. Butenandt, who died in 1995, received the Nobel Prize in chemistry in 1939 for his research on sex hormones and their interactions.

Adolf F. Butenandt was the first to isolate hormones

The Hormone Revolution

As the 21st century unwinds, science is beginning to understand what many scholars have suspected for thousands of years. Hormones have a massive influence over the lives of men, much more extensive than even Steinach could have imagined or science could prove in the early 1990s. Men are controlled by their hormones in every aspect of their lives, at work, at play, and during sex.

Hormones affect the entire life of men

A veritable hormone revolution is now underway in scientific circles.

The new findings are fascinating:

• Estrogen is a prerequisite for male potency
The female hormone estrogen is the basis for male potency and fertility. It is absolutely essential to the mobility of sperm cells. A man who does not have enough estrogen is infertile.

Estrogen is indispensable for the mobility of sperm cells

• Hormones control the aging process
Sex hormones play an important role in the aging of the male skeleton. Not only androgens—male hormones—but also estrogens help prevent osteoporosis. Therefore, the proper prophylaxis will be ever more important in the 21st century.

Estrogen in men prevents osteoporosis

• Lack of androgens makes men fat
In recent years, scientists have identified an important new property of androgens. They help reduce fat. The more androgens a man has, the less fat tissue he has.

They particularly affect the torso fat. Men who have more estrogens have a tendency to gain weight around the hips. After the age of 45, the decline in the effectiveness of androgens begins to show.

• Breast and prostate are very similar

Breast and prostate have almost identical tissue structures

The female breast and the male prostate are very similar in terms of their tissue structure and their response to hormonal influences. Today, there are more men who die of prostate cancer than there are women who die of breast cancer.

• We are all hermaphrodites

The male body is full of female hormones

Men still do not know that their bodies are filled with female hormones. As incredible as it may sound, it is a medical fact that, in terms of hormones, we are all hermaphrodites. The steroids are divided evenly between the two sexes. The difference is just a matter of the quantity of the individual hormones.

Melatonin and testosterone become trendy household words

Since World War II, researchers have paid more attention to the effects of hormones. But interest in investigating their influence on men did not take off until the 1990s. Since then, words like melatonin, serotonin, the growth hormone, estrogen and testosterone have become household terms.

That a deficiency of sex hormones can also cause diseases like osteoporosis in men is now known and scientifically proven. Just ten years ago, only 5% of the population understood the term osteoporosis. Today, 92% correctly associate it with a loss of bone density.

This new awareness makes discussion of hormones and the consequences of hormone deficiency for men easier. The baby boomers are reaching the point in their lives where they have to deal with the effects of aging. But they have a powerful advantage over previous generations. Today's men are not willing, like those of the postwar generation, to simply accept the problems associated with aging as fate. They have come to accept that they can exercise a certain amount of control over the aging process by means of hormones.

The History of Male Hormones

The extension of the life span has been an issue for thousands of years

Cheating the aging process, prolonging life and maintaining manhood and fertility have, for thousands of years, been foremost on the minds of men. Here are a few anecdotes, some of them humorous, to serve as a history of sorts of the study of hormones and aging.

In the course of history, mankind has always tried to achieve eternal youth. Even the biblical progenitors of mankind were driven by the desire to cheat death. Noah begot three sons, Shem, Ham and Japheth, when he was 500 years old. He died at the age of 950. In chapter six of Genesis, the Lord announces that, in the future, man will only live 120 years. And the author of that story, Moses, died when he reached that age.

The First Book of the Kings contains an early example of hormonal stimulation. It is the story of King David, who, old and stricken in years "gat no heat" although he was covered in clothes. "Wherefore his servants said unto him, Let there be sought for my lord the king a young virgin: and let her stand before the king, and let her cherish him, and let her lie in thy bosom, that my lord the king may get heat."

King David's testosterone production had to be stimulated

And they brought to him Abisag, a Shunammite, a fair damsel, who cherished the king and ministered to him. Thanks to her, King David found it within him to settle the fight over the succession between his older son Adonijah, and Solomon, Adonijah's younger half brother. In endocrinological terms, the beautiful Abisag was nothing but an exogenous stimulation of testosterone production in the king.

The Ebers, Passalaquas and Hearst papyri, named after their discoverers or translators and dated around 1600 BC, described stimulating and mobilizing recipes used by the ancient Egyptians. The tanning agents from mulberry plants, to name one example, were used to produce a medication whose substance is similar in structure and effect to adrenalin.

In 1600 BC, Egyptians described adrenalin-like substances

The Passalaquas papyrus also contains the first test, based on hormones, for determining the sex of an unborn baby. "Wheat and barley are moistened with the urine of the pregnant woman everyday. If the wheat grows faster than the barley, the child will be a boy. If the barley grows faster, the child will be a girl."

Hippocrates (460-370 BC), in trying to explain the mental stimulus that goes with the sex drive, believed that the semen of a man came from his brain, sent to the testicles by way of the spinal cord.

Hippocrates suspected that sperm were produced in the brain

In early Christian Rome, the testicles of castrated slaves were traded as a "hot item," to be used as a sexual stimulant.

Medical research into hormones used to be a dangerous endeavor. Andreas Vesalius, a reputable professor in Padua, Pisa, Bologna and Basel, founded the

Vesalius was executed because of his hormone-related discoveries

study of anatomy, and acted as personal physician to Emperor Charles V. In 1553, after publishing his masterpiece, "De Humani Corporis Fabrica," a treatise on the thyroid gland, he was tried by a court of the Inquisition and executed.

The first hormone test for diagnosing fertility was offered in 1696 by Christian Franz Paulini, a doctor from Münster, in the Heilsame Drecksapotheke, or Wholesome Rubbish Apothecary. "If you want to know whether infertility is the man's fault or the woman's fault, take two jars of barley; put the man's urine in one, and the woman's urine in the other. Let both jars stand for 12 days. The blame will rest with that person whose barley has not risen after those 12 days."

But hormonal research was not subjected to scientific constraints until the end of the 18th century. A French doctor, Theophile Bordeu, first suspected that the glandular secretions were moved throughout the body by means of the blood.

In 1762, the English doctor John Hunter, at St. Georges Hospital in London, transplanted a rooster's testicles into its lower abdomen, but he never published any results.

In 1848, hormone research was born

On August 2, 1848, Arnold Berthold, a professor in Göttingen, Germany, repeated the experiment. A half year later, he found that the testicles had not changed. This could be regarded as the birth of what later came to be known as hormone research.

In 1855, French researcher Claude Bernard coined the term "inner secretion."

Prof. Brown-Séquard injected himself with extracts from dog testicles

June 1, 1889, was a historic moment for endocrinology, when professor Charles Edouard Brown-Séquard, a 72-year-old physiologist, announced at the conference of the Societé de Biologie in Paris that had found a cure for aging. After injecting himself with extracts from the testicles of dogs and guinea pigs, he claimed to feel younger and fresher than ever. His findings were contested by other scientists, who attributed the improvement in his condition to autosuggestion. But Brown-Séquard would not hear of it. He repeated his experiment with prison inmates and reached similar results. In order to convince his students of the newly gained potency, he urinated in front of the Sorbonne in Paris, with "a strong and wide stream through the air."

Later, experiments with male gonads became more frequent, and most were crude attempts to restore the virility of castrated test animals, and to rejuvenate animals and old people.

It was in 1905 that Ernest Henry Starling, a physiologist, coined the term "hormone" during a lecture on the chemical interactions of human bodily functions at the Royal College in London. The term was readily accepted and has been widely used in medical research ever since.

It was Eugen Steinach who launched the modern era in hormone research. Then, in 1935, Laqueur and Ruzicka managed to convert cholesterol to testosterone. With the industrial manufacture of testosterone (from the Latin word "testis" = testicles), modern hormone-replacement therapy became possible.

Up until World War II, hormone research focused almost exclusively on men, but things took a dramatic turn. All of a sudden, hormones and their effects were examined only with respect to the female body, a trend that lasted nearly until the end of the 20th century. Men are now coming back into the limelight of endocrinological research. Industry has discovered the potential for economic gain in the aging male driven by his hormones.

Ernest H. Starling coined the term "hormones" in 1905

Laqueur and Ruzicka performed the first successful testosterone transformation

From World War II onward, only female hormones were subject to research

THE DISCOVERY OF HORMONES

● The Old Testament.
King David was treated by means of an exogenous stimulation of his testosterone production.

● The ancient Egyptians.
In the 16th century BC, the ancient Egyptians described, in the Passalaquas papyrus, the first test ever to determine the sex of an unborn baby.

● Hippocrates.
Around 400 BC, he declared that the semen of a man came from his brain and was sent to the testicles by way of the spinal cord.

● Charles Edouard Brown-SOquard.
The 72-year-old physiologist claimed, on June 1, 1889, that he had found a cure against aging after injecting himself with an extract from the testicles of young dogs and guinea pigs.

● Eugen Steinach.
He was the Austrian pioneer of hormone research, and the first to connect a person's mental state with their hormones, ushering in a new era in hormone research.

Hormones as the Body's Email

Hormones give cells clear instructions

What are hormones and how do they work? Hormones function as messengers in an organism, biochemical negotiators that control and regulate the activities of certain organs. Each hormone contains data, specific to certain cells in the body, that trigger particular actions. This entire communication system is highly complex and specialized, and functions at an incredible speed. Put more simply, "A hormone is a molecule that moves to a cell, connects to a receptor and then gives the cell instructions," says Edmund Chein, the US "high priest" of hormones. Comparing the body to a computer, hormones work like email, delivering their information to huge numbers of recipients within a few hundredths of a second.

Hormones reach the target organs within a few hundredths of a second

The word "hormone" has its roots in the ancient Greek word "hormau," which translates into "I activate myself." The science that deals with hormones is endocrinology, the study of the endocrine glands, and their secretions. In simple terms, it is the study of nature's biological communication system.

500 million years ago, cells could not communicate with each other

The evolution of hormones in humans compares with that of the telephone in the last 50 years. Nature, 500 million years ago, had to find a way for a living organism to communicate beyond three or four cells. As long as there were only single-celled organisms, communicating from one end of the cell to the other was not difficult. Bi-cellular organisms had a more complex communication system. In multi-cellular organisms, where all cells perform more or less the same tasks, communication is facilitated by the processes of exocytosis and endocytosis. Information from one cell is extracted and implanted into another. If organisms become too complex, this type of communication is too slow, and the organisms find themselves ill equipped for reacting to external influences. Separate cell systems with specialized functions require a secure information pipeline so that the right information arrives at the right place at the right time.

The Information Pipeline Between Organs

Nature first reacted to the new challenges by building nerves. Nerve fibers, like telephone wires, connect different parts of the body and thus allow for more efficient, faster and better communication. But what happens if even this nervous system becomes overloaded because the cell structures have become too large and complex, and therefore unmanageable? A complex system like the human body would be a muddle of wires and would not be viable. To solve this problem, nature created the hormones, a more refined communication system.

The evolutionary invention of the hormones—there are about 25 hormones in the human body—is the biological equivalent of the development of cell phone technology, with one difference. Hormones are a thousand times more complex than any high-tech data network. Hormones need to be complex in order to sort, filter and screen information. The biological message they carry with them is not meant to be "read" by every cell in the human organism, but only by certain cells.

Man has about 25 known hormones

Ensuring that the hormones reach the targeted cells is the task of receptors located in different parts of the cell. These receptors work like a lock and key. They can only recognize certain hormones. If a cell does not have a lock or receptor for the hormone, the cell cannot respond regardless of the content of the message. The hormone cannot dock and pass along its information to the receptor, which would normally tell the organ to change its activity—for example to produce protein, to store water, and so on.

Receptors are locks for certain key hormones

A hormone can do different jobs. The same biological function may be triggered or influenced by different hormones. For example, to keep the blood sugar at a certain level to ensure optimum brain function, four different hormones are required. In addition to this complex system of hormones that supplement and back each other up, there is also an extensive, sophisticated system of feedback among the hormones. As a result, almost every hormone can reduce its own production and thus the production of other hormones.

Four hormones are required to maintain the blood sugar level

Types of Hormones

Modern medicine distinguishes three types of hormones, based on their method of release into the organism.

1. Endocrine hormones

Endocrine hormones are produced in glands such the pancreatic gland, the adrenal gland or the thyroid gland. From there, they are released into the bloodstream and led to the cells of the target organs, to specific receptors. The bloodstream is a kind of superhighway for endocrine hormones. It allows them to travel swiftly from the location where they are produced to their target. Endocrine hormones require the help of this "third party," the bloodstream, in order to communicate. They are the long-distance transmitters among hormones. Endocrine hormones may be:

Endocrine hormones use the bloodstream as a data highway

- insulin

- cortisol
- glucagon
- growth hormone
- thyroid hormone
- estrogen
- testosterone

The hypothalamus—data center for endocrine hormones

Millions of signals meet in the hypothalamus

The data center for all endocrine hormones is the hypothalamus, a cherry-sized gland in the middle of the brain. It continuously receives signals from the body regarding temperature, blood pressure, glucose and other hormone levels. These signals are picked up by the central nervous system and passed on directly to the hypothalamus.

The pituitary gland produces ten different hormones

The processes within that gland go beyond human imagination. Every second, millions of dynamic input signals reach the hypothalamus, which promptly reacts and releases secretions. These do not have far to travel; they go only as far as the pituitary gland. These messenger substances, which control the pituitary, are called "releasing" or "inhibiting" hormones.

The pituitary gland is located at the base of the brain. Although it is part of the brain, it has direct and intensive contact with the blood system. This small gland produces ten different hormones that are released directly into the blood. Depending on whether the hypothalamus has sent out releasing or inhibiting hormones, some of these pituitary hormones, such as the growth hormone, are released directly into the bloodstream. Other hormones go to the adrenal gland, the thyroid gland and other endocrine glands.

2. Paracrine hormones

Paracrine hormones are released over short distances and over a well-defined path, such as from the hypothalamus to the pituitary gland. These paths are nerves or ducts (intercellular spaces). Paracrine hormones are part of the evolutionary development between the groups of endocrine and autocrine hormones. They do not exist in the bloodstream. In our comparison with a data network, they would be responsible for local calls.

Paracrine hormones may be:
- melatonin
- serotonin
- releasing hormone

3. Autocrine hormones

Autocrine hormones function through the secretion of cells among themselves. They include, for example, eicosanoids. The autocrine hormones were the first primeval hormones, because they passed on their information from one cell to another cell in their immediate surroundings. The autocrine hormones are the most important hormones in the male body. They control almost 60 trillion cells! They influence all the other hormones the way a company like Intel would the computer chips that control your personal computer. Even if the level of endocrine hormones drops as you get older, hormonal communication can be maintained provided the autocrine hormones are protected.

Autocrine hormones control 60 trillion cells

Hormone Classification According to Precursors

There is another way of classifying hormones, based on the substances from which hormones originate—the precursors. Whereas polypeptide hormones (such as glucagon) and neurotransmitters (substances that transmit information from nerve to nerve, such as noradrenaline or adrenaline) are made up of amino acids—the building blocks of protein, steroid hormones (sex hormones like DHEA, estrogen, progesterone, or testosterone) are derived from cholesterol, and eicosanoids from fat.

Precursors are the basic substances of hormones

Another distinguishing feature of hormones is their variation in size. The rule of thumb is that the larger a hormone, the more complicated it will be for the hormone to reach its target tissue. Polypeptide hormones are relatively large. Steroid hormones or thyroid hormones are very small. Some hormones, like melatonin and especially autocrine hormones like eicosanoids are fat-soluble, and do not have to circulate throughout the blood over long distances. They are also quite small, which allows them to get in between the cell membranes.

Melatonin and eicosanoids are fat-soluble

The Effects of Free Hormones in the Body

In order to understand the breadth and complexity of hormones in the human body and their incredible effects, it is important to know first of all that each hormone circulating in the blood is tied to very specific messenger substances, so-called binding proteins. If a hormone, on its way through the body, has been tied to such a protein, it is considered inactive. It is comparable to the inbox in an internet email program, which does not allow messages to be retrieved until the proper code has been entered. Once the hormone has been freed from its connecting protein, thus becoming a "free hormone," it is considered biologically

Only free hormones are biologically active

active. Paracrine and autocrine hormones, however, require no binding proteins, because they are only sent over short distances.

The importance of distinguishing between inactive and free hormones is illustrated by "sex hormone binding globuline," or SHBG. It transports hormones such as estrogen or testosterone throughout the male body. A new study, published by the Mayo Clinic in 1999, provides proof that the SHBG level in men rises significantly after the age of 40, a fact that has so far received little attention. The SHBG level in women, however, remains relatively constant. This finding proves that the estrogen and testosterone levels in men have been measured incorrectly for decades. Why? In the past, it was the entire supply of estrogen and testosterone in the body that was measured. This resulted, in part, in almost identical measurements in 30-year-old men as in 60-year-olds. It was wrongly concluded that the testosterone level of men does not substantially drop with age. Thanks to the separate measurement of bound estrogen, free estrogen and testosterone, we now get the real picture, which reveals a decrease in effective or active hormones with age. In fact, both free testosterone and free estrogen levels in men decrease substantially with age. This correlated, moreover, to a decline in bone density. But what if men could be treated with supplements of estrogen and testosterone?

SHBG sheds new light on testosterone

Free testosterone and estrogen decrease with age

The Principle of Second Messengers

Second messengers work through the cell membrane

Hormones have to deal with periods of inactivity, but they also have to overcome barriers, called endothelial cells. Hormones must find their way past them in order to reach muscular or other tissues. During the aging process, endothelial cells change, which makes it more difficult for the hormones to find their target.

It may also happen that hormones never reach their target cells. This inability to reach the target cell despite higher hormone levels in the blood is called "resistance."

A myriad of substances can impair the work of hormones in the body. One such group of substances is saturated fatty acids. They reduce the quality and quantity of the liquid between the cell membranes and thereby make it more difficult for hormones to interact with the receptors of the target cells. They convey the hormone's information to the cell and stimulate several enzymes, which translate the information into action.

Many hormones do not enter the cell by going between the membranes, but they interact directly with the membranes themselves with the help of so called "second messengers." For his research on the subject of second messenger systems, Earl W. Jr. Sutherland received the Nobel Prize for medicine in 1971.

THE MALE HORMONES

● Endocrine hormones
They are released directly into the bloodstream by special glands (such as the pancreatic gland, adrenal gland or thyroid gland) controlled by the hypothalamus and the pituitary gland. They include insulin, cortisol, glucagon, growth hormone, thyroid hormone, estrogen, testosterone.

● Paracrine hormones
Paracrine hormones are released over short distances and a well-defined path (such as from the hypothalamus to the pituitary). These paths are nerves or ducts. Panacrine hormones include melatonin, serotonin, releasing hormones.

● Autocrine hormones
Autocrine hormones work by direct secretion from one cell to another. They pass on their information to the immediate neighboring cell. Autocrine hormones include eicosanoids.

The most common second messenger is cyclical AMP (adenosine monophosphate). A newly discovered second messenger is nitrogen monoxide. An improper diet will have a negative impact on the function of these second messengers.

AMP is the most common second messenger

Why Do We Age?

Aging as a Process Controlled by Hormones

With the influence of hormones on men so much stronger than previously believed, one essential question comes to mind. What is the role hormones play in the aging process? Besides the telomerase enzyme and the chemical wear-and-tear caused by free oxygen radicals, are there any other mechanisms controlling the fate of cells? Can this biophysical process be influenced by hormones in a way that would enable us to live longer?

Miscommunication among hormones makes us grow older

Recent research in the field of endocrinology has provided us with some incredible findings on the mechanisms of the aging process. The most important discovery is that the molecular changes in the body that make a person age are the result of an increase in hormonal miscommunications, in other words deterioration in the interaction of hormones.

From the age of 30 onward, the male body produces fewer and fewer hormones. If the marvelously complex hormonal system gets out of balance as a result, then the communications between the organism and its various organs will be out of kilter. This is one of the primary causes of aging, and it is a new and almost revolutionary insight.

The Imbalance of Hormones

Balanced hormone levels can slow the aging process

Your body is a powerful and complex biological internet. As a fundamental part of this network, communication among hormones must be harmonized. If hormones are thrown out of balance, the organism will begin to age. Sleep disorders, wrinkles, dry skin, reduced sex drive, depression, chronic pain, obesity, diabetes, cardiovascular disease and cancer are consequences of an imbalance of hormones in the male body. The proper balance of hormones,

---

FOUR POSSIBLE CAUSES OF AGING

1. Too much glucose in the blood
Glucose destroys the cell walls. Too much sugar in the blood leads to an overproduction of insulin, which has to store the glucose in the fatty tissue.

2. Too much insulin
The increase in insulin production may lead to insulin resistance in the cells, which may cause vessel damage and diabetes.

3. Too many free radicals
Free radicals are important to an organism because they kill germs. But an oversupply of them will lead to an attack on the organism's own cells and may cause cancer.

4. Too much cortisol
As stress mounts, the body increases its secretion of cortisol, which raises blood pressure and pulse to very high levels, putting a strain on the organism.

however, can help slow the aging process. It is not so much the lack of certain hormones, but rather the inability of hormones to communicate with each other and to harmonize their effects on the organism that triggers aging.

For now, suffice to say that intervention in the hormone system, by way of hormone replacement or controlling the hormonal enzyme system, can actively slow the aging process. How this works will be explained later in the book. And keep in mind that countering the aging process through the hormones must be accompanied by proper diet, a balanced lifestyle and the minimization of certain risks, as outlined in this book.

Hormone substitution can postpone aging

There are as many different theories of the causes of aging as there are scientists who specialize in aging. All those experts have a different view. But current research efforts focus on four main causes of aging.

Hormonal Factors in the Aging Process

Researchers agree on certain points. Aging is caused by a multitude of external and internal factors. Hormones clearly play a crucial role. Although the endocrine system is complex and sophisticated, only two hormones ultimately have a sustainable influence on the aging process in men—insulin and eicosanoids.

An increase in the production of insulin is probably one of the most important factors in accelerated aging. It exerts its negative influence everywhere. There are markers in the human body, in other words certain tendencies that increase with age, such as insulin resistance (leading to an increased blood insulin level), systolic blood pressure (the first of the blood pressure levels measured), and the buildup of fatty tissue and blood lipids. Other markers decrease with age, such as glucose tolerance (less and less glucose can be used up), aerobic capacity (especially in sports), muscle mass, strength, temperature regulation, and immunological functions.

Insulin and eicosanoids affect the aging process

Too much insulin speeds up the aging process in men

Although these markers cover a variety of physiological changes, longitudinal studies such as the Baltimore Study of Aging (BLSA) consistently name one decisive factor in the aging process: an increase in the production of insulin.

• Insulin—a dangerous aging hormone?

Scientists agree that an increased blood insulin level (also called increased insulin resistance) likely plays a powerful role in the aging process. Insulin has a huge effect on other hormone systems, especially the system of eicosanoids. Every biological function that fails with age is susceptible to an increase in insulin production and its effect on other hormone systems.

Without insulin, cells would starve

It is the task of insulin to store the nutrients we eat, especially carbohydrates, in the respective target cells. If we did not have insulin in our blood, our cells would starve, so a certain level of this hormone is vital to the human organism.

Insulin does not require receptors. It "sneaks" into the cell through a very complicated transport system. Insulin resistance (hyperinsulinemia), or the overproduction of insulin, makes it difficult for the hormone to fulfill its task. Many of the causes of aging, such as increased storage of fat in the body, are direct or indirect consequences of hyperinsulinemia.

• Eicosanoids—key to reversing the aging process

The importance of eicosanoids was recognized only a few years ago. In 1982, the Nobel Prize in medicine was awarded for essential research done on eicosanoids proving that they control nearly every physiological process in the human body. Nonetheless, only a few doctors even know what they are. Eicosanoids are of vital significance to the biological internet. They are, in fact, an essential key to "anti-aging."

Eicosanoids are capable of improving the levels of cyclical AMP—a second messenger—in the target cell, thereby improving communication between the endocrine hormones and the target cell. These second messengers, especially cyclical AMP, are responsible for countering aging, for they are the last important phase in hormonal communication. If communication between the hormone and the cell collapses, no more interaction between them will be possible.

Eicosanoids work through the secretion of cells among each other

Eicosanoids self-destruct within seconds

Eicosanoids are clusters of various substances produced by every cell in our body. They are like microprocessing chips, which turn every personal computer into a technological miracle worker. Just as electrons pass through microprocessors, eicosanoids, too, are ubiquitous. As autocrine hormones, they never enter the bloodstream. They work by intercellular secretion. Eicosanoids are effective in almost unimaginably small concentrations and destroy themselves within seconds. This makes it almost impossible to study them in the body or to measure them. It is also quite difficult, therefore, to replace eicosanoids. Still, pharmaceutical researchers are pouring billions of dollars into analytical studies of eicosanoids.

The Active Agent in Aspirin

Much of our knowledge of eicosanoids derives from research on tissue cell cultures. Until recently, it was a little known fact that the efficiency of one of the most successful medications of this century, aspirin, is based on eicosanoids. Acetylsalicylic acid, which aspirin contains, was even used by the Celts. Concentrations of it can be found especially in willow (salix). The magic potion that Astérix, the hero of the French language comic books, drank before going into battle with the Romans would have contained aspirin or willow extracts. This is just another of the medical surprises to come from early cultures.

Aspirin is equivalent to the extract of willow

The duality we so often encounter in nature, the yin-yang principle, is also found in eicosanoids and other hormones. There are "good" eicosanoids and "bad" ones. The ratio of good to bad eicosanoids is of paramount importance to the aging process and, indeed, the functioning of the entire hormone system.

Yin-yang also applies to eicosanoids

Insulin plays a dubious role with respect to eicosanoids. It increases the production of bad eicosanoids. The more insulin we produce, the more bad eicosanoids we produce at the same time. The consequences are usually high blood pressure and numerous other conditions (various inflammations, diabetes type I, cancer, depression). This could help explain why an increased insulin level is often accompanied by higher blood pressure. As age-related hyperinsulinemia increases, so does the percentage of body fat. However, the production of benign blood lipid, HDL cholesterol, decreases as a result, which raises the risk of cardiovascular disease. If the imbalance deteriorates further at the expense of the benign eicosanoids, the entire hormone system will get out of balance. And this may be an underlying factor in the aging process.

Too much insulin produces bad eicosanoids

Why Eicosanoids Cannot Be Replaced

What can we do to ensure that we have a balance of good and bad eicosanoids? Where do we find good eicosanoids? They cannot be taken as simple supplements. There are no good eicosanoids that we can take as medication. They can only be absorbed indirectly through a proper diet. Maintaing this balance by keeping the production of insulin low can be achieved with a diet low in carbohydrates. This is also the single most important action you can take to maintain the balance of your entire hormone system.

Reducing the intake of carbohydrates is good for maintaining hormonal balance

Another would be ensuring that you always provide your body with sufficient unsaturated fatty acids, which are vital to the production of good eicosanoids.

Fish oil and olive oil contain good eicosanoids

These can be found in fish and olive oil. Eskimos like to eat fatty food, but they have no higher incidence of arteriosclerosis. Why not? Because they eat a lot of fish oil and cod liver oil, absorbing in the process certain elements important to the production of benign eicosanoids.

Excessive overproduction of insulin adversely affects other functions of the body and brings on the aging process as well. A decline in sugar tolerance increases insulin resistance. The body cannot absorb enough sugar from the blood anymore and tries to compensate by producing more insulin.

Aerobic capacity, the capacity of men to exert themselves in sports or other hard physical activities, also succumbs with age. From the age of 20 onward, this capacity decreases by about 1% each year. Eicosanoids play an important role here, too. Benign eicosanoids are bronchodilators. The bad ones are bronchoconstrictors (substances that constrict the bronchi in the lungs).

These consequences of aging concern all men and women. Therefore, every program designed to slow the aging process should focus on reducing the blood insulin level.

Many hormones are secondary parameters of aging

So why are other hormone levels not targeted in the battle against aging? For example, is the reduction of muscle mass not caused by declining production of growth hormones? Yes and no. Production of some hormones drops off with age, but not of all. Some hormones, like insulin and cortisol, may even increase, while others remain relatively constant. In this respect, changes in the hormone levels in themselves are no more than secondary parameters of aging.

As an example, the level of the growth hormone decreases dramatically with age. But if the pituitary gland as the source of the growth hormone is properly stimulated, it is possible to quickly produce the growth hormone at a rate similar to that in a young man. So, it is not reduced production of the growth hormone that manifests itself in lower growth hormone levels, but rather a reduced "response," a diminished reaction to hormonal signals, that is responsible. The decrease in production of the growth hormone as well as the decline in the levels of certain other hormones as a person ages are more the consequence of hormonal imbalance.

Understanding how hormones communicate with each other and pass on biological information, and learning to positively influence this communication are the key to an effective anti-aging program.

THE TWO PILLARS OF ANTI-AGING

Endocrinologists in the US see the following two recipes as the key to countering aging:

1. Eicosanoids keep you young
There are no medications, but eicosanoids are to be found in fish oil and olive oil. They improve communication between the endocrine hormones and the cells. They also create a balance of hormones, which is important in slowing the aging process.

2. Cut down on carbohydrates
With its positive influence on eicosanoids, reducing your intake of carbohydrates is practically a guarantee of a longer life. Dieting or starving would be counterproductive and simply wrong. But too much pasta, pizza and sugar spells death for communication within the hormone system. Excessive glucose in the blood destroys eicosanoids, and the balance collapses.

The Fear of Hormones Is Unfounded

This fear is unjustified, but still widespread. People still have prejudices against hormones, saying that they have not been sufficiently explored. Others think that the danger of side effects is too high.

Attitudes like these have been around throughout the history of medicine. If taken too seriously, we would be in the medical equivalent of the Middle Ages.

Hormones, like any other medication taken improperly, carry certain risks. Improper dosages can lead to damage of the adrenal gland, the thyroid gland or the pancreatic gland. In many countries, even the US, there are hormone preparations blithely sold over the counter in supermarkets or on the internet. This practice is dangerous and should be discouraged. Hormone treatments need to be supervised by an experienced endocrinologist, a doctor specialized in the field of hormone therapies. That would at least render the danger of side effects no higher than in any other drug treatment.

Hormones belong in the hands of an experienced endocrinologist

Testosterone—The Masculine Hormone

When Is a Man a Man?

"Man consists of balls and brain."

Hugh Hefner, founder of Playboy

When Clemens B. visited the department of endocrinology at the university hospital in Vienna, he had a problem that most men would envy him for. His sex drive was insatiable. "I could constantly have sex with three women," he admitted to his doctor. His sex drive, his libido, was uncontrollable. Still, B. complained of a lack of energy to satisfy his needs. Breaking out in a sweat, instability and irritability dragged him down.

A comprehensive hormone analysis confirmed what his doctor had suspected. Clemens B. had a very high testosterone level of 8.5 nanograms, but a very low level of estradiol of only 17 picograms. His hormone system was out of balance.

Testosterone is the most important sex hormone in men

Testosterone is by far the most important sex hormone in men. It is formed primarily in the male gonads, the testicles, from the androstenedione. The male body produces approximately seven milligrams of testosterone per day, the female body only about 0.3 milligrams.

The main switching center for testosterone is in the brain. It triggers or suppresses production, whichever the body requires. The cerebral cortex stimulates testosterone production when we are excited or happy. If we are under stress or angry, our testosterone level drops.

The pituitary gland controls testosterone production in the testicles

The process is always the same. Via the pituitary gland, the hypothalamus controls the production of testosterone in the testicles, where it is produced in the Leydig cells, of which men have about 500 million. The hormones "report" to the hypothalamus on the activity in the testicles. From the testicles, testosterone is released into the blood, and much of it binds to the SHBG (sex hormone binding globuline) protein. Testosterone that is bound to SHBG is inactive. Only about 10% is free testosterone, which can enter the target cell or target organ and bind itself to the receptor in the cytoplasm of

Only about 10% of the testosterone is active in the body

the cell. Once this connection has occurred, it is transported into the core of the cell where it stimulates certain genes, which in turn trigger the synthesis of protein.

Measuring the amount of free, active testosterone in the blood is very complicated. In men, the occurrence of free testosterone, just like free estrogen, decreases with age. But the total amount of testosterone, as of estrogen, does not really decrease, for the level of binding hormone SHBG increases. Nowadays, the level of free hormones is measured when doing a hormone analysis on aging men.

Testosterone in men works in many different ways.
- It is responsible for the growth and the formation of the secondary sexual characteristics, such as body and facial hair, penis, prostate, seminal vesicle and larynx.
- It is responsible for the formation of muscles and the reduction of fat.
- It is of crucial importance to the sex drive, acting like an aphrodisiac with respect to libido and potency.
- Testosterone is also important for spatial thinking. Women who have a very strong deficit of testosterone have tremendous problems, for example, with parking their cars.
- It raises the activity and the capacity of men, but also increases their aggressiveness.

Testosterone is responsible for beard growth, development of the penis, muscle buildup, potency

A study by the National Institutes of Health (NIH) in the United States examined the correlation between the level of testosterone and character traits of 1,700 men. The results clearly indicated that men with a high testosterone level had a tendency to control others. They expressed their views strongly, were highly animated and often threw fits of anger. Men with higher testosterone levels also tend to be more successful, more agile and sexually more active.

Men with a high testosterone level are more successful

Such was the case with Giacomo Casanova, who treated women of the 16th century to his uncommon manliness. He increased his testosterone level without knowing its actual effect on his body by eating raw eggs everyday before going off on his amorous adventures, sleeping with up to ten women daily.

Casanova increased his androgen level by eating raw eggs

A man's life is controlled not only by his testosterone level, however. It is also affected by interaction in his body between the typically female hormone estrogen and the characteristically male testosterone. If the level of testosterone is higher than that of estrogen, perhaps because the level of the latter has decreased, then a condition like Clemens B's will ensue, with the patient suffering from an insatiable libido and becoming more and more aggressive. The diagnosis for these cases may come as a surprise to many men. They lack estrogen.

Sexual Differentiation Starts in Your Mother's Womb

Androgen comes from the Greek word meaning "makers of men"

Androgens—the catch-all name for male hormones—are responsible for male sexuality. The term derives from the Greek and really means "makers of men." One of the primary functions of testosterone is sexual differentiation between males and females. The concentration and the effect of testosterone are essential factors in determining whether we turn into a man or into a woman. Testosterone is also responsible for the different behavioral patterns of men and women. This hormone-related differentiation starts in the uterus. The last third of the pregnancy is characterized by a significant increase in testosterone production. For many years thereafter it falls to a very low level, only to rise again with the onset of puberty. Testosterone decides whether we become a superman or a weakling. Testosterone levels shoot sky high at the end of puberty and drop off slowly with age.

During puberty, the testosterone level jumps

Hormonal imbalances or dysfunctions can make themselves felt in different ways, but mostly in the second half of one's life. Men never experience a drastic drop in testosterone levels the way women do when their estrogen levels fall during menopause. The level of free testosterone, however, drops with age, while the total testosterone level (including the testosterone bound to the carrier protein SHBG and thus inactive) falls off only slightly.

SHBG binds more and more testosterone

One of the essential actions of testosterone, which occurs via the bloodstream, is to build up muscle tissue in the male body and to reduce fatty tissue. It is also responsible for tightening the muscle mass and for so-called body composition, or distribution of fat. A muscular, masculine body is the product of testosterone. This can also be seen in animals, too. A good rooster never gets fat.

Doping agents are mostly derived from testosterone

Testosterone often generates negative headlines due its role in high performance sports and in bodybuilding. The infamous doping agents are largely based on testosterone and misused as an anabolic to artificially raise the testosterone level in the body.

How Does Testosterone Work in Men?

The reductase enzyme transforms testosterone into dihydrotestosterone

In the male body, about 10% of the testosterone is changed into dihydrotestosterone. Dihydrotestosterone is the active ingredient in organs such as the prostate, the seminal gland, or the skin. It is ten times as effective as testosterone and is responsible for baldness as well as for the low, masculine voice. But its most dangerous property is its triggering effect on prostate cancer cells.

It may be possible to beat prostate cancer by blocking the very "aggressive effect" of dihydrotestosterone on the prostate.

The process of changing testosterone into dihydrotestosterone—using the enzyme reductase—or, alternatively, suppressing its production, are of therapeutic importance. Agents that help slow this conversion (e.g., the prostate drug Proscar®) can, for example, stimulate the growth of new hair. Since testosterone triggers the sex drive in the brain, such a drug can often prevent baldness, but it may also, in rare cases, block the libido.

Dihydrotestosterone has little to do with mental state and libido. It is testosterone that works primarily in the brain. Dihydrotestosterone, however, mainly affects the tissues—its effect on the brain is very small.

How Aromatase Turns Testosterone into Estrogen

Testosterone and estrogen are responsible for the development of masculinity in men and femininity in women, and they occur in both sexes, though with some quantitative differences. While a man produces about 25 to 50 times as much testosterone as a woman, she, in turn, produces two to three times as much estrogen as a man.

Men produce 25 to 50 times as much testosterone as women

Testosterone is converted into estrogen by the aromatase enzyme. It is this enzyme that may not have been sufficiently activated in Clemens B., resulting in his relatively high testosterone level and reduced estrogen level. Clemens B., in addition to his elevated testosterone level, also had a low-activity aromatase enzyme.

The aromatase enzyme transforms testosterone into estrogen

But the opposite may happen as well. Rather than of an oversupply of androgens, estrogens may dominate if the enzyme induction of aromatase is too active. Such men usually have no lack of energy, and no potency or erectile problems, but they often complain of not "having been in the mood for sex for some time now" and of lacking a "healthy" degree of aggressiveness, which they need a certain amount of in their jobs or careers.

Some vegetable substances, such as pumpkin-seed oil or its extracts, may be able to activate the aromatase enzyme, important in the treatment of the male climacteric. Royal jelly, produced by bees, is said to have the same effect.

Pumpkin-seed oil activates the aromatase enzyme

Estrogens compensate for the effects of testosterone. If a man experiences an imbalance between testosterone and estrogen, a dysfunction of the enzyme level must be assumed. The diminished activity of the enzyme, specifically of aromatase, becomes a sign of old age.

It is more frequent, however, for aromatase to show a higher activity level, especially if it is in excess supply, because the fatty tissue contains a lot of this enzyme. The more fatty tissue there is, the more estrogen can be produced from testosterone both in men and in women. On the downside, estrogen causes fatty tissue to collect around the hips.

Stress is dangerous for testosterone production

In order to maintain libido, energy and cardiovascular health, the testosterone level in men may not drop too drastically. Stress is fatal to the production of testosterone because it raises the production of the hormone cortisol. While testosterone has an anabolic effect (tissue building), cortisol acts catabolically (reducing).

The best and simplest way to counter the increase in the testosterone level is to build up fatty tissue. Fatty tissue has a high aromatase content, which produces estrogen from testosterone. If you were to lose ten pounds, you would minimize this conversion considerably, which automatically raises your testosterone level.

Sports can raise the testosterone level by 30%

The scientist Alan Mazur was able to prove over a period of ten years that, in men, a 10% increase in fatty tissue brings about a continuous reduction in the testosterone level. Exercise and sports are would raise it again. At the peak of physical exercise, according to US studies, the testosterone level rises by 30%. But the sport must be kept up. Only a few weeks after the end of training, many men experience a decrease to their original testosterone level.

Today, there is much talk about intervention in the workings of aromatase and reductase (inhibiting or activating). Some measures along these lines have already been taken in the search for an active prophylaxis for prostate cancer and baldness.

Testosterone-Replacement Therapy in Men – A Revolutionary Discovery

How can testosterone production be modified in a positive way? Testosterone can be substituted, or replaced. This allows lower testosterone levels to be normalized.

Before starting a hormone-replacement therapy, a patient requires a comprehensive physical examination. The anamnesis needs to be taken right back to childhood, with special emphasis on history of diseases like mumps, or inflammations that may have damaged the testicles and thus the production of testosterone.

Hormone-replacement therapy only through a doctor

The patient has to fill out a long andropause checklist, an extended form of the one used in this book. Following this, an endocrinologist will look for other factors adversely affecting the patient's health, ranging from job-related stress to poor diet. Finally, there is a thorough medical-diagnostic examination of not only the cardiovascular functions, penis, liver and prostate, but also involving a complete blood analysis with special emphasis on the hormones.

After the assessment of the results of these tests, an endocrinologist will discuss all the findings with the patient in a second interview. Hormone-replacement therapy in itself is often not enough to improve a person's life dramatically. A change of lifestyle is usually also necessary. This is completely up to the patient.

Opting for hormone-replacement therapy leaves open several possibilities. Testosterone and other hormones can be replenished by means of injections, tablets, deposits and creams for the skin.

• Injections

As early as the 1940s, patients were given testosterone injections. Initially, their effects only lasted for two hours, and later on, for two to three days. After that, people were injected in their posteriors once or twice a week with doses of 220 to 250 milligrams. This technique is practiced to a limited degree even today.

Injections are effective for only 2–3 days

Injections have a drawback, however. After a few hours, the testosterone jumps up to a level that it is not supposed to reach, with possible long-term negative effects on the liver. Testosterone conversion into estrogen may also be triggered, counter to the original purpose. Finally, the level plummets so quickly that it soon reaches a point below the target level of the therapy.

Many men find it hard to deal with this hormonal roller coaster ride over a longer period of time. Soon, injections will prolong the effectiveness of the testosterone to between one and four months.

• Tablets

The oral ingestion of testosterone has a serious disadvantage in that 40% to 80% of the hormone goes straight down the toilet.

80% of testosterone tablets can end up in the toilet

Methyltestosterone used to fulfill this role, but it has been banned in almost every country in the world except the US, where it is still sold in tablet form. Methyltestosterone, which is the main ingredient lending hormones their "bad name," is extremely dangerous. It damages the liver cells and can cause cancer.

Today, there are several harmless but effective remedies available (Restandol® and Proviron® among others), usually sold in 40-mg tablets. Two to four hours after taking them, the effects reach their peak, so it is necessary to take a tablet two or three times a day. Many men refuse this kind of treatment because it is too much trouble.

• Pellets

Deposits are injected into the fat pads of the posterior

Mostly consisting of crystalline testosterone, these have been used successfully for over 60 years. With local anesthesia, four to ten pellets (usually 180 to 200 milligrams of testosterone) are placed in the fat pad of the posterior by means of a thick needle. This is a painless operation, lasting about 20 minutes, and it guarantees a constant testosterone level over a period of about six months.

• Patches

Patches are a true therapeutic innovation

The testosterone patch, which became available only recently, is a true innovation. It is recommended for men who want a constant testosterone level. The breakthrough came with the product Androderm®, which was successfully put to clinical tests at both Johns Hopkins University and the University of Utah. These patches can be affixed anywhere on the skin of the torso or on an arm.

The path to the development of the patch was long and thorny. There were tests to place the testosterone patch directly on the scrotum, the patch of skin most sensitive to such a treatment. As part of these tests, men were required to place the patch on the shaven scrotum every morning, an unpleasant procedure. The skin of the scrotum is rich in the enzyme 5-alpha reductase, which changed the testosterone into dihydrotestosterone while it was being absorbed.

Natural therapies

An alternative natural therapy would be to adjust testosterone levels using aromatase and reductase. Phytohormones contained in red clover are thought to have an inhibiting effect on aromatase. Extracts of the saba fruit of a certain type of palm tree can inhibit reductase, i.e., dihydrotestosterone. Through the intake of certain plant extracts, we can also stimulate the production of estrogen from testosterone. A very effective androgen can be produced from the ginseng root.

Testosterone-replacement therapy has been tremendously successful. Vitality and virility, energy and potency have been restored in tens of thousands of men. Hair loss has been stopped, and many men have just become happier people.

Hormone-replacement therapy will be one of the most important tools in a man's battle against aging in the 21st century.

How Testosterone Can Activate Prostate Cancer Cells

With all the fascinating positive effects of testosterone on muscle formation, tautness of skin, body hair, and so forth, we must not forget about the downside. Testosterone can have a trigger effect on prostate cancer cells. It would be wrong to conclude that testosterone "produces" prostate cancer, but it can certainly activate it.

This poses a serious problem since, for genetic reasons, one 40-year-old man in four or five has latent, or dormant, prostate cancer cells. Autopsies on 80-year-old men have shown that around 90% of them had a dormant prostate carcinoma. Given all this, it is imperative that men undergo regular screenings for a possible prostate carcinoma after the age of 45.

Any androgen-replacement therapy clearly has to be implemented with great care. It must be "customized" to the individual by specialists after a thorough testosterone-level analysis, with multiple follow-up tests. Mail order testosterone pills and other dubious testosterone treatments are a big no-no. Only a medical doctor should perform testosterone-replacement therapy.

Sex As the Life Elixir of the Male Body

There are new scientific indications that sexual activity and/or erotic impulses stimulate the gonad. This means that frequent sex would automatically boost testosterone/hormone levels.

The more often a man desires sex and the more often he has sex, the higher his libido will be, probably because his testosterone level rises as a result.

Scientific studies have proven conclusively that the secretions of the pituitary gland increase in frequency as the patient watches a pornographic movie. Vienna sociologist K. Grammer was able to draw another correlation in a recent study on testosterone. The shorter the skirt of a woman, the more testosterone is released in a man watching her. The same is true of a see-through blouse.

One could argue to the contrary that single men without, or with diminished, sexual activity tend to have a low sex hormone level. Many of the key symptoms of the male climacteric, such as problems with muscles or joints, could in theory also be consequences of reduced sexual activity. This is why, in vernacular speech, we speak of an "old geezer" and, in the case of a woman who suffers from a chronic deficit of estrogen, of an "old spinster."

Sex is good for you! "The more you get the more you crave" is also true of sexual activity. The stimulation of the gonads and the corresponding increase in testosterone production is ample evidence. Sex is not only exciting, it can actually benefit your health.

THE MALE SEX HORMONES

- Have your doctor determine your hormone status with a blood test. This will tell you exactly which hormones your body has and how many.
- The balance between testosterone and estrogen is of special importance to men.
- Replenishment of hormones through hormone-replacement therapy must be "customized" to each man. There should be regular follow-up examinations.
- Stay away from testosterone pills that can be ordered through the mail. Hormones can, if taken in the wrong dose, pose a health risk. Only a doctor can properly assess your needs and determine the exact quantity of hormones that needs to be added to your body without causing any harm.
- The easiest way to raise your testosterone level is to reduce your weight. Fatty tissue contains a high degree of the aromatase enzyme, which turns testosterone into estrogen. Losing five kilograms (11 pounds) will automatically increase your testosterone level.

Male Estrogens

The Effects of Female Hormones on the Male Body

Estrogen means femininity and female attributes A man without estrogen is not a man, a fact that is not only surprising to men but also hard to accept because they consider it an insult to their masculinity.

Men have an underlying fear of the estrogen hormone because it has been seen for decades as the symbol of femininity and feminine attributes.

Since Eugen Steinach first looked into the workings of the female hormone, and Adolf Friedrich Butenandt received the Nobel Prize for his synthesized hormone, estrogen has been seen as the typical female hormone. In that light, the recent discovery by endocrinologists that this "female" hormone is an important prerequisite for male potency and a series of other male characteristics is especially amazing. The presence of estrogen in the body will not make men grow breasts or lose their potency. This fallacy is now a thing of the past. Estrogen is seen in a different light today.

Estrogen is important for male potency

Do We Have to Rewrite the Bible?

Phylogenetically speaking, estrogen is much older than testosterone. Or to put it more bluntly, if we were to analyze the Bible from the point of view of endocrinology, then God would not have created Adam first, and Eve from one of his ribs. Rather, he would have created woman first with her two XX-chromosomes, and then he would have broken a "branch" off the X to create man with his XY-chromosomes.

The Brain as a Gigantic Hormone Workshop

Estrogen is an endocrine hormone whose production is controlled by the pituitary gland, and which is formed in the testicles, the brain and the fatty tissue of a man. There are only infinitesimally small quantities of it in the body. The ideal level in men is between 20 and 40 picograms per milliliter of blood.

The ideal is at 20–40 picograms per milliliter of blood

The estrogen hormone, in men, is primarily responsible for energy, emotional stability and stress tolerance. It also has a substantial effect on a person's mental state and on the brain, which recent research has shown to be a gigantic hormone "production facility." The male brain is teeming with estrogen and testosterone receptors. Eugen Steinach suspected this much in the 1920s when he spoke of the "eroticization" of the brain, but he could not prove it.

Whenever hormone specialists talk about estrogen, they are usually referring to 17-beta-estradiol, which is the exact term.

17-beta-estradiol is the most important estrogen in men

Estrogen reaches the hormone-sensitive tissues in the body through the blood, but only a relatively small amount is needed for reproduction. Sex hormones only account for about 20% of male sexuality. The vast majority of tissues that are dependent on sex hormones are extragenital; that is, about 80% of their work is geared to organs and body parts that have nothing to do with the reproductive process. Rather, they act upon the brain, bones, skin, hair and cardiovascular system.

It is responsible for the mobility of sperm cells

Estrogen is important to men for various reasons.
- Estrogen is responsible for male fertility.
- It is essential for the mobility of sperm cells. The less estrogen the male body has, the less mobile its sperm are.
- Risk of cardiovascular disease decreases with a normal estrogen level.

Estrogen prevents osteoporosis

- Estrogen supports the buildup of bones in men and helps to prevent osteoporosis.

The fatter a man, the higher his risk of feminization

The more fatty tissue men have, the more estrogen they produce. Fatty tissue contains large quantities of the aromatase enzyme, which turns testosterone into estrogen. The fatter a man is, the greater his risk of feminization. If there is poor balance between estrogen and testosterone levels, men will become more aggressive, break out in a sweat or experience sleep disorders. If a man lacks estrogen, then his stress tolerance will be lower. A 55-year-old man who starts to cry over touching scenes in a movie is likely to have a very low estrogen level.

Estrogen Is Essential to Male Potency

Estrogen is responsible for sexual potency during the sex act

Estrogen has an essential function in male sexuality. Alongside testosterone and DHEA, it is important for the potency of men. A man who has a high testosterone level, but low DHEA and estrogen levels, will be a frustrated man. He has a very strong sex drive but cannot act on it.

Estrogen provides the basic energy for sexual arousal. Testosterone triggers eroticism and is responsible for the libido. However, the sexual strength, the endurance in the sexual act, is equally dependent on estrogen.

One could say that a woman's sexuality, which is more estrogen-controlled, is different from a man's sexuality, which is controlled by estrogen and androgen as well as by short term, instinctual, impulses.

To reiterate the importance of the female estrogen hormone for men, consider the case of the anamneses of two patients who suffered from an extremely rare endocrinological mutation. One had an extremely defective aromatase enzyme and could not produce estrogen from testosterone. The other had a normal estrogen level, but had completely defective receptors, which resulted in the estrogens having no effect at all. Both men lacked the benefits of estrogen, and they had two things in common. Their bone density was very low and, because of a strongly diminished mobility of the sperm cells, they were both infertile.

Without estrogen, men would be infertile

Estrogen as Protection From Heart Attacks and Osteoporosis

Estrogen serves not only a sexual purpose, but also has other benefits for men. It has long been known that estrogen provides women with protection from heart disease. A woman undergoing proper hormone-replacement therapy is less prone to cardiovascular disease than a woman without such therapy. If, and to what extent estrogen provides this type of protection to men is still not clear. There are clinical trials underway to see if estrogen can also help prevent Alzheimer's in men.

Can estrogen prevent Alzheimer's in men?

A clinical study of osteoporosis in men was carried out at the Vienna General Hospital a couple of years ago. A direct comparison was made between men who suffered from osteoporosis and those who did not. One essential difference was discovered. The men afflicted with osteoporosis had a significantly lower estrogen level.

Men Are Lost Without Receptors

Estrogen becomes effective through receptors that activate the cells. We have known for only a short time that there are, in fact, two different estrogen receptors—alpha and beta. It is quite likely that more subgroups will be discovered in the near future. Receptors differ from one person to the next. For example, 17-beta-estradiol connects both to the alpha and the beta receptors, and can have an extremely positive effect on bone density, elasticity of the skin, hair density, and more. But if the dosage is too high, it can stimulate the tissue of the mammary gland in men, or induce gynecomastia, a female fattening of the hips, especially through its effect on the alpha receptor.

Estrogen has alpha- and beta-receptors

Why Men Become More Feminine With Age

As they progress in years, men and women become more similar endocrinologically speaking. It has been scientifically proven that women after menopause tend to become masculinized, and men often develop female charac-

Men and women become more similar with age

teristics. Because the testosterone level remains constant while the estrogen level declines during the climacteric, a woman experiences an excess level of androgens. She becomes virilized, which may, for example, result in beard growth. Men experience the opposite process. Their legs become thinner, and they gain weight in the hips.

A 30-year-old man has more estrogen than a 60-year-old woman

The androgens in men decreases in favor of estrogens. During the climacteric, the estrogen level in women drops within a short time from an average of about 100 to about 10 picograms. As a result, a 30-year-old man has more estrogen than a 60-year-old woman.

Men may suffer from gynecomastia in old age

Aging men often end up with excess estrogen. Too much estrogen, disproportionate to the level of testosterone, or for endogenous reasons (i.e., production is too high or there is too much external intake), may have undesirable feminizing effects, such as typical female fat distribution (hips and posterior) and gynecomastia, the growing of breasts.

Balance Is Everything

What can be done about it? The most important findings and their practical consequences for the field of endocrinology—the replacement of hormones in men and women—are not mere theories. They result from the constant observation of reality. Andropause in men and the influence of hormones on their lives are two new areas of medical research that are still *terra incognita* for many doctors.

Experience has shown that men exhibit different types of endocrinological change as they grow older, changes that are different for each individual and that must be assessed individually. It would be hard to find two men with exactly the same hormone levels. For each, the balance of hormones has different effects on, and consequences for, his body.

The balance between testosterone and estrogen is decisive

A proper balance between the levels of testosterone and estrogen in the male organism is vital to the health and well-being of his mind and body.

A primitive form of estrogen replacement was practiced as early as the 19th century. Young men, primarily from the rural population of the Austrian province of Styria, sucked on combs from a hive of bees before going to see their girlfriends. Those combs, where the queen bees mature, were said to have a potency enhancing effect. But that ritual, if taken too far, had an undesirable side effect. The young men grew breasts. They did not know that the royal jelly in those combs contained about 20–30% of substances that act like estrogen, namely isoflavon, a high-grade substance that queen bees feed on.

Royal jelly contains the estrogen substance isoflavone

The effects of these substances are fascinating. Genetically, all bees are equal. They decide somewhat randomly, the way Tibetans choose the Dalai Lama, which of the eggs will be used for queen bees. These eggs are then given special food, the royal jelly. This ensures that the queen bee not only lives 30 times longer, but also becomes 40 timers bigger than all the other bees.

The ancient Egyptians already knew about the incredible effects of royal jelly. The substance was added to the grave of King Ramses the Great. Ramses is said to have been over 90 years old and to have fathered more than 200 children. He must have been acquainted with the oldest anti-aging substance in the world.

Thanks to royal jelly, Ramses II was over 90 years old when he died

The First Designer Estrogen for Men

What can be done today if a man's estrogen level is too low? The secret is to achieve an ideal replacement, to choose the right estrogen substance and the proper dosage while eliminating any undesirable side effects.

Endocrinologists had their first experience with this type of treatment with transsexuals, who demanded a hormonal change from man to woman.

The hormone 17-beta-estradiol, which is mainly used in female hormone replacement, is not recommended for male use because of its feminizing side effects.

17-beta-estradiol is not suitable for men

In the next decade, a new development will open up new estrogen-therapy possibilities for men. The Berlin pharmaceutical group Schering presented the first designer estrogen for men at a press conference in the spring of 1999. This non-feminizing estrogen, 17-alpha-estradiol, promises improved results.

The genistein in soybean and red clover may also replenish diminished estrogen levels in men. An added advantage of these phytohormones is that they stimulate mainly the beta receptors, with positive effects on the vessels, skin, hair and bones, but none of the feminizing effects. Red clover lowers the concentration of beta-estradiol, which feminizes men, but, being an estrogen substance, it acts on the beta receptors, which is beneficial to men.

Genistein in soy and red clover may supplement estrogen

Estrogen-replacement therapy in men is done only by means of tablets. Sometimes, estrogen patches are used with women, but the effects on men have not yet been fully explored.

GDR Leaders and Estrogen Therapy

Medical hormone-replacement therapies used to carry unidentified risks, but modern research is advancing at warp speed. In the former German Democratic Republic (GDR), hormone replacement was quite common among the leaders. East German scientists experimented intensively with sex hormones during the Cold War. For athletic competitions such as the Olympics, GDR athletes used a lot of performance-enhancing drugs. In order to fool the drug testers, experts had to create medical means of concealment, often with remarkable results.

Erich Honecker and other GDR bosses received estrogen supplements

In the course of their research, GDR doctors soon stumbled onto the preventive and protective effects of estrogen with respect to cardiovascular disease. A decision was made to have the entire East German political hierarchy undergo hormone-replacement therapy in order to keep them alive to run the country as long as possible. They were given estrogen preparations. According to a secret medical bulletin that was uncovered after the collapse of the GDR in 1989, these politicians reported a feeling of invigoration. Even today, many of the former GDR bosses are in good health. After all, they had been treated with estrogen over a long period of time.

Is There Any Help for Pavarotti?

A decline in vocal range points to menopause

For an example of the extent to which a lack of estrogen can affect a man, let us look to the arts. The nightmare of any opera diva, the apocalypse of any soprano, has got to be the sudden inability to reach the C-note two octaves above middle-C. The fear of being booed when the voice fails on stage for the first time is not the worst of it. Rather, it is the onset of old age. The decline in the range of the voice, as a rule, is the first sign of the incipient climacteric. The first organ to react to an estrogen deficiency is the voice box, the vocal chords.

Men experience this problem with one striking difference. This loss of vocal range has not been attributed to the onset of the male climacteric. Famous opera singers such as Caruso, Gigli or Pavarotti experienced problems later in life with changes creeping into the voice. It usually happens around the age of 55.

Even a slight shortage of estrogen may lead to severe vocal problems in men. Hormone dysfunctions are not the only causes, but they certainly play a considerable part.

Estrogen deficiency may lead to vocal problems in men

MALE ESTROGEN

- Estrogen is responsible for male fertility.
- The less estrogen a man has, the less mobile are his sperm cells.
- Estrogen can protect a man from heart attacks.
- It promotes the buildup of bone in men and helps prevent osteoporosis.
- A 30-year-old man has more estrogen than a 60-year-old woman.

DHEA—The Energy Hormone
Opponent of the Aging Process

Rudolf S. was for many years the successful manager of a large company. He was feared by his enemies and had the humble respect of subordinates. Behind his façade of a tough professional, there was a mind full of doubt. Rudolf S. suffered from depression, which the public did not know. Sometimes he would need half a day to bring himself to pick up the phone and make an unpleasant call. His secretaries were ordered to make excuses for him. He became more and more withdrawn.

Rudolf S's public reputation was that of an energetic leader. He reached a point where he could no longer bear the depression and indecision, so he consulted several doctors.

Several leading doctors could not find the cause of his problem. But then, Rudolf S. went to see an endocrinologist. Results of analysis of his hormones readily explained his condition. Through the process of chemotherapy he had undergone in his fight against cancer, his gonad and adrenal gland functions had been damaged. As a result, he lacked the essential hormones DHEA and estrogen. Only after receiving DHEA replacements did Rudolf S. regain his old energy. After this successful treatment, he thanked his endocrinologist and said, "You have given me the gift of a new life. I never thought that a man could depend this much on his hormones. Yesterday, I was actually able to play golf for ten hours—it is a magnificent feeling."

Dehydroepiandrosterone–The Male Power Hormone

DHEA is the most commonly produced male hormone

Dehydroepiandrosterone (DHEA, for short), the substance with the unspeakable name, is considered the power hormone of man. No other hormone exists in the human body in such large quantities. Almost 25 to 30 milligrams a day are produced in the male adrenal gland. Like any other hormone in the group of steroids, it is derived from cholesterol.

The larger the brain, the more DHEA

It is interesting to note that the DHEA level increases in proportion to the size of the brain. Studies on rats have shown that they have hardly any DHEA in their blood, while primates (more advanced apes) have a DHEA level comparable to that of humans.

DHEA prevents the formation of cortisol in the organism

DHEA has several characteristic features in the male body. Among its most important properties is an ability to prevent the production of cortisol. Cortisol, with its 10 to 20 milligrams per day, is the hormone produced in the second greatest quantity in men. One of the conditions most dangerous to the human organism, stress, triggers its release.

It fights stress, reduces the energy consumption of the body

DHEA can connect to the cortisol receptors and fight cortisol's negative effects, thereby protecting the body from unnecessary loss of energy. Cortisol inhibits the utilization of glucose, which normally would result in an increase in the blood-sugar level and the release of insulin. But DHEA provides active protection from these effects as well as from aging. Cortisol also has a tissue-reducing effect on bones, muscles and skin, and dehydroepiandrosterone prevents that too.

If a man's body does not produce enough DHEA, cortisol production, with its very real threat to the organism, will increase. The ratio of cortisol to DHEA is therefore an essential element in the aging process.

Low DHEA level points to diminished production of eicosanoids

Recent studies raise the possibility that a low DHEA level may be connected to a diminished production of eicosanoids. Low DHEA levels must therefore be equated with low production of eicosanoids, which are important to the male body.

American studies have named a series of positive effects DHEA has on the body.

• More power and energy
By inhibiting cortisol production, DHEA reduces unnecessary energy con-

sumption in the body. Men with a high DHEA level not only exhibit more energy and strength, but their mental functions, such as memory retention and other cognitive skills, are positively influenced and reinforced by the neurotropic (directed at the nervous system) effect of DHEA.

The neurotropic effect has a positive influence on the brain

• Lower risk of cardiovascular disease

The risk of cardiovascular disease decreases if the DHEA level is normal or elevated. The mortality rate, too, is lower than in men with an insufficient DHEA level.

The cardiovascular mortality rate declines when DHEA rises

• Fewer pounds or no excess weight at all

DHEA supports the body by reducing fat tissue.

• Improved immune system

The immune system of a man is strengthened by dehydroepiandrosterone.

The immune system is strengthened by DHEA

• Stress reduction

DHEA prevents the release of the stress hormone cortisol, which causes the blood pressure and pulse to take a jump.

The Production of DHEA in the Body

Just like its opponent, cortisol, DHEA is produced primarily in the adrenal gland. Its production is triggered and controlled by the same hormone that also triggers the production of cortisol, the pituitary hormone ACTH (adrenocorticotropic hormone). The effects of ACTH are governed by so-called cyclical AMP (adenosine monophosphate), a second messenger.

ACTH controls DHEA production

DHEA secretion is greater if the level of cyclical AMP is raised or even within healthy parameters. When the adrenal gland produces a corresponding level of cyclical AMP, the first step in DHEA production is activated. This includes the release of cholesterol from the adrenal gland.

This free cholesterol moves to individual cells and enters the mitochondria, the "power plants" of the cells. A series of reactions produces pregnenolone, an interim step in the creation of steroids. The pregnenolone is immediately converted into three different hormones: progesterone, cortisol and DHEA.

The free cholesterol enters into the mitochondria

Diminished DHEA production with age is surely caused at least in part by a decrease in cyclical AMP, without which no DHEA can be produced. If the

Reducing calories raises the DHEA level

cyclical AMP level decreases, then the production of benign eicosanoids must be encouraged. The easiest way to do this is by reducing calories. Tests with rhesus monkeys have clearly shown that DHEA production rises significantly with calorie reduction. It is important, therefore, to take in those substances that are precursors of eicosanoids, that is, polyunsaturated fatty acids (found in fish oil or olive oil).

Before a man starts taking DHEA as part of his hormone-replacement therapy, he should first try to reduce his intake of calories and add fish oil or olive oil to his diet.

How Does DHEA Affect Men?

In men, DHEA is transformed into estrogen

Men and women process DHEA differently. Its high concentration in the organism is probably due to the fact that it synthesizes testosterone and estrogen in the body. In women, DHEA in tissue is mostly converted into the male testosterone hormone. The process in men is the exact opposite. DHEA is transformed mostly into estrogen.

DHEA can help with erectile dysfunction

First and foremost, DHEA is responsible for a man's energy. Studies done in San Diego, California, show that men who had a low DHEA level felt better after hormone replacement. DHEA, however, has no effect on the libido because it does not significantly raise the level of androgens that men need for their sex drive. In a new study, published in the scientific journal Urology, Werner Reiter and Johannes Huber, two doctors in Vienna, Austria, were able to prove that DHEA can reverse the erectile dysfunction of impotent men in 30–40% of cases.

Research done by French scientists shows that high levels of DHEA in older men can lower their risk of cardiovascular disease. The extraordinary fact is that women have not been shown to experience the same positive effect. How is that possible?

The answer, found only recently, is that men and women process the hormone differently. In men, DHEA creates more estrogen, which protects the vessels. In women, DHEA produces more testosterone, which does not have the same positive effects.

These findings are new, as is the fact that DHEA has a significant influence on cognitive thought and on the immune system of the organism.

Can DHEA Be Used to Fight AIDS?

Research into DHEA is only in its infancy. Scientists continue to come across new, positive effects of DHEA on the human organism. Recent studies in the US prove that the defense cells of the body, the lymphocytes, have their own receptors for DHEA. This way, DHEA can enter the immune system of the body directly and fight viruses, bacteria, and so forth, from within the cells.

Lymphocytes have their own DHEA receptors

This allows for completely new methods of treating diseases. Feverish attempts are underway to put DHEA to work against AIDS, to find a way to introduce it into the lymphocytes. Up until now, this was medically impossible. There is real hope that the DHEA hormone may hold the key to effectively fighting AIDS.

DHEA Therapy—Too Much of a Good Thing

DHEA therapy in Europe is different from that in the US. In Europe, the principle is to measure what's there and replace what's missing.

In the US, DHEA has become a trendy hormone

In the US, however, practicing a policy of "the more, the merrier" raises concerns. DHEA is often administered without checking the dosage. DHEA, like melatonin, has already become a fashionable hormone. In spite of its various positive properties, the application of DHEA needs to be monitored more closely than is the general practice in the US.

DHEA can be taken in different forms, the most common being tablets with 20 to 100 milligrams. Most patients receive an average of 50 milligrams. But DHEA can also be applied as an ointment.

Usually tablets of up to 50mg are prescribed

It is very important to have regular follow-up appointments with a doctor. The therapy's goal is to optimize the DHEA level, to come as close as possible to the concentration found in the body of a 20-year-old male. Since the DHEA level of a 50-year-old is usually only one quarter of that, full replenishment is possible only through regular checkups and a monitoring of hormone levels.

The goal of therapy: the DHEA level of a 20-year-old

The effects of an overdose of DHEA are still unclear. But the motto "too much of a good thing" applies.

The reason that DHEA is still shrouded in mystery is that dehydroepiandrosterone cannot be patented. Major pharmaceutical companies, therefore, are

DHEA cannot be patented

reluctant to invest larger sums of money in research. As a result, it may take several years before large scale studies confirm the advantages of DHEA.

THE ENERGY HORMONE DHEA

- Anti-stress. It reduces the production of the stress hormone cortisol.
- More power. It provides men with more energy and positively affects, through its neurotropic effect, mental skills such as memory retention.
- Less fat. It promotes the reduction of fat tissue.
- Improved immune system. It supports the immune system of the organism.
- Lower risk of cardiovascular disease. It lowers the risk of cardiovascular disease.

Melatonin and Serotonin

Hormones for a Long Life

Melatonin—The Anti-Aging Hormone

Melatonin controls people's biological clocks

Our biological clock controls our entire life. Melatonin is the battery in the clock. It is one of the most effective substances available against sleep disorders and jet-lag, but at the same time it is one of the strongest antioxidants ever discovered. Melatonin lowers the bad LDL-cholesterol level, fights cancer and strengthens the immune system.

Like a vampire, melatonin is active only during the night

It is produced in the pineal gland in the brain, in response to serotonin impulses. Like a vampire, melatonin becomes active at night and disappears during the day. At nightfall, the pineal gland starts producing melatonin, which is strongest in complete darkness. Light perception is passed through the visual nerve of the eye and the spinal cord. From there it gets to the pineal gland, the timing device of the brain. Thus, the pineal gland receives constant feedback on the processes in the outside world and can signal to the cells of the organism by recognizing the change from light to dark to go into "economy mode" or reduce the energy output.

It lowers the body temperature

But melatonin also reduces the body's temperature. As a result, the organism requires less energy (energy = heat), and all cells in the body that need not be active during the sleep phase can regenerate.

One of the main functions of melatonin is to control the so-called circadian rhythm, the day-night rhythm of the body, to which many hormones—cortisol, testosterone and the growth hormone—are subject.

While testosterone and cortisol are secreted mostly in the early morning hours, the release of growth hormones peaks during sleep, just before the REM phase.

The circadian rhythm of hormones influences a multitude of physiological functions. For example, heart attacks are twice as likely to happen in the morning as during the rest of the day. That the birth rate is highest between one and two o'clock is also due to the circadian rhythm. If you have a heavy meal, you will see that your weight gain is far smaller in the morning than in the evening. Pharmacokinetics, the effects and functions of drugs on the body, may also be different. For example, aspirin has a longer half-life if taken in the morning.

> Heart attacks are twice as likely during the morning hours

These rhythms, which may differ from person to person, can be thrown off balance by melatonin dysfunctions. A lower level of melatonin or a dysfunctional rhythmic secretion can cause an imbalance in all the hormones that depend on melatonin.

> Melatonin dysfunctions wreak havoc on the entire body

Melatonin Prolongs Our Lives

The special power of melatonin was first proven in animal tests, which revealed that the life expectancy of the test animals increased sharply with the addition of melatonin. The lengthening of the life span using melatonin supplements was about 20% to 25%. While reducing the supply of calories concurrently, it was possible to raise the melatonin level by almost 100%. Rats with a reduced caloric intake had a melatonin level twice that of rats on a normal diet. In other tests, the pineal glands of older rats were transplanted to younger ones and vice versa. Young rats given the pineal glands of older rats exhibited signs of accelerated aging, while older rats with the pineal glands of younger rats appeared to be rejuvenated and remained more active throughout the rest of their extended lives.

> In animal tests it prolonged life by 25%

It appears that the internal, biological clock affects the life expectancy of humans. And maintaining the circadian rhythms is of immense importance in the battle against aging. The Russian researcher Vladimir Lesnikov claimed, following animal experiments, that an internal clock in the hypothalamus, the superior control center in the brain, actually sets the pace of the aging process.

> Maintaining circadian rhythms helps against aging

Perhaps that clock in the hypothalamus is also accelerated by declining melatonin levels.

A 1995 US study provided scientific proof that melatonin can strengthen the immune system, especially in patients who have undergone chemotherapy for cancer. In these cases, the results were particularly positive. An Italian study at the San Gerardo Clinic in Monza significantly improved the "one-year survival rate" of patients with metastasizing lung cancer. Another study of 200 patients in the advanced stages of cancer with perhaps six months to live showed that a combination of melatonin and immunotherapy could bring about a complete reversal in the growth of the tumor in 2% of the patients, a partial turnaround in 18% and at least a stabilization of the condition in 38%. Melatonin may also play an important role in the prophylaxis of breast cancer and prostate cancer, for patients with these types of cancer usually show especially low melatonin levels.

In cancer patients, melatonin may cause a reversal in tumor growth

It counters the stress hormone cortisol

Moreover, melatonin levels, like those of many other hormones, drop markedly with age. At the age of 80, the melatonin level is only about 10% of the level of a 20-year-old. The body, in advanced age, can no longer reduce its temperature at nighttime.

Melatonin maintains the eicosanoid balance

Each reduction in melatonin also affects the production of eicosanoids, with disastrous consequences for the aging process. Melatonin plays a crucial role in maintaining the balance of eicosanoids, which is considered the key to retarding the aging process.

Melatonin As an Antioxidant

Constant bombardment by so-called free radicals, the waste products of nutrition and oxygen, is a substantive factor in the aging process and the source of cardiovascular disease, cancer and autoimmune diseases. Melatonin is one of the toughest opponents of free radicals known. It attacks the radicals on the outside membrane of the cell, which is rich in lipids, as well as on the cell's interior, which is filled with water.

Melatonin destroys free radicals

In 1993, it was discovered that melatonin is an antioxidant with a series of unique properties. In the course of evolution, humans have lost the capability to produce some important antioxidants—vitamin C, E or beta carotene—that render free radicals harmless. Other antioxidants, like melatonin and some enzyme systems, have survived. They form a strong defense against the extremely destructive hydroxyl-free radical. Of all free radicals, the hydroxyl-free radical is the most active and thus the most dangerous. Antioxidant enzymes, like vitamin C, work together to prevent the production of the hydroxyl-free radical. But melatonin is also very effective in the binding of this hydroxyl-free radical.

The hydroxyl-free radical is the most dangerous

These radicals pose the biggest threat to the cells, especially those of the brain. The brain, 50% of which consists of fat, a third of polyunsaturated fat, is quite receptive to free radicals. Located in the center of the brain, the pineal gland is ideal for the synthesis and secretion of melatonin for binding the dreaded hydroxyl-free radicals. Melatonin, as it were, is the last defense against these free radicals.

Radicals attack the cells in the brain

The body needs melatonin in order to protect the essential fatty acids and to transform these into the benign eicosanoids it requires to maintain the corresponding levels of cyclical AMP and to transform serotonin into melatonin.

Melatonin to Fight Jetlag

Other properties have led melatonin to be used widely in medicine and therapy in the past few years. Melatonin is one of the most effective agents against jetlag after long flights across time zones. The quality of our sleep depends directly on the amount of melatonin that we secrete during sleep. Older people suffering from sleep disorders have only half the melatonin level of younger people. The decline in the level of the growth hormone, too, contributes to lack of sleep.

Melatonin helps against jetlag

Studies have shown that even low doses of melatonin (0.3 to 1 milligram) not only shorten the time it takes to fall asleep, but they also significantly extend the total time spent sleeping.

Used in this way, melatonin can "reset" the internal clock of the body after flights across different time zones or after shift work. In more than 50% of cases, it reduces the degree of exhaustion, mood swings or disorientation.

The Proper Dosage

The most effective dose whether as a soporific or to fight jetlag varies from person to person. Some people can do with relatively low doses of 250 micrograms; others may need 70 milligrams to feel any benefit. Up to the age of 60, it is usually not necessary to take additional melatonin. It suffices to sleep in a completely dark

Melatonin substitution not before the age of 60

room. Make sure that no light gets into the bedroom; otherwise, melatonin production will be reduced.

From 60 onward, a person should begin hormone supplements in low doses, between 0.5 and one milligram. Take a tablet between 45 minutes and two hours before going to sleep. Within the first 30 minutes of taking the tablet, most men get drowsy. If you feel bushed after waking up, then you should reduce the dose. If you still have problems falling asleep, increase the dose to 5 to 10 milligrams. Should you want to stop taking melatonin, you should not do it abruptly, but stretch it out over at least one week. Your doctor, whom you should consult first and foremost, will give you more exact recommendations.

Warnings

No melatonin in case of depression, autoimmune diseases!

Melatonin should not be taken by men who suffer from mental conditions, such as depression, allergies, autoimmune diseases like multiple sclerosis, or cancer of the immune system (e.g. leukemia). Melatonin production rises in the winter because of the long periods of twilight and darkness. This permanently increased production of melatonin may lead to winter depression, which is characterized by constant fatigue, listlessness and exhaustion.

Melatonin should never be taken during pregnancy or by nursing mothers. Children, or women who want to have children, should not take it either (high doses have a contraceptive effect).

Seratonin—The Hormone of Bliss

"True bliss can be achieved only by making one's feelings independent of fate."
Wilhelm von Humboldt

Happiness is a momentary positive sensation

What is bliss in the lives of men? As defined by psychophysiologists, it is an arbitrary emotion that lasts only a few seconds. It is a positive sensation, be it the moment of reaching orgasm or a bite of chocolate bar. Everything we feel and think, consciously or not, is the result of complex processes in the brain. The ability to perceive bliss is largely a chemical process between hormones and nerves. In the human body, our good mood primarily comes down to the serotonin hormone and the dopamine neurotransmitter.

Serotonin is the male hormone of bliss. The more serotonin the body produces, the happier, more positive and more euphoric we are. It plays an essential role in psychological stability and affects eating behavior, the circadian rhythm, mood, sexual behavior and the perception of pain. Lack of serotonin may lead to listlessness and sleep disorders because serotonin also helps control sleep. Serotonin is created from the amino acid L-tryptophan in body tissue such as the brain. It acts as a transmitter in the gastrointestinal tract and has substantive functions in hemostasis, or blood clotting.

The more serotonin, the more euphoric we get

Just like noradrenaline, serotonin transmits signals from nerve cell to nerve cell. As soon as a neuron is stimulated electrically, it will produce serotonin at its synapses (its connections to other neurons) and then secrete it. Receptors on the external membrane pick up the hormone and transmit the chemical impulse into the cell's interior. There it is converted into an electrical potential. The more receptors that are occupied, the stronger the signal will be. Studies have shown that depressed men produce an insufficient amount of serotonin. Other studies have attempted to prove that depressed people have fewer nerve cells that use serotonin as a transmitter. But depressed patients may show more receptors for their transmitters. This endocrinologists interpret as compensation for the deficiency. Estrogen can trigger the release of serotonin and also prevent its depletion.

Depressed men have too little serotonin

Serotonin as Antidepressant

The most important property of serotonin is its antidepressant effect. New drugs, so-called Selective Serotonin Reuptake Inhibitors (SSRIs), inhibit the uptake of serotonin and noradrenaline from the synaptic gap, which raises their concentration (e.g., Fluctine®, Seropram®).

A study conducted at the psychiatric clinic and polyclinic of the Benjamin Franklin University Hospital in Berlin, tested 70 patients who had survived attempted suicides. The study showed that they all had a low level of serotonin. Faulty regulation of serotonin on the biochemical level could be a contributing factor in a person's committing suicide. Currently, feelings and emotional impulses are being explored in the context of serotonin. "It will probably be possible in the 21st century to prevent suicides with medication," says Bernd Ahrens, in charge of the Berlin study.

Suicide candidates have a low serotonin level

Blissful Chocolate

Formerly, L-tryptophan, a precursor of serotonin, was used in the treatment of depression. Tryptophan is also contained in chocolate, which explains why men tend to eat chocolate under stress. Chocolate increases the blood serotonin level. In the summer, the bright daylight prevents serotonin from being reduced in the body. In the winter, on short and cloudy days, our body breaks serotonin down. Chocolate, with all its negative ingredients, such as fat and sugar, prevents the degradation of serotonin in the body.

Chocolate prevents reduction of serotonin

Serotonin is the reason that we feel stable and balanced. The fat in the chocolate mobilizes endorphins, which can trigger feelings of euphoria.

Serotonin is responsible for weight loss

Another effect of serotonin, according to the Medical Sciences Bulletin, is weight loss. Even in the late 1980s, a connection between serotonin and eating disorders like bulimia was suspected. The theory was that dietary food would be transformed into sugar that would stimulate the pancreas to produce insulin. Insulin increases the level of the amino acid tryptophan, a precursor of serotonin. Serotonin regulates our mood and produces a feeling of happiness or bliss.

Undesirable Side Effects

Does serotonin make men sleepwalk?

A new study in Utah seeks to prove that serotonin encourages sleepwalking at night. Also, increased levels of serotonin are said to diminish a person's concentration and memory. But these effects have not been confirmed by any other studies.

The effects of adrenaline, noradrenaline and cortisol on men and women have long been known (therefore, they are not dealt with in this book), but the discovery of the effects of melatonin and serotonin on men is something new. Both affect the mental and physical well-being of men, their strength and energy level, and their longevity.

The Growth Hormone

Fighting the Aging Process

David Rudman managed to make men younger by 10 to 20 years

On July 5, 1990, the world of medicine seemed to stand still for a moment. The renowned scientific journal, The New England Journal of Medicine, published a clinical study of a hormone that seemed to hold the key to the fountain of youth. David Rudman, a scientist at the Medical College of Wisconsin, had treated twelve war veterans between the ages of 61 and 81 with the Human Growth Hormone (HGH). Rudman achieved results that he described in a manner unusually brief for a journal of such stature. "The effects of the growth hormone after six months brought about a change that made the bodies ten to twenty years younger." Gray hair turned black, wrinkles on the hands and face disappeared, the libido was back in such force that the wife of one of the participants in the study said in an interview that, although she was 15 years younger than her husband, she had a hard time keeping up with him sexually.

His study launched a worldwide boom

Rudman's trailblazing study started a worldwide boom in hormone-related research, especially HGH. Since then, thousands of studies worldwide have analyzed the growth hormone and its influence on aging. The National Institute of Aging in the US, for example, is conducting a five-year study at nine different clinics to find out whether HGH could slow, or even stop, the aging process.

The All-Around Hormone—From Immune System to Blood Pressure

Since then, numerous properties of HGH have been identified and confirmed by clinical studies. Among them are:
- strengthened immune system
- massive reduction in body fat
- increase in muscle tone and strength
- fewer wrinkles
- better memory retention
- higher energy level
- lower blood pressure
- stronger bones
- faster healing of wounds
- thicker skin
- more "good" HDL cholesterol, less "bad" LDL cholesterol
- more fulfilled sex life
- sounder sleep
- fewer chronic diseases

After six months, the participants in the study who had been given the growth hormone had average muscle growth of 8.8% without exercising in any way. At the same time, they lost approximately 14.4% of their fat without going on any special diet. HGH builds muscle mass, reduces fat tissue and makes the skin thicker. Aging men, however, are not the only ones that use the versatile hormone. It enhances performance and cannot be traced in doping tests.

Muscle growth of 8.8%, fat loss of 14.4%

HGH can stop cell death after a heart attack

HGH deficiency: double the mortality rate in case of heart disease

The effects of HGH on a number of diseases are quite amazing. It can stop cell death following a heart attack. Tests with rats in whom heart attacks had been induced showed that fewer cells died immediately after the rats had been given HGH than was the case in the control group without HGH. As for serious lung disease, the University of North Carolina School of Medicine in Chapel Hill found that patients who had been on HGH for three weeks not only had an improved pulmonary function, but also better overall prospects. A study done at the Sahlgrenska Hospital of the University of Göteborg, Sweden, involved 333 patients who all suffered from a severe HGH deficiency. The study showed that their mortality rate in instances of heart disease was twice as high as that of patients with a normal HGH level. And there are many similar examples.

But the Human Growth Hormone may have one property that is even more fascinating. If there really is a hormone against aging, the growth hormone has the highest potential of being the one.

The Growth Hormone Exists for Only a Few Minutes

The growth hormone has a half-life of 5 to 6 minutes

HGH production starts with an impulse from the hypothalamus in the pituitary gland and is released directly into the bloodstream from there. It is one of the few hormones that the pituitary gland secretes directly into the blood. The growth hormone is released in rhythmic intervals, but its half-life is only five to six minutes. Therefore, it cannot stay in the blood very long, but there is enough time for it to be absorbed by the fat cells and the liver. There it is transformed into, among others, the insulin-like growth factor-1, IGF-1, also known as somatomedin-C. IGF-1 is responsible for most of the positive effects of the growth hormone.

75% of HGH is released during sleep

HGH reaches its highest level during the growth phase of puberty, and 75% of it is released during sleep. Its concentration is highest during phases of deep sleep. The saying, "You grow in your sleep," has endocrinological support.

At 80, men have only 1/20 of the peak HGH level

With age, HGH production steadily decreases. The secretion of the growth hormone drops by 10% to 15% with each decade of your life. After the age of 60, the HGH level is not even a quarter that of a 20-year-old. A 20-year-old produces an average of 500 micrograms of HGH everyday. At 80, men produce only around 25 micrograms. Although the receptors on the pituitary gland are fully functional regardless of age, the decline in second messengers such as cyclical AMP seems to diminish the secretion of hormones.

This is all the more surprising as studies so far have shown that aging people could very well produce as much HGH as young people, provided that its production could be properly stimulated. The cause of the rapid decline must therefore lie in the regulating processes between the pituitary gland, the liver and IGF-1.

It May Cost a Bundle, but It Helps

As far as we know, many effects of the aging process can be traced back at least in part to a growth hormone deficiency. This deficiency is a natural process in the organism and results for example in changes in the body's proportions. But to what extent these processes can be reversed by means of grow hormone substitution has not been clearly established.

Today, many different growth hormone preparations are commercially available to help replenish the "missing" hormone. Nutropin AQ®, for example, is available as a vaccine to be injected. It contains 192 amino acids (one more than the HGH in the body). Other products are Norditropin®, Genotropin® or Humatrope®.

The growth hormone suits the American mentality. Any medication must be powerful and act immediately. This helps explain the HGH boom in the United States, which is only held back by the high cost of the growth hormone and the method of application—injection. HGH therapy can run up bills of 700 to 1,500 dollars. The growth hormone may only be replenished by an experienced hormone specialist. The interaction of hormones works through a complex system in the body. The substitution of a single hormone, like HGH, automatically has repercussions on other hormones that need to be considered. The doses used by Rudman in his legendary war veterans experiment were too high by 50% to 75% and had undesirable side effects, such as the growth of breasts.

HGH, as hormone substitution, is mostly injected

75% of Rudman's doses were too high

If, for the time being, hormone-replacement therapy is to be avoided, the growth hormone can also be stimulated through diet, especially through the intake of arginine, ornithine and galanine—amino acids that are contained in vegetables.

The growth hormone can be stimulated by vegetables

It is not yet clear to what extent HGH can slow the aging process in people, but all indications point to this conclusion. Most age researchers and endocrinologists agree that the maximum age people can reach is currently 120. But some scientists, like Dr. Ronald Klatz, president of the American Academy of Anti-Aging Medicine, think a life span of 150 or more years is possible.

Anti-Aging president Ronald Klatz believes 150 years is possible

All such estimates have a fundamental flaw, however. The effects on the aging process can only be confirmed in experiments with animals, namely with mice, who have short lives. The effects on humans will not be clear until 2050 when today's 30-year-olds are 80. But tests on mice have already shown that those treated regularly with HGH do live longer and exceed the life span typical of their species.

The long-term effect can only be tested on animals

Undesirable Side Effects

Nothing in life is without its price. HGH, too, has certain side effects that do not always occur, but which cannot be fully discounted either.
- The growth hormone can lead to acromegaly (enlargement of the head, nose, hands, etc.).
- It can cause edemas (accumulations of fluid in tissue).

HGH also acts as a doping agent

- HGH is not an anabolic steroid, but its effects are similar to those of doping agents.
- Although there is no scientific evidence yet that the growth hormone stimulates the growth of malignant cancer cells, there are some indications that HGH might, under certain circumstances, increase the risk of cancer.

THE SUPERHORMONE HGH

The growth hormone has a half-life of only 5 to 6 minutes in the blood. Seventy-five percent of it is released during sleep, and it reaches its production peak during puberty. HGH-replacement therapy is very expensive (up to $1,500 per month).
- The growth hormone lowers the risk of heart attacks.
- It can stop cell death following a heart attack.
- It supports the buildup of muscles and reduces fat.
- It strengthens the immune system.
- It makes the skin thicker and tighter.
- It improves memory retention.

The Thyroid Hormone

Regulator of the Body

The thyroid gland is the supreme regulator of the hormone system. This is why every modern endocrinological screening program should include tests for the thyroid hormone, or more particularly the TSH level. The thyroid gland is a butterfly-shaped organ that is located below the larynx. It weighs barely 20 grams. Its most important task is to produce hormones from iodine and other substances and to release them into the bloodstream.

The thyroid gland weighs only 20 grams

The thyroid hormones regulate all the metabolic processes in the male body and keep them in balance. They control:
● the body's temperature and heat production
● growth and development of the body
● the metabolism
● brain growth in the newborn
● behavior

It regulates the body's temperature

How Does the Thyroid Gland Work?

The thyroid gland contains so-called follicles whose cells produce the two thyroid hormones triiodothyronine (T3) and thyroxine (T4). For this purpose, it requires iodine, which is absorbed from the blood if the person's nutrition contains sufficient amounts of it (e.g., iodized salt). Thyroxine is the prohormone, while triiodothyronine is the actual active hormone. After their production, they are stored in the colloid of the follicles, bound to a protein, thyroglobulin.

The thyroid gland produces thyroxine and triiodothyronine

Triiodothyronine is between three and eight times stronger than thyroxine. Unfortunately, thyroxine has a much shorter life span in the blood than T3, i.e., it disappears sooner.

The thyroxine hormone quickly disintegrates in the blood

Most of the work of the thyroid gland is done by the triiodothyronine in the blood. As is the case with most endocrine hormones, the process begins in the hypothalamus. Depending on the environmental influences on the hypothalamus, it will release a small quantity of a peptide called TRH (thyroid-releasing hormone). The binding of this TRH to the receptor in the pituitary gland causes the secretion of TSH, the thyroid-stimulating hormone, into the blood. TSH connects to receptors in the thyroid gland. The second messenger in this process that triggers the biological activity in the thyroid gland, is, again, cyclical AMP (the "lubrication" in hormone-related processes). It is only through the activity of cyclical AMP that thyroxine can be formed, which is then sent out to the target organs in order to act as triiodothyronine there.

Since thyroid hormones are not really soluble in water, they must be tied to binding proteins for transport through the bloodstream (TBG, thyroid binding

Thyroid hormones need binding proteins

The hormonal loop: hypothalamus–pitui tary gland–thyroid gland

globulin). As is true of cortisol, estrogen, progesterone and testosterone, here too, it is only the free hormone that is biologically active. This free thyroid hormone sets up a feedback mechanism to the brain in order to prevent the next release of TRH in the hypothalamus. This is the basis of the hormonal loop: hypothalamus–pituitary gland–thyroid gland.

When the free thyroid hormone enters the cell, it connects to the receptor and is then sent to the cell's core. This produces RNA, which, in turn, triggers the production of certain proteins in the cell and ensures that additional proteins will be produced later if they are needed.

Hyperthyroidism and Hypothyroidism

Having too many hormones "jumpstarts" the metabolism

Hyperthyroidism leads to an increased secretion of the thyroid hormones thyroxine and triiodothyronine. This starts up the entire metabolism: fat is burnt and energy released. The organism is working flat out, the body temperature and heart rate increase, and tachycardia often occurs. The results of this condition may be sleeplessness, shaking, sweating, indigestion, but also increased appetite without weight gain. The most common cause of hyperthyroidism is that certain areas in the thyroid gland do not respond to the control of the pituitary gland and produce an excess amount of thyroid hormones. But it may also be caused by an autoimmune reaction, which prompts the immune system to produce substances that stimulate the growth of the thyroid gland and thus, increase the production of hormones. This often includes the growth of a goiter.

Basedow's disease: eyeballs protrude

In the case of Basedow's disease, the eyeballs protrude as well. Only about 20% of the diagnosed cases of hyperthyroidism affect men. The condition can be controlled quite well with the proper medication, vitamins-rich foods and by avoiding foods containing iodine (e.g., fish). Some patients may also be treated

Hyperthyroidism is treated with radioactive iodine

with radioactive iodine in order to destroy the thyroid function altogether. The missing hormone would then be supplied by means of thyroid-replacement therapy for the rest of one's life.

Hypothyroidism is a systemic error

Hypothyroidism is based on a systemic error. The body lacks the thyroid hormones thyroxine and triiodothyronine often because the diet does not contain enough iodine to produce sufficient quantities of the hormones. As a result, the blood hormone level drops. This deficiency is passed on to the pituitary gland, which in turn sends a signal to the thyroid gland to increase its hormone production. In an

The thyroid gland gets bigger and bigger

attempt to adapt to the situation, the thyroid gland becomes bigger and bigger to enable it to track down even the most minute amounts of iodine in the body and to use them for hormone production. And the thyroid gland grows. Even though this growth does not cause any problems in the beginning, from a certain stage onward, nodes in the neck become sensitive to touch as the thyroid gland expands and requires more space in the throat. Because of the missing thyroid hormones, the body produces less energy, and all the processes are slowed down. This often goes hand in hand with lack of concentration, fatigue, diminished fitness and feeling cold. In many instances, hypothyroidism may be accompanied by depression. It frequently happens that doctors do not diagnose these signs in men correctly. The most common causes of hypothyroidism are insufficiently developed glands (which may be congenital), iodine deficiency or a dysfunction of the regulation of the release of thyroid hormones. From the age of 50 onward, the production of hormones in men usually plummets. A possible treatment is hormone substitution.

Depression and fatigue occur

Why Is the Body Temperature 36.8 C?

ATP (adenosine triphosphate) is the stored energy in our body cells that produces heat when burnt. This heat is the main source of temperature control in the body. Its function is to maintain a constant body temperature of 36.8 C. But why not a lower temperature that would save energy? One of the main reasons is that the body's enzymes, which are responsible for the biochemical processes in the brain and the nervous system, work best at this temperature. At higher temperatures, their structures collapse. At a lower temperature, our cardiovascular system would fail. The human body works best within a limited temperature zone. This is the price that we, as warm-blooded beings, have to pay.

At a higher body temperature, the enzyme structures fall apart

Is My Thyroid Gland Still Working Properly?

Body temperature is one of the best ways of checking the condition of the thyroid gland. Just take your temperature in the morning by placing a thermometer in your armpit. If it is lower than normal, it could be a case of hypothyroidism, and you should see a doctor. The reason for the low temperature is that the effects of the thyroid hormone do not fully reach the fat cells, and that reduces heat production, and less fat gets burned. As a result, men often also gain weight.

A low body temperature in the morning points to hypothyroidism

What Can the Doctor Do?

Until now, hormone substitution for women to fix problems with the thyroid gland has received too little attention. As far as men are concerned, it has been totally ignored. The adjustment of a dysfunctional thyroid gland requires a lot of skill and experience. Much fine tuning is necessary in the treatment of hormonal dysfunctions and hormone-related conditions.

For years, it was common knowledge that gaining weight was a result of not burning enough fat, i.e., hypothyroidism. Today, it has gone out of fashion, but hypothyroidism is still a problem. For example, in 1997, 36 million prescriptions for thyroid medication were filled in the US. This makes it the second most prescribed medication. Only 4% of the aging population suffers from a diminished thyroid function, but many more have been prescribed thyroid hormones. The assumption is that these medications are effective even for patients with "normal" blood levels. Current research promises to answer some of these questions soon.

The thyroid hormone level hardly decreases

How can people measure their thyroid hormone level? While other endocrine hormone levels decrease dramatically with age, the blood-thyroid hormone level never seems to decrease by very much. If there is a hormone system that can be observed by patients themselves, it is the thyroid hormone with its typical symptoms. Sir William Osler said, at the beginning of the 20th century, "If you let the patient talk long enough, you will probably have a diagnosis just like that."

How well your thyroid hormones work is something you can find out for yourself by observing and describing your symptoms. A blood test or urine test can confirm your suspicions.

Analysis: 24-hour urine sample required

Men can sometimes show normal results while exhibiting symptoms of a diminished thyroid function. Therefore, many experts recommend collecting urine samples for a period of 24 hours. The adrenal hormones should also be analyzed. The functioning of the adrenal cortex needs to be checked as well, since cortisol is important in the conversion of thyroxine to triiodothyronine. So, if the function of the adrenal cortex is diminished, this could also pose a problem for the thyroid gland.

In cases of severe hypothyroidism, there are clear symptoms, including weight gain, dry skin, thinning hair, brittle nails, articular pain, weakened immune system, slow wound-healing, depression and reduced sexual functions. Hyperthyroidism leads to frequent recurrence of the following symptoms: extreme restlessness, a feeling of being driven, weak concentration, and irritability.

Here are a few tips for protecting your thyroid hormone and maintaining the hormone level.
● Reduce your intake of carbohydrates by at least 50%. This way, you can

increase the cyclical AMP, triggering an increase in the TSH and the release of thyroxine from the thyroid gland. This would also lower insulin levels raised by increased production of triiodothyronine, the active form of the thyroid hormone.

● Avoid stress. In doing so, you will avoid the release of cortisol. If the cortisol level rises, thyroid production will drop. Elevated cortisol levels also signal hypoinsulinemia.

Allowing your body to control its development and metabolism more naturally will enable you to feel fully energized and healthy.

Phytohormones

Nature's Miracle Substances

It was the miracle cure of the aboriginal tribes in the Amazon Basin. Passed on over centuries, the bark of a special tree brought members of the tribe a worry-free life of lust. Taken orally, the bark would serve as a contraceptive for women. They could not have known that they had discovered what would later be called the anti-baby pill. Their remedy was as reliable as its current, synthesized, counterpart. This changed the entire life of the tribe. Aware of the contraceptive effect, these Amazon tribes indulged in free love. Ethnologists who later analyzed their language found out that the tribes had 70% more erotic or pornographic expressions than tribes that did not have access to this natural contraceptive.

From the Daisy to Romeo

Young men who experience a burning passion are said to "feel their oats." But did you know that similar sex hormones make plants like the daisy grow?

Only in the 20th century was it discovered that the sex steroids or hormones, the stuff of reproduction in simple plants and in humans, had hardly changed over the course of evolution. From the very beginning, they were one of nature's masterpieces, a brilliant new turn of evolution, which did not have to be especially adapted or modified. The occurrence of sex hormones in plants and mammals has not really changed over time, which opens up very interesting therapeutic and prophylactic possibilities for substances found in plants that are similar to sex hormones.

Phytohormones have effects similar to testosterone

The great old medical schools of Asia, especially those in China, knew thousands of years ago that phytohormones, natural hormones like ginseng, have effects similar to hormones like testosterone. Chinese doctors treated the upper class with hormone substitution as a selective anti-aging strategy. How far had the Chinese come thousands of years ago? Upon analyzing a substance found in distilling flasks of a "cosmetics manufacture," it was found to consist of conjugated estrogen, similar to the active ingredient in Premarin®, in use around the world for 50 years.

Hippocrates discovered an ancient abortion agent

Phytohormones were also very popular at the time of Hippocrates (around 400 BC). The Greeks had vegetable products that they used to perform abortions. The Hippocratic oath still contains a sentence to the effect that it is not permitted to "give a woman a pessary" to procure an abortion.

Old growth forests hold "untold hormone treasures"

The natives of North America used certain plant mixtures of phytohormones as an anti-aging component of their diet. The actual effect of so-called phytohormones has been analyzed only since the middle of the 20th century. The more sophisticated the analysis becomes, the more surprising scientists will find the diversity of hormones and their various effects that nature has given us. Old growth forests, endocrinologists are convinced, have an abundance of undiscovered treasures.

There are many phytohormones. Here are just a few examples:

• Oats

Oats have androgen-like substances that are similar to male sex hormones in structure. People have long known about these factors. "Feeling one's oats" has for many years been associated with feeling giddy and sexual.

• Clover

Clover contains estrogen-like substances

If horses eat only clover, their coats will have a very intensive sheen. The reason for this is the so-called extragenital effect of sex hormones. Clover contains the estrogen-like substances, isoflavones.

• Ginseng

The best known example of a plant with rapid results is ginseng, a substance similar to the male hormone and with a similar effect.

A ginseng root takes seven years to become ripe. The region where it is planted determines how rich it is in hormones. In the last ten years, more and more studies have confirmed its numerous benefits. The effect of ginseng corresponds to that of a male hormone like testosterone or androstenedione. But in terms of the balance of desired and undesired effects (e.g., on prostate-cancer cells), it seems to have an advantage over pure testosterone or androstenedione. With ginseng, nature might have given us a "natural, selective steroid." The ancient Chinese worked intensively with different phytohormones for therapeutic uses, and ginseng is certainly one of the best known and most effective.

Ginseng is a natural selective steroid

The basic reason that phytohormones have not made it big in today's modern world, even though their effects have been known for thousands of years, is that natural substances have only a small or non-existent industrial lobby to promote them. That also explains why little research has been conducted on them so far. But many pharmaceutical companies can no longer afford to close their eyes to this trend toward natural cures. They have recently created "bio-lines" of products. In the next two decades, biological agents will probably experience a veritable boom.

Industry has had no interest in phytohormones so far

There are many examples of the effectiveness of phytoestrogens. For example, hops were shown to have estrogen-like effects on Bohemian hop-pickers, who often experienced mid-cycle menstruation, for hops and of course beer contain phytoestrogens.

Beer contains estrogen

Estrogens and estrogen-like substances can best be absorbed through foods. Every Chinese pharmacy used to have an inn that offered "functional food." Functional food is now becoming fashionable for nutritional corrections and therapies. Prescribing a special diet for gastric disease is now taken for granted. We should pay a lot more attention to the possibilities afforded us by nutrition and diet as natural alternatives to therapy and hormone replacement (e.g., soy used for dry skin and tension of the breast).

Every Chinese pharmacy had its own inn

Phytoestrogens in Soy and Red Clover

One of the best known phytoestrogens is soy. The role of phytoestrogens from soy, as part of a healthy diet, was proven in a comprehensive study done in Japan. Japanese women usually have fewer menopause-related problems than women in the West. The same is true of Japanese men. The mortality rate due to prostate cancer is significantly lower in Japan. The study further showed that the state of health of Asians who emigrated to the US adjusted itself to Western levels within a few years. It would appear that lower mortality rates have nothing to do with genetics. Recently, red clover was identified as an important source of phytoestrogen. The binding effect of a red clover preparation (menoflavone) on the estrogen receptor was then compared to that of soy extracts. The findings of the test were surprising. The red clover extract showed a binding effect on the estrogen receptor that is up to 100% stronger than that of soy extracts used up to that point. It was also proven that red clover, but not soy, inhibits the aromatase enzyme, which brings about a slight increase in the precursor testosterone. Substitution of red clover extracts, therefore, affords men all the desired effects on the estrogen beta-receptor (e.g., strengthening of bones, positive effect on the brain), but excludes the undesired ones such as the growing of breasts or fat distribution typical of women. Red clover extract is seen as a natural, selective estrogen for modulating the receptor.

Red clover inhibits the aromatase enzyme

One argument often raised against phytohormones is that they are mixtures of different substances that we do not know enough about, and that the effects of each of these substances have not been evaluated in proper studies. But the most commonly applied hormone substitution, Premarin®, is a mixture of steroid substances, many of which have not been subjected to rigorous testing. Yet they work wonderfully.

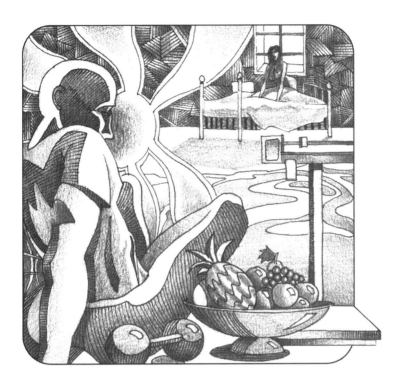

Maximizing Manhood

Forever Potent

Sex–Eroticism–Hormones

It should be 10 inches long, as hard as steel and ready for action at all times. The mere sight of it should make women lose all inhibition and pleasure it immediately.

The ultimate dream: 10 inches long and always ready for action

This is the typical wishful thinking of the average man about his 'best friend.' But reality is quite a different story.

You know the problem. Everyone knows it, even though many of us hate to admit it. Our reliable friend leaves us hanging, and usually in situations when we need it most of all. About 450,000 men in Austria between the ages of 40 and 70 suffer from severe and medium-to-severe erectile dysfunction. Another

700,000 Austrians have an erectile dysfunction

250,000 have this problem at least sometimes. Even young men are experiencing it more and more often.

Although lust, sex, potency and impotence have become hot topics of discussion in our society today, only a small number of medical studies have been done, and data about male sexuality is limited. It is no coincidence, therefore, that the few studies that have been carried out, such as the Kinsey report or the Massachusetts Male Aging Study of 1994, have become staples in the research of sexuality.

One in Two Men Has Potency Problems

52% of men have potency problems

The numbers contained in the Massachusetts Male Aging Study are alarming. Fifty-two percent (over half) of men between the ages of 40 and 70 suffer from potency dysfunctions and feel impaired as a result. Of these, 10% were completely impotent, 25% complained of severe problems and 17% of slight erectile problems.

A breakdown by age group would look as follows:

- 40-year-old men: 16% slight
                       17% moderate
                       5% complete erectile dysfunction
- 50-year old men: 16% slight
                       23% moderate
                       9% complete erectile dysfunction
- 60-year-old men: 17% slight
                       28% moderate
                       12% complete erectile dysfunction
- 70-year-old men: 18% slight
                       34% moderate
                       15% complete erectile dysfunction

Why Does Your Buddy Not Stand Up for You Anymore?

Hormonal disease may be the cause

The causes of potency problems are manifold. Erectile dysfunction is primarily caused by systemic vascular diseases (arteriosclerosis, diabetes), cardiovascular diseases, conditions affecting the kidneys or liver, conditions of the nervous system like Parkinson's disease or multiple sclerosis, hormonal conditions (hyperthyroidism/ hypothyroidism, hypogonadism and hypoprolactinemia) and depression.

DRUGS THAT COULD LEAD TO IMPOTENCE

- Hypotensive drugs (beta blockers, Reserpine, Dihydralazine, Clonidine)
- Dehydrating drugs (spironolactone, hydrocholorthiazid)
- Cardiac stimulants (digitalis, verapamil)
- Anti-lipid drugs (clofibrate)
- Antidepressants (tricyclic antidepressants, lithium carbonates)
- Tranquilizers (benzodiazepine)
- Soporifics (barbiturates)
- Stimulants (amphetamines)
- Migraine drugs (dihydroergotamine)
- Weight-loss preparations (fenfluramine)
- Corticosteroids (cortisone preparations)
- Opiates
- Estrogen and gestagen
- Cytostatics

But the chronic use of alcohol and cigarettes, increased lipid levels in the blood, and obesity can heighten the risk. The real catastrophe occurs when several risk factors come together.

Too much alcohol leads to erectile problems

Certain prescription drugs could as a side effect also cause impotence.

What Happens in the Body of an Impotent Man?

Is impotence only in the head? Or do hormones play an essential role?

In general, impotence is defined as a man's inability to perform sexual intercourse, which is due to an erectile dysfunction. But this has nothing to do with infertility.

Erectile Dysfunctions

Impotence does not cause any physical pain. Still, it can have great psychological significance. Every man, no matter how old he is, wants to be able to have sex at all times. Among the age group of 18 to 35, as many as 10% state severe erectile problems, and 30% complain of early ejaculation.

Impotence is painless

There are erectile
and ejaculatory
dysfunctions

This type of sexual problem is not easy to define. The line between short-term problem and pathological affliction is blurred. There are different forms of impotence. Depending on the phase of intercourse, it could be an erectile dysfunction or an ejaculatory dysfunction. The latter mostly has to do with early ejaculation. Apart from organ dysfunction, impotence may be caused by psychological problems, such as depression or stress, exaggerated expectations, performance orientation or anxiety.

A distinction is made between psychogenic and physical impotence.

Psychogenic impotence
- Acute occurrence
- Only in certain situations
- Only with a certain person
- Morning erections still happen
- Masturbation is possible

Physical impotence
- Slow onset
- Chronicity
- General continuous deterioration
- Morning erections happen rarely or not at all
- Masturbation is not possible anymore

What Makes the Penis Hard?

Neurotransmitters
relax the penis
muscles

The erection of the penis depends on the smoothe muscle of the cavernous body (corpus cavernosum). Chemical neurotransmitters relax the muscles in the penis. This enlarges the arteries, and more blood can flow back into the penis. At the same time, the smooth muscle cells stop the blood runoff, while the blood platelets seal off the veins and prevent blood from flowing back into the body. If everything works well and simultaneously, an erection will occur. The whole process is controlled upstream. In addition to an intact mental state, normal hormone levels, a functioning nerve supply and an unhindered blood flow are the prerequisites for an erection.

But for an erection to happen, several complex processes must unfold in the brain, processes necessary for the stimulation of the 'sex centers,' especially the hypothalamus and the limbic system. This stimulation releases neurotransmitters that trigger an erection, in particular dopamine, ACTH, NO, oxytocin and serotonin.

These impulses are transmitted from the brain to the erection center through the spinal cord. From there they travel as reflexes to the penis through neural pathways and are finally released as nitrogen oxide (NO), a neurotransmitter. Nitrogen oxide is a protohormone, which does not require any receptors and only travels over short distances before it breaks down. It is one of the smallest molecules that we know of, a so-called free radical. In the smooth muscle cells of the cavernous body, it increases the production of cyclic guanosine monophosphate (cGMP), which leads to an erection by relaxing the muscle cells.

Stimuli are released as nitrogen oxide

Cyclic guanosine monophosphate triggers erections

The occurrence and maintenance of an erection are attributed to an increased flow of blood into the cavernous body and from there into the penis.

Viagra—The Magic Pill

What does the date March 27, 1998, mean to you? Nothing? Nevertheless, it is a day that changed the lives of men more than any other.

Viagra was first approved on March 27, 1998

On that date, fast-track approval by the Food and Drug Administration (FDA), usually adopted only for cancer medication, gave Viagra the official green light for sale as a drug in the US.

In the first year or so after Viagra's introduction on the market, about 35 million pills had been prescribed to approximately three million patients in the US alone. The number of men who bought it on the black market, or who were healthy but curious enough to try it, is even higher. No other drug has ever created that kind of worldwide furor.

"Sildenafil," the chemical name for Viagra, actually started out in the mid-1980s as a major flop. At the time, researchers at Pfizer, one of the giants of the pharmaceutical industry, were looking for a new drug for angina pectoris, but the results of a pilot study on a substance that was supposed to improve blood circulation in the heart were nothing short of sobering. A number of the voluntary test subjects reported strong but unexpected erections.

At first, Viagra was a colossal flop

It would be another couple of years before researchers finally understood the key role played by nitrogen oxide (NO) in triggering the erections. Nitrogen oxide is essential to blood circulation and the ability to have an erection. The Nobel Prize in medicine was only recently awarded for research done on nitrogen oxide.

Sildenafil is an effective and selective inhibitor of the cGMP-specific phosphodiesterase (type 5 PDE 5) in the cavernous body of the penis, where it is responsible for the reduction of cGMP. When, under sexual stimulation, the NO-cGMP metabolic pathway is activated, the PDE 5 inhibition induced by sildenafil raises the cGMP level in the cavernous body. Sexual stimulation results and sildenafil achieves its desired effect.

The maximum level is reached after 60 minutes

Sildenafil is absorbed quickly and reaches maximum levels in the blood within 60 minutes. The absolute bio-availability is at 40%. The binding of protein occurs at a high rate of 96% and may cause interaction with other drugs. Sildenafil's half-life, i.e., the time it takes for half the substance in the body to break down, is about four hours. If taken several times a day (not recommended), an accumulation may occur. According to observations, however, the effects are diminished if it is taken together with fatty food.

Increased blood levels in patients over the age of 65 may be the result of a diminished catabolism, liver damage or a severely impaired renal function. Clinically important interaction occurs with drugs like cimetidine (gastric-secretion inhibitor), erythromycin (antibiotic), ketoconazol (anti-fungal agent) or even grapefruit juice. The preparation has been shown to be effective for erectile dysfunctions, both organic and psychogenic.

Placebos also showed effects during tests

Sildenafil is available in doses of 25, 50 and 100 milligrams. According to studies, the success rates of 25 mg were between 60% and 67%, for 50 mg between 78% and 84% and for 100 mg between 86% and 100%. One surprising result from a study on 100 mg pills showed that 12% to 20% of the men who received placebos (useless substitutes) also had some sexual success. Merely believing in miracles can work wonders.

Viagra Also Helps Diabetics

78% of diabetics feel an improvement

Viagra can help men with quite different medical problems. A study published in the spring of 1999 showed that the sexual functioning of diabetics could be improved with Viagra. Between 35% and 75% of male diabetics suffer from erectile dysfunction. After a twelve-week treatment, the patients in the study improved their erectility by 78%. Of the men treated during the study, 61% had successful intercourse at least once, with the attempt to have intercourse successful four times as often as among the untreated patients.

The magic blue pills, however, can also have undesired side effects. The most common are headaches, facial blush, gastric complaints, stuffy nose and problems of the respiratory tract, urinary tract infections, impaired vision, indigestion, drowsiness and skin rashes. These conditions are usually slight or moderate and of a short-term nature. According to experience so far, the side effects depend on the dosage and cause no lasting damage.

"Magic pills" can cause dizziness

Another substantive side effect is the lowering of the blood pressure to about 10 mm/Hg, while the heart rate climbs by about 10%. The hypotensive effect is reinforced when taking medication that also affects the nitrogen system, particularly nitrates and molsidomine. A scientific study has revealed that some patients who suffered from a stable angina pectoris showed a maximum reduction of the systolic blood pressure to 50 mm/Hg by taking their standard medication together with 50 mg sildenafil.

Who Should Take Viagra?

Since September 1998, Viagra has been available to European men. Along with the warnings with regard to side effects come the jokes as well. "Are you fit for Viagra?"

But it is no laughing matter. Men who suffer from one or more risk factors, or from heart disease, need to find out whether they are physically fit enough for the exertion that comes with sexual activity. They should visit their doctor and undergo a general physical examination. It is possible to get a rough idea of your physical condition using a bicycle ergometer (see the chapter "Fit for Life").

Viagra can be dangerous if you suffer from heart disease

There is already a growing misuse of Viagra. In the red light districts of big cities, for example, prostitutes sell Viagra to their older customers, who take it without giving it a second thought. Another trend on which there is no agreement is for young people in the drug scene to take sildenafil together with amyl-nitrite sprays that have hallucinogenic effects, so-called "poppers." This increases the exhilaration, but may result in a life-threatening drop in blood pressure. The chapter "Engine of Life" contains recommendations for patients with heart disease.

128 deaths since
the introduction of
Viagra

Currently, people with an allergy to Viagra, or who are simultaneously taking drugs of the nitrate or NO-donator group, are warned off Viagra. Patients with the eye disease retinitis pigmentosa should never take it either. Older men and patients with liver damage, deformations of the penis or conditions that could lead to priapism (painful continuous erection) should be very careful when taking Viagra. People with blood-clotting disorders or an acute gastric or duodenal ulcer should not take Viagra under any circumstances while suffering from such conditions. Since its introduction in the US, 128 deaths have been reported in connection with Viagra. But whether there is any causal connection is still unclear in most of these cases. It has also been impossible to prove Viagra at fault from the physical exertion that goes with sexual intercourse.

How Do I Take Viagra?

Start with a dose of
25 milligrams

It should be taken in a gradual fashion, but never in doses exceeding 100 milligrams. A patient should start with 25 milligrams. Only if there is no effect should the dose be increased to 50 or 100 milligrams. Anyone suffering from heart disease should be very careful with increasing their intake. The pill should be taken one to four hours before the intended sexual intercourse—Viagra usually becomes effective after 25 minutes. It should be taken only once in a 24-hour period.

What Else Can I Take to Increase My Potency?

Since the stock prices of the pharmaceutical group Pfizer went through the roof on the New York Stock Exchange, other pharmaceutical companies have been working feverishly to introduce their own potency medications.

Apomorphine will
be the potency pill
of the 21st century

The Japanese chemical group Takeda has filed an application with the FDA (Food and Drug Administration) for a substance called Apomorphine®. This new potency pill is now being tested clinically in North America. Apomorphine does not work through the blood vessels, but through the sexual stimulation of the central nervous system. The manufacturers hope that this treatment, which is intended to affect the sex center in the brain, will be of interest to women, who have been disappointed by Viagra.

Apomorphine is supposed to have an effect within minutes. The initial results, which were leaked to the public, show an effectiveness of about 70%. However, about one in six users complained of nausea and, in some cases, vomiting. So far, Apomorphine has been tested only on patients with psychogenic impotence. No tests have been carried out yet in cases of physical impotence. In the US, the effects of Apomorphine in cases of female sexual dysfunction is also being looked into.

70% are said to become potent again Vasomax vs. Viagra

Since the drug has not been fully tested, we do not yet have a clear idea of its side effects or long-term consequences. It remains to be established whether it is to be classified as a medicinal product or just a lifestyle drug.

Another drug that, like Viagra, aims at the blood flow in the penis is a substance called phentolamine, which is sold under the name of Vasomax®. This medication belongs to the category of alpha-2-receptor blockers. It inhibits the sympathetic nervous system and its negative effect on penile erection. Initial results of the study showed a 100% improvement in sexual performance in comparison tests using phentolamine versus placebos. Vagomax is manufactured by a company in Texas, Zonagen Inc., in cooperation with another pharmaceutical giant, Schering. Like Viagra, Vasomax is to be taken about half an hour to an hour before sexual intercourse.

Natural Potency Preparations

For thousands of years, people have known of substances with well proven effects on potency. As the pharmaceutical giants race each other to market with chemical solutions to impotence, natural remedies are experiencing a tremendous rebirth. The difference now is that they are finally being tested scientifically.

It is wrong to think that everything that Mother Nature has given us must be without risk. Some of these potency boosters can be dangerous. And most natural remedies or aphrodisiacs can help the problem, but cannot eliminate it.

• Ginseng

The best known treatment is ginseng. The ginseng root contains, among its numerous active ingredients, ginsenosides. It is assumed that these substances trigger the release of the body's own hormones, probably testosterone, and thus increase the libido and potency. It should be noted, however, that ginseng is only effective when taken regularly. Other substances may dilute the effects of ginseng. Therefore, when you buy a ginseng product, make sure that it contains at least 15% ginsenosides. The most common side effects of ginseng are skin rashes, hypertension and a feeling of tightness in the thorax area.

Ginsenosides increase libido and potency

• Yohimbine

Yohimbine is the most recognized aphrodisiac

This extract from the bark of the African yohimbe tree is one of the oldest aphrodisiacs. Even the ancient Egyptians used it. Among the aphrodisiacs currently available on the market, yohimbine certainly gets the most scientific credit. It has even been officially approved as a drug.

Studies done in Germany in 1997 showed that 71% of impotent men taking the yohimbine extract had noticed a change in their potency. The assumption is that yohimbine causes the blood vessels to expand and thus improves the blood flow in the pelvic region. It has a stimulating effect on the nervous system in the lower spinal cord. This is of great importance for sexual stimulation. Yohimbine seems to be especially suited for patients with erectile dysfunctions caused by stress and fear of failure.

But nothing comes without side effects: 20% to 40% of those taking yohimbine reported a number of side effects. For this reason, preparations with a high yohimbine content are classified as prescription drugs. Frequent side effects include shaking, tachycardia (with too high a dose), nervous disorders, increased irritability, sleep disorders, high blood pressure and anxiety.

• Royal Jelly

Royal jelly stimulates sperm production

Royal jelly comes from bee pollen. It is an extract that bees produce and feed to the queen bee. Scientific studies have shown that royal jelly stimulates and increases the production of sperm. This probably helps to boost sexual desire and libido. Allergic people should be careful because these preparations contain pollen, which could trigger allergic reactions such as asthma attacks, skin rashes, and allergic shock.

• Gingko biloba

Gingko biloba helps you "get it up" again

Gingko biloba relaxes the arteries and thus improves the circulation to all organs. By increasing the supply of blood to the penis, it is said to help with potency dysfunctions caused by impaired circulation. In one study, 50% of the men reported daily erections after six months of taking 60 milligrams of the gingko extract. Follow-up studies, however, failed to repeat these results. The vegetable ingredient should be taken in daily doses of 60–80 mg, and never exceeding 200mg. Gingko is a fairly safe herbal remedy, even though it may occasionally cause stomachaches or headaches. It should never be taken with aspirin or other blood thinners.

• Muira puama

Muira puama is also known as "potency wood." It is made from the inner bark and the grated wood of the eponymous South American tree. The daily dose is about 1 to 1.5 grams. The preparation is said to be sexually stimulating, and there are no known side effects.

• Pumpkin seeds

Pumpkin seeds are often used in the treatment of prostate problems. The seeds contain large amounts of vital substances, such as zinc and vitamin E, which can have a positive effect on the genital organs. The scent of pumpkin is rumored to have a stimulating effect on men.

Pumpkin seeds have a positive effect on the genitals

• Pheromones

Love is an olfactory sensation, and it is no secret anymore that the olfactory sense is important to having erotic feelings. Pheromones take center stage here. These substances are not picked up by the actual olfactory sense, but by the so-called vomeronasal organ, or VNO.

Pheromones are the scents of lust

Tests on very different animals, such as lizards and hamsters, have shown that, if the VNO is surgically removed prior to its first intercourse, the male was no longer able to copulate. Scientists concluded that the VNO is crucial to learning sexual activities. Meanwhile, the study of pheromones has become a science in its own right. It has been discovered that every animal species has its own stimulating secretions—scents that only work on members of the same species. Pheromones are typically secreted through the skin, which is covered in sweat glands. An especially high concentration of sweat glands is found in the armpit, the hollow of the knee, the groin and on the back. Another area that produces a lot of pheromones is the tiny spot between the nose and the upper lip. In 1980, human pheromones were isolated for the first time, and their existence proven. The VNO has already become commercialized. For some time now, special skin gels have been available (Phenomenal Gel in Germany, for example) containing artificial pheromones intended to have an effect on the opposite sex. Phenomenal Gel is a moisturizer enriched with sandalwood extracts. No scientific studies have been conducted on these products yet, but it is almost inevitable that pheromones will experience a veritable boom. New perfumes made from scented oils and pheromones will promise to make the wearer "irresistible."

Penile Injections

An erection may also be achieved by injection of a substance produced in the body called "prostaglandin E1" (prostaglandin is an artificial coinage derived from prostate and glans, the tip of the penis) into the cavernous body. It can be accomplished by self-injection as well. This therapy is successful in 70% of all cases. However, it should be closely monitored by a doctor because mistakes in administering the injections can result in damage to the cavernous body.

Penile injections help in 70% of all cases

Penile self-injections can involve different substances, but all require that special attention be paid to side effects, such as persistent erections. In 10% of these cases, the result is damage to the cavernous body, with severe scarring.

Besides prostaglandin E1(sold under the name of Caverject®), there is also papaverine, sold as Androscat®. Another, fairly recent, product is the hormone VIP (vasoactive intestinal polypeptide), which was released in Denmark in 1998 as Invicort®.

Vacuum Pumps and Penile Implants

A method that has been around for more than 30 years is the penile vacuum pump. This can be used to achieve an erection. A rubber ring around the root of the penis prevents the blood from flowing out of the cavernous body.

Penile implants are becoming less popular

There are also penile implants, which have never become very popular. They come as hydraulic penile prostheses, consisting of one, two or three parts. They are controlled by a pump inside the scrotum, invisible from the outside.

If you experience only an occasional problem, do not worry. It is normal and can happen to the best of us. If it happens, talk to your partner about it. But before the whole thing turns into a domestic drama, contact your physician for a prescription for Viagra to restore your self-confidence. If the problem should still persist, then go and see a specialist.

Cycling can cause potency problems

Be careful when you go cycling. Urological studies have shown that, among more than 700 middle-aged cyclists who spend at least four hours a week on the bike, 4% experienced in some cases, substantive potency problems. The more hours they spend on the bicycle, the more frequent the recurrence of symptoms. A control group of runners showed only 1% having the same symptoms as the cyclists. Urologists say that the hard saddle causes the nerves and the bloodstream in the penis and testicles to be shaken. It is important to reduce the pressure on the lower abdomen in order to better absorb the shocks. Also, take a break every 30 minutes.

FOREVER POTENT?

- Reduce the bad LDL cholesterol. Over time, it leads to impotence.
- Stop smoking because nicotine constricts the blood vessels in the penis. The chances of a smoker's becoming impotent are twice as high as of a non-smoker.
- Watch your blood pressure.
- A normal blood sugar level is especially important. One in two diabetic men eventually becomes impotent.
- Watch out for vasoconstriction and sclerosis, the most common causes of physical impotence.
- Regular sex raises the level of testosterone. Therefore, you should have sex as often as possible. Sex to the penis is what recharging is to a battery.

The Right Nutrition
The First Step Toward a Healthy Lifestyle

Michael W., a university graduate, is 32 years old and works for IBM. He is single. Whenever he gets a free minute between preparing listings or testing new programs, he likes to eat sweets. He always keeps a 500-gram chocolate bar within reach next to his computer. In his briefcase, he carries a box of chocolates, preferably an assortment of truffels. And for a snack in the evenings in front of the TV, or on the weekend, in his car or on his way to work, he has a weakness for a new kind of chocolate ball filled with nougat cream and apricot flavor. He likes food rich in calories—TV dinners and fast food, but he eats small portions at a time in order not to attract attention. Michael W. is obese and has become socially isolated as a result. He hates his body and stays clear of mirrors. In the words of his dietician, everything he eats is "too sweet, too fattening, too unhealthy."

You Are What You Eat

Michael W. is not an isolated case. More and more men are overweight, and this trend will continue. According to the World Health Organization (WHO),

Obesity will be a major problem in the West

being overweight will be the biggest nutritional problem in the Western world in the future.

Germans and Austrians eat too much fat

The food we eat every day is the source of our energy. If our diet is not balanced, the whole organism will be adversely affected and, by extension, so will our lives. The first step to becoming the "Power Man" of tomorrow, therefore, is to carefully control our diet. Eating too much fatty food brings on diet-related diseases like cancer, arteriosclerosis or diabetes. In Austria alone, there are probably half a million diabetics. The high sugar content in most foods threatens to destroy our teeth and our waistline. Men take in way too much cholesterol everyday—on average, 421 milligrams (300 would be considered normal)—and this puts a major burden on the body.

The MTV generation prefers burgers and French fries

In primeval times, the most powerful man in the tribe, the chief, received the richest meals. In the postwar years, Europeans eagerly consumed what they had been denied before—sausages, ham, cake and chocolate. In the 1980s, people went for a quick burger and french fries so they could get back in front of the TV and the VCR. Only in the 1990s did people become more nutrition-conscious and attempt to change their ways somewhat. More and more overweight people are willing to battle their excess baggage. They go on diets, take appetite suppressants, new miracle pills, and laxatives. They will even undergo surgery.

Do You Know What You Eat?

In the spring of 1999, the Austrian Federal Ministry of Labor, Health and Welfare commissioned a report that revealed the "sins" of many adult Austrians as far as nutrition was concerned. The biggest problem with their diet is the huge consumption of meat, a lack of vitamins D, B1, B2 and B6 and the minerals calcium, magnesium, zinc and iodine. In contrast to Mediterranean countries—only one adult in 16 is overweight in Italy—Austrians eat too much red meat and not enough fruit, vegetables and cereal products. The other nutrients appear to be balanced.

80% of men eat meat everyday

Older people need more vitamins B6 and D, and their intake of vitamin C, folic acid and beta-carotene needs to be increased. A look at their consumption patterns revealed that 80% of Austrian males eat a mixture of foods everyday, but always in combination with meat. Only about 2% of men are vegetarians. Significantly more women are reducing their consumption of meat, while men prefer to stick with the traditional diet.

Age is an important factor. Of the younger participants in the study, 6% said they were vegetarians, but 75% opt for standard fare. Less than 20% make a conscious effort to eat healthy or to try to cut down on meat.

Only 20% of young people eat right

People with a lower level of education prefer traditional foods. Better-educated people, by contrast, prefer a diet low in meat. The differences in habits become obvious when one looks at various body-weight groups: 92% of the vegetarians have a normal weight, and only 8% are slightly overweight. Of those consuming standard food, 67% have a normal weight, 27% are slightly overweight, and 6% are severely overweight. Approximately 20% of the people who prefer a diet low in meat are overweight.

27% are overweight, 6% are obese

As part of the same research project, people's nutrition awareness was tested. The findings showed that women are better at assessing their awareness level than men. But with respect to daily energy requirements, most people underestimated their actual needs. One third of those surveyed were unable to even guess at their needs. Among the different dietary groups, vegetarians had the best results, followed by the more health- and diet conscious. People who consumed a standard mix of foods had the lowest level of awareness.

These results are proof that people do not really think about what they eat. What is worse is that such a low level of dietary consciousness rarely goes hand in hand with healthy eating habits. Without knowing about proper nutrition, it is impossible to effectively improve one's diet. Many of those questioned complained that the dietary recommendations available to the public were confusing. Most of the information came from radio or television and was often contradictory.

Even those who know about proper nutrition do not necessarily eat right

In order to feel good, fend off disease and live as long as possible, the body needs a balanced diet. Many chronic conditions in Western civilization, especially heart attacks, cancer and stroke, are usually brought on because people eat the wrong things or eat excessively. So, what is a balanced diet? Nutritionists name five elements as essential to good health:

Diseases like cancer or heart attacks are linked to our diet

1. energy balance
2. nutrient balance
3. fluid balance
4. electrolyte balance
5. balance of vitamins and trace elements.

Do You Eat Right?

Many conditions, even a number of life-threatening ones, can be traced back to unhealthy eating habits. Here is a test to help you learn more about your diet. Professor Kurt Widhalm, Austria's leading expert on nutrition, along with dietician Monika Koch, compiled the following test. Are careful or negligent in the treatment of your body? Let's find out.

1. How many meals do you eat a day?
2	☐	1 point
3	☐	3 points
More	☐	5 points

2. What do you normally have for breakfast?
Rolls, jam, eggs	☐	3
Whole wheat bread with a spread, muesli	☐	5
I don't eat breakfast	☐	1

3. Which is your main course?
Fish, lean turkey or chicken, unbreaded schnitzel (beef/veal)	☐	4
Potatoes, vegetables, corn, salad	☐	5
Offal, fried schnitzel, sausages	☐	0

4. Which makes up the largest portion of your main course?
Meat or fish	☐	1
Side orders (potatoes, rice, vegetables, salad)	☐	5
A balanced mix of the two	☐	3

5. Which type of fat do you primarily use?
Butter, lard, coconut fat	☐	1
Sunflower oil, corn oil	☐	3
Cold-pressed olive oil, pumpkin seed oil, thistle oil	☐	5

6. How often do you eat fish?
Twice a year	☐	1
Twice a month	☐	3
Twice a week	☐	5

7. What do you like to eat for a snack?
Baloney sandwich, hamburger, pastries, snack food	☐	0
Fruit, low fat dairy products, whole wheat rolls with a spread	☐	5
Readymade fruit yogurt, muesli bar	☐	4

8. How often do you eat fresh fruit?
Once a day	☐	3
A few times a day	☐	5
Not every day	☐	1

9. How much liquid do you drink a day?
3 glasses or large cups	☐	1
6 glasses or large cups	☐	3
More	☐	5

10. Which drinks do you prefer when you are thirsty?
Fruit juice, lemonade   ☐ 3
Tea, water, concentrated fruit juice   ☐ 5
Coffee, beer   ☐ 1

11. How often do you add salt to your meal?
Seldom   ☐ 4
Frequently   ☐ 1
Never   ☐ 4

12. Do you smoke cigarettes?
No   ☐ 5
Yes, but no more than 5 a day   ☐ 3
Yes, more than 5 a day   ☐ 1

13. How often do you exercise or play sports?
Regularly (at least twice a week)   ☐ 5
Not regularly, but climbing stairs, walking   ☐ 3
Very seldom   ☐ 1

14. How often do you drink alcoholic beverages like beer, wine or tea with rum?
Every day   ☐ 1
3-5 times a week   ☐ 3
Never, except for special occasions   ☐ 5

15. How do you usually eat ?
On the run   ☐ 1
Taking your time   ☐ 6
While watching TV   ☐ 1

16. When do you eat?
When I'm with friends (even when I'm not hungry)   ☐ 1
Only at meal times when I'm hungry   ☐ 5
When I watch TV, read or when I'm angry   ☐ 0

Total Score

EVALUATION

65 to 80 points

Congratulations. You are aware of what you eat. A proper diet can have a positive effect on conditions such as arteriosclerosis, heart disease or diabetes. Stick to your eating habits and keep an open mind about new healthy diet ideas.

40 to 65 points

Your diet is an important part of your life. There is room for improvement though. Follow the recommendations in this book and try to eat more fruit, vegetables and whole wheat products. By making conscious choices about fats and oils, you will be able to improve your cholesterol level. When it comes to choosing your main course, try to go with vegetables more often rather than meat.

Less than 40 points

You are not really concerned with your diet. This can be a fatal mistake if you want to remain healthy. Many conditions are caused by the wrong diet. But you can take action now. Try to change your eating habits following the recommendations in this book.

Your Personal Energy Balance

Energy balance is crucial for your strength and performance

In today's world, the word "balance" is of great importance. Wall Street deals with balance sheets, and governments are concerned with the trade balance. And then, there is the energy balance of the body. Men need it for their strength and performance. The energy balance shows how many kilocalories we use per day. It can be calculated easily: Total energy consumption consists of the base metabolic rate, the performance-related metabolic rate and the exercise-related increased metabolic rate. The base metabolic rate per day of a slim 70 kg (155 lb) "normal" man is calculated as follows:

Body weight (in kg) x 24 hours x 1 calorie = base metabolic rate

In our example: 70 x 24 x 1 = 1,680 kilocalories

The energy consumption of people when performing sedentary work increases by about 30% of the base metabolic rate. Therefore, the performance-related metabolic rate is equivalent to the basal metabolic rate multiplied by 1.3. As for medium physical exertion, such as walking over a longer distance, painting a house or fence, the base metabolic rate shoots up by 200% for the duration of the activity. In other words, the performance-related metabolic rate corresponds to the base metabolic rate multiplied by three. Be careful not to calculate it for one day, but only for the duration of its actual performance.

Sedentary jobs require a 30% higher energy metabolic rate

The total metabolic rate (= base metabolic rate plus performance-related rate) every 24 hours for a normal man with an 8-hour working day is approximately:
- light physical activity: 2,000 kilocalories
- medium physical activity: 2,700 kilocalories
- heavy physical activity: more than 3,500 kilocalories

How You Can Improve Your Lifestyle

How can I recharge my batteries? A proper diet requires a good balance of nutrients, and plenty of them.

Sources of energy: carbohydrates

Slow carbohydrates (e.g., pasta) increase performance. Complex carbohydrates (e.g., beans, lentils) improve exercise tolerance, which is especially important in sports. These are the findings of a study done at San Jose State University in California. Cyclists had to eat a meal containing complex carbohydrates a half hour before training. As a result, their training performance improved because complex carbohydrates are transformed into glucose—the fuel of muscles—more slowly and evenly.

But what are carbohydrates? The main function of carbohydrates is to provide a continuous supply of energy to all the cells in the human organism. They fill you up and stay with you longer. They also increase performance. One major advantage is that they can reduce a person's craving for sweet and fatty foods. But also of importance are the low-sweet carbohydrates, so-called monosaccharides such as dextrose and fructose, which can be absorbed without any further breakdown. Disaccharides (ordinary sugar) and polysaccharides (starch and cellulose) are also low-sweet carbohydrates. About 50% of the calories we consume are derived from carbohydrates. One gram of carbohydrates supplies 4.3 kilocalories. Carbohydrates should make up between 55% and 60% of the body's total energy consumption.

Carbohydrates supply cells with energy

Half of our caloric intake comes from carbohydrates

The good and the bad: fatty acids

Basically, there are two types of fat—saturated and unsaturated fatty acids. Fats from plants are generally unsaturated, while saturated fatty acids are usually of animal origin. The latter can be found in butter, fatty meat, sausages and some fatty cheese. They are the main culprits when it comes to gaining weight. In fact, one gram of fat results in 9.5 kilocalories and thus has more than twice as many calories per gram as protein or carbohydrates. For adults, the ideal daily intake for each kilogram of body weight should be less than one gram of fat in the event of medium physical activity. On average, fat should only make up 20% to 25% of our total calories. But as the 1998 Austrian nutrition report shows, the average Austrian—and the numbers are similar for Germany—gets more than 40% of his daily intake of calories from fat. Unsaturated fatty acids that the body cannot produce by itself are especially recommended. They are found in cold-pressed oils like olive oil or rapeseed oil, but also in fish. Unsaturated fatty acids can help pre-

Unsaturated fatty acids protect against heart attacks

vent cardiovascular disease and thus heart attacks. Olive oil contains approximately 70% of monounsaturated oleic acid and about 12% of polyunsaturated linoleic acid. These unsaturated fatty acids reduce the bad LDL cholesterol level in the blood, while increasing the proportion of the good HDL cholesterol.

The building blocks: proteins

Proteins, which are composed of different amino acids, are the most important building blocks of cells, including human cells. Of the 20 amino acids that form all the known proteins, eight essential ones must be taken in with one's food (e.g., milk and dairy products). But they must already be complete at this point because they cannot be assembled from other substances through metabolism. One gram of protein supplies 4.3 kilocalories. It is crucial that the proteins we eat have a balanced content of amino acids because the lack of these acids results in serious health problems.

Eight of twenty amino acids are found in our food

Fiber

Fiber, or bulk material, is a component of vegetable foods (especially whole wheat such as rye or corn, vegetables such as peas, as well as beans, lentils and fruit) that cannot be broken down by intestinal enzymes. It increases salivation and regulates the bowel function. Fiber also delays gastric emptying and thus increases the time during which food remains in the stomach. As a result, we feel satiated longer and take in fewer calories. Our diet is rich in fiber-free animal nutrients, but low in natural fiber. Many conditions of the gastrointestinal tract result from this lack of natural fiber.

Fiber regulates intestinal function

Salts of life: minerals

The human body absorbs two groups of minerals, in differing quantities:
1. Macronutrients
These are minerals that must be consumed in large quantities. They include sodium, potassium, calcium, phosphor and magnesium.

There are micronutrients and macronutrients

2. Micronutrients
These minerals are often referred to as trace elements. They occur only in very small quantities, and include iron, copper, manganese, nickel, selenium, silicon and vanadium.

The German Society for Nutrition (DGE) has worked out guidelines for daily mineral requirements, which is shown in the table "Fit Through Vitamins" in this chapter. It is important to have a sufficient supply of the right minerals. Hair, fingernails and toenails especially depend on them.

Some of these minerals, such as sodium, are indispensable for water metabolism in the human body. Others, like calcium, are necessary to achieve proper bone density. Many minerals also play an important role in the body's immune system, and they support many different metabolic and cell functions. Iron, for example, is vital for the transport of oxygen and the functioning of the red blood cells. A lack of iron typically results in fatigue, weakness, pallor and anemia.

Minerals strengthen the body's immune system

If you decide to take mineral supplements, you should make sure it is well-balanced and that you avoid any extreme overdoses of individual elements. 'More is better' can be dangerous in the case of some minerals. If we are to believe the advertisements and the health magazines, then "superpills" containing vitamins, minerals and trace elements could help us fight any condition whatsoever—heart attack and hair loss, fatigue and sleep disorders, the flu and the hangover the morning after, deafness and lack of concentration.

Biological active ingredients the cure-all
Biological active ingredients are becoming more and more important. There are about 10,000 such substances known to us (pigments, bitter principles, enzymes, flavors, etc.). They are found in vegetables as well as spices. And they can neutralize free radicals that destroy cells, have a positive effect on the cholesterol level and support the excretion of environmental toxins. Biological active ingredients will be the focus of much attention as the millennium unfolds. The most important biological active ingredients are:

Biological active ingredients act as antioxidants

• Carotenoids
Carotenoids stimulate the immune system, prevent cancer, and are important antioxidants. They can be grouped into lycopenes, luteins, alphacarotenes and betacarotenes. They are found in orange-colored fruit and vegetables, tomatoes and grapefruit.

• Terpenes
Terpenes are important for cancer prophylaxis. They include menthol, citrus oil and carvone. They are found primarily in mint, caraway and lime.

• Sulfides
Sulfides can truly work miracles. They act as antioxidants, prevent cancer, stimulate the immune system, inhibit inflammation, lower the blood sugar level and support digestion. They are found primarily in garlic.

Sulfides prevent cancer

• Polyphenols

Polyphenols are also important antioxidants. They stimulate the immune system and prevent cancer. They are found, for example, in red wine, grapes, onions, green beans, corn, blueberries, raspberries, red cabbage and kale.

Vitamins

The end of the 20th century marked a new era in vitamin research. Medical researchers discovered the value of vitamins as a prophylaxis against cancer, as protection from stroke and as treatment for aging-related problems. Vitamin E can even be used to prevent heart attacks. According to a study of 300 Alzheimer's patients, vitamins can slow down the mental degradation that comes with advanced age. In the old days, an apple a day was supposed to keep the doctor away. The American National Cancer Institute now recommends five portions of fruit and vegetables every day. It says that these quantities provide optimum protection. The German Society for Nutrition (DGE) also issued recommendations in 1999 calling for higher vitamin intake than ever.

Vitamins slow down Alzheimer's

Vitamin C

Vitamin C protects the cell layer of blood vessels

Patients with a circulatory disturbance of the coronary vessels (coronary disease) will probably profit from a long-term intake of vitamin C (ascorbic acid). American scientists were able to prove that a daily supplement of 500 mg of vitamin C could significantly improve the controlled expansion of the brachial artery necessary to the flow of blood. Apparently, long-term treatment with ascorbic acid has a sustained beneficial effect on the functioning of the inner cell layers of blood vessels. Vitamin C also supports the immune system and fights many different diseases.

Vitamin E

Vitamin E lowers the risk of suffering a stroke

Vitamin E is quickly becoming a multipurpose cure. A study done by scientists in New York and published in April 1999 confirms that regular ingestion of vitamin E can lower the risk of suffering a stroke. They concluded that the ideal would be a combination of vitamin pills and a healthy lifestyle. The study showed a clearly lower risk of stroke for the group that took the most vitamins.

Folic acid, vitamins B6 and B12

In January 1999, the US Society of Cardiology added folic acid (primarily in lettuce, green vegetables and legumes), vitamins B6 and B12 to their list of substances that, besides vitamins C and E, provide protection from heart attacks and strokes. They did this in response to a group of heart patients who, despite having normal cholesterol levels and normal weight, had been shown to have a higher level of the amino acid homocystein—the cause of 10% of all heart conditions—in their blood. Giving such patients folic acid and the two B-vitamins provides an effective prophylaxis by reducing the homocystein level.

Folic acid lowers the homocystein level

Vegetables or Pills?

The five portions of vegetables and fruit recommended by the National Cancer Institute in the US are unrealistic even for health fanatics. Among other things, this kind of advice has led to the vitamin-pill craze, "vitamin mania." In the US, there are vitamins for adult men, young men going through puberty, women and athletes. Vitamins are touted as brain food, stress relievers, potency enhancers and everything else. But many important issues are being ignored.

1. Vitamins can be overdosed just like drugs. Quite often, the line between benefit and harm is a fine one. A recent study of women in Sweden showed that taking a daily overdose of vitamin A significantly increased the risk of suffering a hip fracture.

Careful: it is possible to overdose on vitamins

2. Is there a difference between natural and synthetic vitamins? In principle, no. Synthetic vitamins are pure and their structure is identical to that of their natural counterparts. Still, nutritionists say that most vitamins reach their true potential only in combination with others. They also warn that there is a chance that the body may process vitamins from food differently than their artificial counterparts in spite of their identical chemical structure. Recent studies conducted at the University of Michigan confirm that vitamin E has a positive effect on cholesterol metabolism, but this is only the case if the vitamin is taken naturally (in food). Vitamin E pills did not show the same results.

Which Vitamins Do I Need?

A vitamin deficiency often causes depression, lack of concentration and fatigue later in life. When we have a cold, our body requires more vitamin C, as it does for physical exertion or harsher climactic conditions.

Not only competitive athletes but also everyone else who engages in sports require more vitamins C, E, betacarotene and vitamin B because of increased energy and carbohydrate metabolism. The daily recommendation for athletes is 2 to 4 milligrams of betacarotene, 150 to 200 milligrams of vitamin C, and 20 to 50 milligrams of vitamin E. For every 1,000 calories of increased energy consumption, a person needs an additional 0.4 milligrams of vitamin D.

Smokers use up more vitamin A

Smokers need more vitamin A, which is considered an anti-cancer vitamin. Studies have shown that vitamin C can lower the risk of lung cancer and that smokers generally need 40% more vitamin C, and up to 50% more vitamin E (120–150 mg of vitamin C and 30 mg of vitamin E everyday).

B-vitamins are helpful in cases of high alcohol consumption

The B-type vitamins can help in cases of excessive consumption of alcohol. In Australia, where alcohol is often consumed for breakfast, vitamin B1 is added to alcoholic drinks.

Teenagers, who often skip a meal or eat fast food, typically require more vitamins. They should take multi-vitamin and -mineral supplements.

Vitamins as Antioxidants

In heart patients, vitamins C and E strengthen the body's vascular protection system. To help prevent heart attacks, you should take 100 to 200 milligrams of vitamin E and 250 to 500 milligrams of vitamin C everyday.

Vitamins act as antioxidants

Studies in the US say that alcohol and smoking create more free radicals—highly reactive spin-offs of oxygen molecules, which are chemically rather inert. These radicals attack the cell walls and are instrumental in the development of cancer and vascular disease. Vitamins can act as antioxidants here because they neutralize the free radicals. People who smoke and drink and are frequently under stress can take a mixture of vitamin C, folic acid and vitamin E.

The diet of aging men is often poor and unbalanced. Older men do not get enough of vitamins B2, B6, and B12, as well as vitamins C and D, and folic acid. It may also happen that, when on medication (analgesics), they do get enough of vitamins B and C. Stomach medication inhibits the intake of vitamin C, antibiotics are bad for almost all vitamins, and cholesterol drugs affect vitamins A, D, E and K.

Vitamin D can prevent osteoporosis

During the winter months, to make matters worse, the intake of vitamins drops even further. Men, and women too, should take vitamin C to prevent osteoporosis. The recommended daily doses are 2 to 4 milligrams of betacarotene, up to 0.1 milligram of vitamin B12, 150 to 200 milligrams of vitamin C, and 20 to 50 milligrams of vitamin E.

Vitamins: Cancer Prophylaxis 2000

"A Vitamin Revolution Is Coming," appeared recently right on the cover of the American news magazine Newsweek, usually a pretty sober publication. The title is from an inside story containing the most recent findings about vitamins. It is based on a mega study of 30,000 people that resulted in the first conclusive proof that vitamins can probably be used to prevent cancer.

The number of cancer-related deaths among the group with a high vitamin intake was 13% lower. The general mortality rate declined by 9%. The rate of gastric and esophageal cancer even dropped by 21%. The antioxidant combination of vitamin E, betacarotene and selenium proved very successful.

Vitamins can help prevent 13% of cancer deaths

Another study from Harvard University took a look at the eating habits of 80,000 US nurses. A clear connection was drawn between vitamin-rich nutrition and prevention of breast cancer in women in their pre-menopausal years. Women who ate more than five portions of fruit and vegetables everyday had a 23% lower risk of breast cancer than women who received these same vitamins less than twice a day.

It is still not possible to identify one specific vitamin or mineral as protection against cancer. Usually, natural substances do not come "packaged" individually. Foods always contain several active ingredients, and it could well be a combination of different vitamins that helps fend off cancer.

The vitamin trend continues, with no end in sight. Vitamins have also crossed over into cosmetics, where they are used as active ingredients in skin- and suntan lotions, and hair care products for men. After all, even sunlight creates aggressive free radicals that trigger an oxidation process in the skin, leaving its mark by accelerating the aging of the skin. That is why there are now "power cosmetics" for men, promising them skin like a baby's. Vitamin A and betacarotene are used in anti-wrinkle creams, which are designed to counteract the aging process of the skin by forming collagen. The B-vitamins are used in hair care products. They promote the formation of keratin, the most important building block of hair. Vitamin B3 is believed to strengthen the hair fiber from within. Vitamin E, in combination with vitamin C, is said to smoothen and moisten the skin. Another "hair vitamin" is vitamin H or biotin.

The cosmetics industry has discovered vitamins for men

FIT THROUGH VITAMINS RECOMMENDED DAILY DOSES FOR MEN

Vitamin A (retinol)	1 mg
Betacarotene (precursor of vitamin A)	2–3 mg
Vitamin B1 (thiamin)	
(from the age of 60 on up to 10 mg)	1.3 mg
Vitamin B2 (riboflavin)	1.7 mg
Niacin	18–30 mg
Pantothenic acid	6 mg
Vitamin B6 (pyridoxin)	1.8 mg (in some cases, up to 50 mg daily)
Vitamin B12 (cobalamin)	0.003 mg
Vitamin C (ascorbic acid)	75–120 mg
Vitamin D (calciferol)	0.005 mg

Attention: higher vitamin-D doses only after consulting your doctor

Vitamin E (tocopherol)	15–20 mg
Vitamin H (biotin)	0.03–0.1 mg
Vitamin K (phylloquinone)	0.08–0.1 mg
Folic acid	0.4 mg

When the German version of this book went into print, the German Society for Nutrition (DGE) was about to issue its own recommendation with respect to vitamins B6 and B12 as well as folic acid. These will probably include higher doses in order to lower homocystein levels and the risk of heart attacks.

Important: Vitamins or minerals, when taken in excess, can cause nausea or a range of other conditions. This is also true of eating too much raw food and isolated fiber, of which an excessive amount can impair resorption and thus diminish the supply of minerals and trace elements.

Food as the Medicine of the Future?

Functional food is the key to a good health

Food can be an effective medication. A new field of research, which will probably experience a boom in the coming years, deals with "functional food," a branch of pharmacology that focuses on the medicinal uses of food. As Professor Berthold Kolezko of the Department for Metabolism and Nutrition at the Hauner Clinic in Munich explains: "Functional food has an additional health benefit, apart from the usual nutritional value, which we call 'added value.'"

By 1997, the US Food and Drug Administration (FDA) had confirmed ten connections between food or food ingredients and a lower risk of disease. These include a reduced risk of osteoporosis through the intake of calcium, a reduced risk of coronary heart disease through low-fat foods containing low-saturation fatty acids and cholesterol and/or a low content of soluble fiber from oats. The lower risk of tooth decay via sugar alcohol is well recognized.

Currently, studies are underway in the US on the possible anti-cancer benefits of a variety of substances, from the root of licorice to flaxseed. The first results are expected in 2000/2001.

For years, scientists have been studying omega-3 fatty acids. They discovered that Eskimos, in spite of their considerable consumption of fat, suffer few heart attacks, and that Eskimo blood agglutinates very slowly. The most likely reason is that they get most of their fat from seafood, which contains a high concentration of omega-3 fatty acids. Omega-3 lowers the cholesterol level and the blood pressure. It also thins the blood. Omega-3 fatty acids are found in mackerel, sardines, redfish, eel and sole.

The Eskimos' secret: omega-3 fatty acid

Those Extra Pounds and Their Consequences

Excess weight is one of the risk factors in hypertension and heart disease. This has long been known. But less known is the influence that a moderate, but steady, weight gain can have over a longer period of time. A study at the university hospital in Göteborg, Sweden, published in the European Heart Journal in 1999, shows that even a slight gain of only 4% to 10% between the age of 20 and the "middle" years can increase by a factor of 1.5 the risk of suffering a heart attack or dying from heart disease. Of the participants in the study, 80% had gained an average of ten kilograms over the specified period of time.

Even a weight gain of 4 to 10% can increase the risk of heart attacks

Men who had gained more than a third in the course of their lives saw their risk of suffering a fatal heart attack increase threefold. According to information from the World Health Organization, obesity in Europe has increased by up to 40% in the last ten years. About 40% of all cases of obesity and 25% of those that are slightly overweight suffer from cardiovascular disease in contrast to 13% of those with normal weight. Overweight people are three times as susceptible to hypertension as people with normal weight. There is a direct correlation between rising blood pressure and weight gain. Excess weight increases the risk not only of hypertension and coronary heart disease, but also of diabetes, increased serum lipid levels, gallstone trouble, apnea, cancer and degeneration of the joints.

Overweight people are three times as likely to have hypertension

My Ideal Weight

The long term goal of any man has got to be achieving his ideal weight and maintaining it. The current scientific method of calculating normal weight, overweight and obesity—6% of Austrian men are affected by it—is the body mass index (BMI). Body weight alone is not a sufficient parameter. With the BMI, the weight is defined in relation to a person's height. The BMI is calculated on the basis of the weight in kilograms divided by the square of the height in meters.

The BMI is the ratio between weight and height

The BMI readings are:

Up to 18.4:   underweight
18.5 to 24.9:   normal weight
25 to 28:   overweight
Above 29:   obesity

Here is an example:

A man weighs 88 kilograms (about 194 pounds) and is 1.82 meters (5'11'') tall. His BMI is calculated as follows (There are about 2.2 pounds in a kilogram and 39 inches in a meter):

88: (1.82)2 = 88 : 3.3124 = 26.5668
This man is overweight, but not obese.

Abdominal fat deposits have a higher cell count

Another indication of excess weight besides the BMI is the distribution of fat tissue. A good measurement is the girth of the hips. So-called apple-shaped people (abdominal fat) and pear-shaped people (fat hips) are distinguished in terms of their risk profile. The first would be the male type and the latter, the female.

Apple-shaped people or androids, the male type, have a markedly higher risk of concomitant conditions. The accumulation of abdominal fat is different from other fat deposits inasmuch as there are a higher number of cells per measurement unit, a higher number of receptors for cortisone and male hormones (androgens) as well as a higher rate of dissolution of fat induced by the stress hormone catecholamine. On the other hand, the pear-shaped female type with fat deposits on the hips (often perceived by women as a cosmetic problem) is more difficult to influence, either by changing eating habits or through exercise.

A simple method for assessing abdominal fat deposits is measuring the abdominal girth. If the abdominal girth of a man exceeds 94 centimeters (about 37 inches), he will have an increased risk of metabolic disease. If the girth exceeds 102 centimeters (about 40 inches), that risk will be significantly higher.

A girth of more than 94 cm? Increased risk of metabolic diseases

The Austrian nutrition report, which we have already mentioned, points out that the different methods of and products for weight loss make up the third largest segment of nutritional advertising. In health magazines, 11% of all ads and up to 17% of content deals with this topic.

The message that printed media are spreading is that it is possible to lose weight within a short time and that it should be done for cosmetic reasons. This reinforces the standards of slimness that are so prevalent in our society today, and that doctors believe to be part of the problem to say the least. The report states that 80% of all weight loss ads and one-third of the methods that are promoted in those articles cannot bring about any lasting reduction in weight. What is more, the information contained in articles on dieting is incomplete. The reader ought to have the complete picture in order to properly assess the benefits of the diets recommended. Such diets promise to take off, on average, 2.5 kilograms (5.5 pounds) a week, which is considerably more than doctors recommend (one kilogram or 2.2 pounds at most).

"Trying to lose weight in a record time is useless," says Professor Michael Kunze, an expert in social medicine. Everyday sees the advent of miracle cures and crash diets. But buyer beware! Especially beware crash diets that promise the greatest weight loss in the shortest possible time. They either have no effect beyond the medium term or may actually be acutely harmful. Programs that are based on diets rich in protein and low in carbohydrates, especially when combined with anabolic agents, have often resulted in death, even among bodybuilders.

Trying to lose weight in record time is useless

Proper diets are always based on the same principle. Eat less while maintaining a balanced diet. Follow some of the examples set by Mediterranean and Asian cultures.

Five Pointers for Losing Weight the Right Way

1. Take it slow

Fasting may be "in" and have a meditative quality to it, but it is absolutely the wrong thing to do if you want to lose weight. Try to match your daily base metabolic rate of about 1,680 calories.

2. The best way to lose weight is by exercising

The best method for losing weight is stamina training with the right intensity of physical exercise. A recent US study carried out by the Mayo Clinic in Rochester, Minnesota, shows that it does not take much to work off excess calories. Moving your fingers, frequent getting up and sitting down, climbing stairs, and so forth will even accomplish it.

You start losing weight once you burn 2,000 calories/week

The American National Weight Control Registry conducted longitudinal studies on people on weight loss programs. It found that almost all the men who lost at least 15 kilograms and were able to maintain that weight burnt a minimum of 2,000 calories a week playing sports. This can be achieved by slow running (jogging), which affects the lipid metabolism. This is said to be the ideal way, with a heart rate of about 60% of the maximum rate—about 120 heartbeats per minute. Slow running burns fat at a rate of 80% and carbohydrates at 20%. The energy turnover is about eight kilocalories per minute. If you run at medium speed with a heart rate of 75% to 80% of the maximum heart rate (150–160 beats per minute), your energy consumption will be significantly higher (about 15–18 kilocalories per minute), with 50% to 60% of that energy coming from the burning of fat and 40% to 50% from the burning of carbohydrates. Approximately nine fat calories are burned every minute. This means that, during the same period of time, more energy (calories) is consumed, which is important for losing weight, but the body also burns about 33% more fat.

3. Losing weight in your sleep

Losing weight means reducing body fat, the decisive factor in which is not so much the fat reduction during training, but the so called "after burn," and the total fat reduction within a 24-hour period. Total energy consumption per day must be higher than the energy supply, or the supply must be lower than the consumption. Each additional kilogram of muscle tissue, as a result of training, burns up 150 to 200 calories a day, even while you are asleep. Stamina train-

The body taps the energy reserves of fat tissue at night

ing will also use up more energy because of the increase in muscle mass. The human body gets its required energy from the fatty tissue during sleep. So, while you are resting, your body is burning fat.

4. Avoid alcoholic beverages

Two glasses of beer a day = 13 kilograms of fat more each year

Drinking alcohol not only piles on the calories (two glasses of beer a night amount to 13 kilograms of fat per year), but also stimulates your appetite. People who have an alcoholic aperitif before a meal usually eat more. You should also keep in mind that many alcoholic beverages, and even many non-alcoholic drinks, are in fact "calorie bombs."

- Sparkling wine · · · · · · · · 10 calories
- Cocoa · · · · · · · · · · · · · 80 calories
- Red wine · · · · · · · · · · · 74 calories
- White wine · · · · · · · · · · 70 calories
- Milk · · · · · · · · · · · · · · 66 calories
- Coca-Cola, Pepsi · · · · · · · 57 calories
- Beer · · · · · · · · · · · · · · 47 calories
- Apple juice · · · · · · · · · · 46 calories
- Orange juice · · · · · · · · · 42 calories
- Iced tea · · · · · · · · · · · · 29 calories
- Coca-Cola, Pepsi (light) · · · · 4 calories
- Coffee · · · · · · · · · · · · · · 1 calorie
- Mineral water · · · · · · · · · · 0 calories

So, as you can see, it would be better to have water or mineral water with or before your meal.

5. Stay away from crash diets

If the body suddenly has to go without the amount of food it is used to, it will automatically shift all systems into low gear. In crash diets, the caloric base metabolic rate will drop after a few days. The body learns to do with fewer calories while on the diet. People usually return to their old eating habits with a vengeance at the end of such a diet, and put the pounds right back on. And the body will convert the excess calories to fat pads even more than before. Therefore, it is not worth denying yourself the food you really like. Forget about resolutions like "Starting tomorrow, I won't eat chocolate anymore." The important thing is to eat slowly, chew your food carefully and savor every bit of it. Also, drink a lot of water before meals. This way, the stomach gets full and can send the corresponding signal to the brain. It usually takes about 15 minutes.

Crash diets are dangerous

Is There a Miracle Diet Pill for Men?

There is no slimming pill without any side effects, nor will there be any time soon. Researchers are working intensively on the fat gene, the leptin hormone, which is supposed to reduce the fatty tissue. There is also the newly discovered substance orlistat (Xenical®), which is supposed to block the absorption of fat from the intestines, and new serotonin-like preparations (e.g., Reductil®) that act directly on the satiety center in the brain.

A diet pill without side effects remains a pipedream

Preliminary findings, however, show that the fat-absorption blocker orlistat only works for obese people with a body mass index over 30, and in combination with a strict low fat diet. Other medications still have to undergo clinical testing to find out whether they are effective and free of side effects.

TEN TIPS FOR A HEALTHY DIET

- Have five small meals every day, instead of three large ones.
- Avoid fatty foods.
- Eat more fruit, vegetables and whole grain products.
- Prepare food carefully in order to retain the vitamins.
- Reduce your consumption of meat.
- Regularly eat fresh fish.
- Do not salt your food excessively.
- Drink at least two liters of fluids every day.
- Make sure you have a sufficient vitamin intake.
- Cut down on sugar and sweets.

Fit for Life

More Power for the Male Body

"Three minutes... two... go for one more! Done. That's it for now." The personal trainer crosses the imaginary finish line next to his client, Dr. Albert N., a 45-year-old surgeon from Vienna, without losing a beat and without having worked up a sweat. The doctor, flushed and sweating, is a wreck following the 20 kilometer (12.5 mile) run.

It is 6:30 in the morning, and there is a fog hovering over the Danube Canal. Doctor and trainer have been running along the Danube for 90 minutes. It is all part of the doctor's stamina training. They head back to the fitness studio for strength training.

Some days, the doctor prefers "spinning" to running. This is a super-aerobic training with a mental element. On a special exercise bike—the next generation of the home trainer—the modern ergometer, he pedals to loud music, surrounded by other spinning aficionados.

The balance between body and soul is important

Sport is part and parcel of life. Maximum personal performance and professional achievement are greatly facilitated by a lifestyle that consists of an optimized balance of mental, physical, emotional and spiritual well-being.

Albert N. is the typical modern West European man whose job leaves him little time for himself. Still, he has managed to integrate sports into his life. His philosophy is that of a new generation of power men: "Feel good about yourself and remain active even in old age."

The interaction of body, mind and soul was recognized by the ancient Greeks. And Leonardo da Vinci gave us an impressive depiction of it in his "The Vitruvian Man." The original can be seen at the Accademia in Venice. That famous study placed the human body in proportion to basic geometric shapes, the square and the circle. But many say that it is an expression of the harmonious coexistence of body and soul.

Our modern concept of fitness goes back almost thirty years to a former Air Force officer whose idea circled the globe and revolutionized fitness for the rest of the 20th century. Dr. Kenneth H. Cooper created a special kind of stamina training that he called simply "aerobics," from the Greek word for "air" and "oxygen." Aerobics involves movements that balance the supply of oxygen with the burning of fat, and stimulate the oxygen metabolism. At first, his method completely changed the way Americans, and then the rest of the world, looked at sports. Today, Ken Cooper controls a fitness empire and runs his own clinic, the Cooper Institute for Aerobics Research in Dallas, Texas, as well as a chain of Cooper fitness studios. At his studios, prospective customers are subjected to a thorough medical examination using state-of-the-art diagnostics and sports medicine equipment and techniques before they are allowed to begin training. Their blood and urine samples are subjected to as many as 50 different tests in the laboratory. Doctors check cardiac and pulmonary functioning, vision and hearing, and if requested, will even check for signs of cancer. After an exercise tolerance test, a fitness program geared to the age of the person and the mobility of the spinal cord, as well as to the composition of the body fat, is designed. While aerobics has gone out of fashion in Europe, Cooper's method has undergone further development under different names and remains the dominant fitness program in the world.

Ken Cooper started the fitness boom with his "aerobics"

At the Cooper Clinic, but also in Austrian and German fitness studios, two-thirds of the clientele are men. Their ages tend to range between 32 and 45. Three out of four think that they are fit and healthy, but they nevertheless want to counter the small signs of change in their bodies. One trend that is growing is the method that Dr. N. chose, a personalized training program that can be pursued either at a fitness studio or at home. Having a personal trainer is the latest craze. People go jogging with their personal trainers two to three times a week or work out in a gym under the supervision of such a personal trainer.

Two-thirds of people at gyms are men

The latest trend: a personal trainer

It does not matter what type of sport you go in for. The important thing is to have the right attitude toward your body. Has stress turned your body into a ticking time bomb? Do you have problems sleeping? Do you spend your weekends eating pizza and drinking beer in front of the TV? How long has it been since you last went out of your way to do something healthy?

The goal must be active prevention

Most men pay no attention to their body until they have, or a close friend or relative has, serious health problems to contend with. Only then are they willing to take some kind of action. This attitude allows medical problems to gradually worsen until there is a full-blown crisis of cancer, stroke, heart disease or diabetes. The goal of modern men has to be active prevention of disease rather than just a knee-jerk response to serious breakdowns.

Many men blame their poor exercise- and dietary habits on a lack of time. Time is money. This may be true, but can you afford to be sick?

Lack of Exercise Can Be Life Threatening

"You must exercise your body if you want to succeed intellectually. New ideas and innovations usually require that the body and mind are equally fit."

Niki Lauda

25% of men never exercise

In 1996, the World Health Organization (WHO) and the World Association of Sports passed a resolution to the effect that half of the population of the world is physically inactive and wastes important potential. They maintained that inactive people are putting their lives on the line. According to the resolution, more than 60% of adults do not do the recommended level of physical activity, and 25% are completely inactive and engage in no sports whatsoever. Older adolescents are significantly less active than younger ones. "Adults should engage in moderate physical activity for at least 30 minutes everyday, e.g., by walking at a fast pace, hiking or climbing stairs," the WHO wrote in its recommendations.

The WHO recommends that we exercise 30 minutes a day

There are many ways to get started. But you have to be willing to take the first step. The growing interest in fitness, health and well-being is the result of a fundamental social change. We use our bodies differently than did our Stone Age ancestors or our great grandparents. Prehistoric men were predominantly hunters who had to be in top condition to survive and were constantly faced with physical stress. But this has changed over the course of time. Even our great grandfathers did hard physical labor from early childhood onward. They

Our great grandparents suffered from typical degenerative diseases

often suffered from typical symptoms of wear-and-tear. Being healthy meant surviving first and foremost. Only a few people lived past 50, many being felled by infectious diseases. With the scarcity of medical resources, many people accepted disease as a fact of life.

But the 20th century ushered in a brand new era. Machines started to replace human labor, taking a huge load off people, but in the process causing them to become less active. Hunched over a desk for hours everyday, commuting long distances and then sitting in the front of the TV trying to unwind is more and more a day in the life of a typical man.

The increasing pressure to be successful, or the struggle just to hang on to a job, increases psychological stress. Modern lifestyles, coupled with smoking, drinking and excess weight, lead to stress, which in turn leads to the number one cause of death, cardiovascular disease. In our service-oriented world with its 'marvelous' conveniences such as fast food, drive-thru service and home delivery around the clock, we are being deprived of even the minimum amount of activity necessary to be fit and healthy and to keep up our performance level.

Modern lifestyles are responsible for cardiovascular disease

Physical inactivity and the aging process eat away at the capacity to perform physical work in the first place. If we retreat from activities that require strength, skill and agility, it will be increasingly more difficult for us to perform them as we get older. We will be more likely to get injured or sick.

In the past ten years, medical scientists, especially in the fields of sports medicine and physiology, have gained valuable new insights. There is no doubt anymore that stamina training can help prevent heart attacks and cardiac death. Strength training can improve performance and body coordination even in 60-year-olds. It is never too late to get fit. But consult a physician before you begin.

Exercise can help prevent heart attacks in many cases

What are the benefits of regular physical exercise? It all comes down to the right balance of stamina, agility, strength and quickness. This will keep you healthy and slow the natural aging process. Stamina training leads to the lowering of the pulse rate and the blood pressure, while intensive training increases the cardiac volume. The heart is strengthened, the strain on it is lessened, and it requires less oxygen.

Sports are good for the circulation and the gas exchange in the lungs, thereby improving the oxygen supply to the entire body. The blood flow properties are

A NORMAL HEART VERSUS AN ATHLETE'S HEART

The magazine Men's Health drew parallels between a normal heart and an athlete's heart.

	Normal heart	Athletic heart
● Size	The same as a person's fist	Up to 100% larger
● Amount of blood pumped	6 liters/minute	Up to 30 liters/minute
● Heart rate	60 to 75 beats/ minute at rest	30 to 55 beats/

The healthy HDL cholesterol level increases with sports

also improved, and the sensitivity of certain tissues to hormones is improved. Also important is the effect on the metabolism, especially on the serum lipid levels. The total cholesterol level is lowered and the beneficial HDL cholesterol rises in direct proportion to the kilometers run. The blood sugar level of men can be lowered even by sports pursued only as a hobby. The immune system is enhanced, and the body mass, which is lost with age, can be increased by up to 1% every year if you engage in regular strength training. This is so important because the number of muscle cells drops 20% to 40% in men by the time they reach the age of 70. Strength training can put the brakes on aging.

After the age of 20, muscle cells decrease by up to 40%

Sports Will Bring You Better Sex

Athletic men are generally more relaxed

Recent studies show that exercise causes massive changes in the body. Athletic men have a deeper sleep, are usually more relaxed and enjoy sex much more. The well known magazine Nature published a study that found that trained rats showed signs of nerve growth in memory-related structures. It would appear that there is a positive connection among movement, intellect and memory. If this can be confirmed and applied to humans, another new fitness wave will circle the globe.

"No pain, no gain" is a fallacy

But beware too much of a good thing. This is especially true for people new to sports. Overexertion and poorly planned training can lead to physical exhaustion in beginners and amateurs. "No pain, no gain" or "If I train harder, I'll be faster than the rest," are common fallacies. Of athletes with exhaustion syndrome, 80% can develop depression. It is important for people of all age groups to consult a general physician before embarking on a regular stamina-training program or, if they have athletic ambitions, an expert in sports medicine.

Aerobic Versus Anaerobic Training

Aerobic training, which, literally translated, means "training with oxygen," is when you continuously move large muscle groups such as your legs. This type of exercise challenges the heart, lungs and muscle cells. Such training enables the body to make better use of oxygen. And it is not so intensive as to inflict pain, which would normally result from the buildup of lactic acid in the muscle.

Aerobic training improves the use of oxygen

Anaerobic exercise (training without, or with reduced, oxygen supply to the muscle tissue) uses up the entire oxygen supply in the course of the exercise, which overstrains the muscles. This leads to the formation first of lactate, and then of lactic acid. It is the lactic acid that causes the muscles to be sore. Anaerobic exercise is recommended for top athletes only. It is not suitable for overly ambitious people who go to the gym for the first time and think they can lift the heaviest weights.

Lactic acid causes sore muscles

In the January 1999 issue of The Sports Medicine Bulletin, which can also be found on the Internet (www.acsm.org), published a set of recommendations together with the American College of Sports and the United States Olympic Committee on how to design an individual fitness program for athletes.

The authors distinguish between health-associated and fitness-associated physical activities. Health activities are supposed to have positive effects on one or more health-related variables, such as blood pressure, stress, body fat, risk of cardiovascular disease, cancer, diabetes, etc. Fitness activities are targeted at improving performance in certain athletic areas, such as stamina, timing, etc. The two sometimes overlap. Many fitness activities also improve health variables but not always. Let us look at a simple example. If your primary goal is to reduce stress, it would not be the right thing to start jogging with a group of experienced runners who take part in competitions. This may actually increase the stress, even though it improves your aerobic fitness.

Fitness activities improve health-related variables

EXERCISE IS VITAL

- Stamina training helps lower the blood pressure and pulse rate.
- Exercise makes the body more sensitive to hormones.
- Regular exercise lowers the cholesterol and blood sugar levels.
- Fitness strengthens your immune system.
- Exercise can slow the natural aging process.

Harder Is Not Necessarily Better

The factors that are important when setting up an exercise regime are age, body weight, current physical condition, and others. You should always consult your physician before starting out on a training program. "Harder is not necessarily better" is the message here.

● Blood pressure

Exercise increases the blood pressure to 300/150 mm/Hg

Normal blood pressure, according to the World Health Organization (WHO), is 135/85 mm/Hg. During extreme exercise, it may rise to 300/150 mm/Hg temporarily. This should not be problem for people who do not suffer from arteriosclerosis or cardiovascular disease.

● Training frequency

Exercising three to five times a week is best

The health benefits increase steadily with the frequency of training. The ideal training frequency is between three and five days per week. Fewer than three will not do much for you. If you exercise more than five days a week, you will see some additional benefit, but there is an increased risk of muscle and bone injury.

● Intensity and duration of training

The target heart rate should be 60% of the maximum rate

Recent research proves that it is easier to overcome a lack of willpower and stay with a program if it is low intensity. The target heart rate should be about 55% to 60% of the maximum heart rate. Another study showed that a non-stamina program in four ten-minute installments has the same positive effect as a 40-minute endurance exercise. Low intensity exercises that are done for at least 30 minutes a day continuously or in ten-minute sequences have a considerable health benefit. The key to such positive results may lie in the total energy consumption. Another option is to reduce the intensity and compensate by increasing the duration of the training so that the total consumption of calories remains the same. As an example, 30 minutes of walking at a speed of 6 km/h (almost 4 mph) or 40 minutes of fast walking at 4.3 km/h provide the same results. The lower speed can be compensated for with a greater distance, and the energy consumption will be the same.

Other physical activities:
● Less intensive, but longer: 45 minutes of volleyball; 30–45 minutes of gardening; walking 2.8 km in 35 minutes; 30 minutes of basketball or shooting hoops; cycling 8 km in 30 minutes; energetic dancing for 30 minutes.
● Medium intensity: walking 3.2 km in 30 minutes; 20 minutes of water aerobics or swimming

- More intensive, but shorter: 15 minutes of basketball; cycling 6.4 km in 15 minutes; jumping rope for 15 minutes; running 2.4 km in 15 minutes; shoveling snow for 15 minutes; climbing stairs for 15 minutes.

Moderate activity uses up about 150 kilocalories of energy per day or 1,000 kilocalories per week.

• Type of training
The American College of Sports Medicine stresses the importance of choosing the right kind of sport. You can reduce your risk of injury if you choose low impact sports (such as cycling or swimming) especially if physical exercise is something new to you. High impact sports would be running, advanced aerobics, and so on.

"Sport is a like drug: the right dose can cure you; too much of it will kill you," says Dr. Boldt, an expert in sports medicine and director of the State Institute for Sports Medicine in Berlin. Every athlete does simple stretches to warm up. You should choose your endurance routine on the basis of your physical condition rather than your personal preference.

Too much sport can kill you

- If you are extremely overweight, you should stay away from jogging.
- If you tend to have back pains, you should strengthen your abdominal muscles and forgo cycling.
- If you have knee problems, avoid squash. But you could strengthen your muscles and circulation by swimming.

Overweight people should not go jogging

A large scale study of 17,000 university graduates carried out by Harvard University has shown that intensive exercise, such as two hours of tennis or four hours of cycling per week, can increase your life span.

Intensive exercise increases the life span

The following is a chart of the most common sports and their advantages and disadvantages.

Sport	Advantages	Disadvantages
Jogging	Ideal stamina training No overexertion possible because the body reacts with massive fatigue	High level of exertion on the joints (esp. of the knees and feet) Jogging on concrete over a longer period of time can damage the locomotor system Not suitable for overweight people

Swimming	Optimal stamina training Activates almost all muscle groups Ideal for overweight people	Practically none
Cycling	Very good stamina training there may be circulatory problems	Careful in case of back problems Ideal for overweight people In case of extremely long distances,
Bodybuilding	Selective buildup of muscles	No stamina training Risk of pulling or rupturing ligaments and muscles No positive effect on the heart Careful in case of hypertension
Tennis	Stamina training Improves body coordination and skill	Abrupt stop-and-go is bad for knee joints and ligaments

Five Rules for Beginners

1. Consult your physician if you are over 40 years old

If you are older than 40 and have never exercised regularly, or if you suffer from a chronic disease, such as hypertension, heart disease, diabetes or kidney disease, consult your doctor before you start the program.

2. Go slowly

As a beginner you should not overdo it

Rome was not built in a day. Do not overdo it. Start by going for 20-minute walks. Later, you can start running slowly. After the first month, increase each training unit by a distance 10% longer than the previous one. If you paused between October and February, like one-third of all recreational athletes, then forget everything you were able to do six months before and start from scratch. Increase your volume by 10% to 15% each week. Even after a break of only two weeks, the body loses 10 to 15% of its strength and 25% of its stamina. Never try to compensate for what you missed. Instead, reduce your speed by 10% during the first week after a break.

3. Choose the program that is best for you

You should choose a sport that you enjoy. Walking, jogging, swimming, cycling, squash, inline skating, tennis, dancing, skiing, cross country skiing and aerobics are all ideal for sensible and efficient circulatory training.

4. You must exercise regularly

At a minimum, 20 minutes three times a week, i.e., 60 minutes a week. The ideal would be at least 30 minutes five times a week.

5. Stick to your individual program

You do not have to become a top athlete or Superman. Do not set yourself unrealistic goals. Ideally, get a pulse meter for a controlled, risk-free exercise program.

How Fit Is Fit? How to Exercise Properly

The goal of the ideal exercise program is to increase your endurance. It allows your body to restore its level of adenosine triphosphate (ATP) during physical activity and thus maintain your performance level. It also makes you more resistant to fatigue during periods of exertion and increases your ability to recover after such physical exertion.

The body restores its adenosine triphosphate (ATP)

In other words, a particular activity can be pursued longer and your body recovers much faster. So, how can you measure your stamina? The easiest way is a bicycle or treadmill ergometer. You can do this test at almost any fitness club. Your blood pressure, heart rate and EKG will be measured under physical exertion for subsequent analysis.

Test your performance on an ergometer

You will begin with a light exercise of 25 watts, which will be increased by another 25 watts every two minutes until you become exhausted and the test is stopped. The performance at the time the test was stopped is your actual maximum performance ("wattmax"). In the case of younger or physically fit people, it is permissible to start at 50 watts and raise the level 50 watts every two minutes. But the test must last at least eight minutes. There are standard levels for the wattmax depending on the sex, age and height of a person, and they can be calculated as follows:

Age of man (in years)	25	35	45	55	65	75
Wattmax/kilogram	3.0	2.76	2.52	2.28	2.01	1.77

In order to determine the individual's normal wattmax level, the corresponding value of wattmax/kilogram is multiplied by the body weight. Finally, the individual wattmax is computed as a percentage of the normal level. Thus, the deviation from the normal level, the training state, can be quantified as a percentage. The normal performance level of each age and weight is always 100%. The normal range is between 90% and 110%. If it drops below 90%, the performance is considered below average. If it is over 110%, it is said to be above average. Using a bicycle ergometer is certainly the most precise and reliable method of measuring a person's performance, and everyone should have this done. You can contact your family physician or a sports medicine specialist.

The normal performance level is 100%

The American College of Sports Medicine recommends the following:
1. Training frequency: 3 to 5 days a week.
2. Training intensity: 55/65% to 90% of the maximum heart rate (HRmax) or 40/50% to 85% of the maximum oxygen uptake. The low intensity levels, 40% to 49% of oxygen uptake and 55% to 64% of maximum heart rate, are ideal for men who are not very fit.
3. Duration of training: 20 to 60 minutes of continuous exercise or spread across several units of at least ten minutes each.
4. Type of activity: any activity that moves large muscle groups and that can be done in a continuous, rhythmic and aerobic manner outdoors, such as walking, hiking, running, jogging, ice skating, cycling, cross country skiing, jumping rope, rowing, climbing stairs, swimming, etc. The best measure of the intensity for which you should aim is not the degree of physical exertion involved, because this varies from one activity to another. Rather, the desired intensity is a training heart rate (HRtr) of about 60%. Because the training heart rate is the ratio between intensity and the heart rate (pulse), it remains constant, whatever the activity.

20 to 60 minutes of training is ideal

To determine the individual training heart rate, you will have to know the maximum heart rate, which is taken at the time that the ergometer test is stopped, and the heart rate at rest, which is measured after a few minutes of resting on your back. The individual HRtr is calculated as follows: HRtr equals HRrest plus (HRmax minus HRrest) multiplied by 0.6 plus 5 beats per minute. The HRtr must be checked for each exercise. The current level of exertion must be adjusted each time so that the set HRtr can be maintained. The best way to do this is to use an automatic miniature pulse meter. Controlling the intensity is based not on a certain speed or lactate level, but on the individual HRtr. This way it is possible to maintain the same intensity even when exercising outdoors in an area with various inclines. In case of a slight incline, unfit or older people can achieve the right HRtr simply by walking.

The Joy of Running

No other sport has experienced a boom the way running has. The thing about running is that you can do it wherever you are. Beginners can typically start by going for a staggered endurance run once a week (30 minutes of alternating fast walking with slow running, each for a minute), a 20-minute endurance run (at an even pace) once a week and, using a pulse meter, doing "freestyle" exercises for 30 minutes once a week. Such freestyle exercises involve walking and running while alternating the pace at will.

Start endurance running in intervals

This weekly program will progress systematically. The walking time remains at one minute, but the staggered endurance run is increased to a total of 60 minutes, and the running time is gradually raised to five minutes. For endurance running, the running time is increased to 60 minutes, and the freestyle exercise may also be extended to 60 minutes. The maximum pulse rate if not calculated following the method explained earlier can be calculated using this rule of thumb: The maximum pulse is 220 minus your age. This maximum should never be exceeded.

Keep in mind that you should not engage in sports for one to two hours after eating. You should also do warm-up exercises before your training and cooling-down exercises afterwards. By running slowly for five to ten minutes, you can bring your muscles up to "operating temperature." You should follow up by stretching your muscles to make them more resistant to mishaps such as sprains. The stretching improves their elasticity and makes them more flexible. The movability of the joints is also improved. Try touching your feet with the tips of your fingers while keeping your knees and back straight. Stay in this position for a few seconds.

Do not exercise up to two hours after a meal

After running, you should relax the muscles with a period of cooling down by running slowly and stretching your muscles. Also helpful after the training would be a bath or a shower (alternating cold and hot), a sauna, steam bath or massage.

Jogging or Running?

The origin of the word "jogging" is not quite clear. Some say that it is a mixture of "jump" and "go." In fact, jogging denotes slow running, comparable to walking extremely quickly. Thus, jogging is aerobic running.

Glucose and fatty acids supply the body with energy

The body needs energy to work the muscles. The "fuel," so to speak, is a mixture of sugar (glucose) and fat (fatty acids). Its mixing ratio depends on the intensity of the running. The energy for the muscles comes from sugar and fat in the muscles as well as from the intake of oxygen through respiration. The faster you run, the greater the physical exertion, and consequently the more sugar is mixed into the fuel. The lower the level of exertion (slow jogging), the more fat there will be in the mixture. If the sugar supply has been used up completely, we feel exhausted. It is, therefore, the goal of jogging to burn fat, not sugar. Physically unfit people often have more sugar in the mixture when they reach 50% of their maximum training intensity, so it is important for them to take it slow.

Thirty minutes of jogging at 9 km/h burns up 300 calories

If we jog or run faster, and our body cannot take in enough oxygen for the increased energy consumption, we enter the phase of anaerobic (no oxygen) running. The consumption of calories for 30 minutes of endurance running at a speed of 9 km/h (about 5.5 mph—there are about 1.6 kilometers in a mile) amounts to 300 kilocalories. At 15 km/h, this comes to 385 kilocalories. By way of comparison, look at the consumption rates for cycling. Thirty minutes result in 70 kilocalories at 10 km/h and 235 kilocalories at 20 km/h. Thirty minutes of walking at 5 km/h consumes 95 kilocalories.

It does not matter whether you run for competitive or health reasons. Almost every regular jogger points out that jogging gives them mental balance. "I'm calmer and more easy going," "I'm not feeling so restless anymore," "Jogging gives me the balance I need in my life," "I'm not so crazy and hectic."

Frequent jogging can become an addiction

Running improves your ability to cope with stress. It has even been said that jogging can eliminate anxieties and that some people even manage to "run away" from their depression and psychosomatic problems. Many joggers say that running can be addictive. In a study of runners, more than 50% considered themselves addicted to running. Generally, we should only speak of addiction if the runner disregards warning signals from the body— feeling pain and taking painkillers, cortisone or drugs rather than adjusting the exercise routine. Addiction may be an apt term in the sense that jogging can bring about a change in a person's mental state, and this, of course, refers to the secretion of the body's own happiness and stress hormones, endorphins and catecholamines.

Healthy jogging cannot trigger the release of endorphins. In order to reach that level, you would have to run between 30 and 45 kilometers every day, which is what happens in a marathon. Many runners are tough, but they make the fatal mistake of ignoring pain. Pain can mean only one thing: there is a problem that needs attention.

Endorphins are secreted only during a marathon

TIPS FOR BUSY MEN

Men with heavy work schedules often have no time to engage in sports on a regular basis. Still, here are a few suggestions for things you could do:
- Do knee bends while brushing your teeth in the morning and evening.
- Do not use elevators, and make it a principle to take the stairs.
- Do not take the car short distances. Walk.
- Walk briskly.
- Do stretches while waiting for your computer to load the operating system.
- Contract your gluteal muscles now and then while sitting at the desk. Keep them contracted for ten seconds, then relax them. Then start over.
- While driving, tense different groups of muscles for about five to ten seconds, then relax them again. Repeat the exercise for each muscle at least ten times.

These exercises burn about the same amount of fat as a light fitness training session, according to a study of the Cooper Institute of Aerobics Research in Dallas. Even the levels of blood pressure, body fat and cardiac function can be improved. Surely you can spare five minutes a day?

Mental Fitness
How to Use Your Brain Power

The department of neuroscience and neuropsychology of the National Institutes of Health (NIH) in Bethesda, Maryland, is as secure and shielded as the grounds of a federal maximum security prison. Behind the walls of this leading biomedical laboratory, scientists and researchers are trying to unlock the secrets of the brain and its amazing abilities. Many of the findings gained in Bethesda are used by the CIA and the FBI against foreign intelligence services. Some have even been applied in military operations.

Brain research for the FBI

Begun as the one-room Laboratory of Hygiene in 1887, the National Institutes of Health today is one of the world's foremost biomedical research centers. Almost all trailblazing research and development of innovative treatments in recent decades—new forms of cancer therapy or new findings in the field of molecular biology—originated, at least in part, at one of the 25 institutes of the NIH in Bethesda.

Currently, the researchers are working on risk minimization and treatment of heart attacks, cancer, Alzheimer's and mental disorders, as well as on the aging process and possible ways of slowing it down. The analysis of brain functions is another area of research. The budget of the National Institutes of Health was $15.6 billion in 1999. "We will be able," predicts NIH director Harold Varmus, "to embark on a new type of medical science based on the findings of genome research in the new millennium."

Going After Intelligence

In order to understand all the facets of human intelligence, the research teams in Bethesda perform intensive studies of memory and related structures within the brain.

"Memory clinics" deal with memory-related problems

The memory test that scientists at the Memory Clinic of the NIH developed looks, at first sight, like those simple intelligence tests that personnel consultants have used for decades to test the ability of a potential secretary or sales manager. But the highly complex computer program that the researchers at NIH have developed is a far cry from those tests. Within minutes, it can determine whether a subject has memory problems, and in many cases, it provides detailed information on the exact nature of the problem.

Harsh animated graphics appear on a screen, followed by the faces of men and women of different ages. They all say their names and addresses. At the end of it, the screen is filled with 36 heads, and the patient is asked to reproduce the name and address that go with each face.

Within seconds, the task is changed. A large number of common items—apartment key, gloves, hat, umbrella, coat, briefcase and much more—is to be spread around a virtual apartment on the touch-sensitive screen. Then the phone rings, and different phone numbers are shown on the display, which the patient has to repeat. Suddenly the synthesized music stops, and the screen shows the faces of the people from the beginning of the test. The patient is questioned about the faces shown and asked to recall their names and addresses.

"Most men," explains NIH director Varmus, "that have come to the Memory Clinic for help are not so much afraid of being diagnosed with a severe memory dysfunction. Rather, they are more concerned about being below average intellectually."

Men are afraid of being below average

These tests, which were developed in Bethesda under the guidance of the NIH, have meanwhile come to be used in various "memory clinics" around the world. After all, the number of people who doubt their mental abilities and suspect advanced Alzheimer's, before even seeing a neurologist, is rapidly increasing. Often, the cause of memory impairment is not physical, but simply a side effect of stress or depression.

Memory dysfunctions are often caused by stress

To be able to effectively increase your brain power, you should first look at the structure of this miracle of evolution.

The Brain—The Center of Life

The human brain is a fantastic organ. It weighs about 1.4 kilograms and consists, on average, of 125 billion nerve cells, which makes it more efficient than any modern computer. The fascinating thing about it is that it is a vital organ whose functions and performance constantly adapt to changing circumstances. Indeed, it is possible to train the brain.

The human brain consists of 125 billion nerve cells

We still know very little about this "switching station" of the human body, which not only controls all vital functions, but is also home to our consciousness. Its complexity is unprecedented. Every single one of its nerve cells can communicate with 2,000 to 200,000 other neurons within fractions of a second. Its magnificent versatility is based on "division of labor" and "joint operations." Each of its numerous segments is responsible for a specific task, but most also take part in the joint control of the entire organism.

If we compare the brains of reptiles, birds and dogs to the human brain, we get a clear picture of the amazing evolution of the brain over the last 500 million years.

Only about four million years ago, when our ancestors, hominids, roamed the earth, their brain weighed about 300 grams. The first true member of the human species, homo habilis, appeared on the scene about two million years ago with a brain weighing about 600 grams. Homo erectus, one million years ago, had a brain weight of about one kilogram (2.2 pounds); the

About four million years ago, the brain weighed only 300 grams brain of Neanderthals, who lived 100,000 years ago, weighed 1.3 kilograms.

The male brain is approximately 100 grams heavier than the female brain

Homo sapiens—the current human species to which we belong—appeared between 35,000 and 50,000 years ago. Average brain weight is now 1.4 kilograms. The average male brain is approximately 100 grams heavier than a woman's brain. This is primarily due to the larger muscle mass of the locomotor system that the brain has to supply. There are other differences too.

- More men than women are left handed.
- Generally, girls start talking before boys.
- Girls are also better at learning foreign languages.
- The average writing skills of girls are usually more developed than those of boys of the same age.
- Boys are generally better at arithmetic.
- Spatial thinking is better evolved in boys.

There is no scientific data to explain all this. Again, hormones probably play a vital role here. As a result, the concept of "nurture" is losing ground in scientific circles.

Fighting Alzheimer's With Estrogen

Viktor Handersen, an American doctor at the University of Southern California, made an incredible discovery in 1994. Women who had been taking estrogen pills regularly for their menopause-related problems or as a preventive measure against heart disease and osteoporosis had a 40% lower risk of developing Alzheimer's.

Estrogen protects against brain degeneration

Other studies involving rats showed that estrogen indeed provides a certain degree of protection from this type of brain degeneration. Estrogen stimulated the nerve cells of the rats in the very regions that are affected by Alzheimer's in the human brain.

The female sex hormone, however, serves a second purpose. It stimulates the formation of an enzyme that produces the neurotransmitter acetylcholine. While the estrogen level drops significantly in women during menopause, men are less affected by it. In their brains, estrogen is formed by the conversion of the male sex hormone testosterone. This could explain, at least partially, why not as many men as women get Alzheimer's.

In 1999, researchers at Yale University, using functional magnetic resonance imaging (fMRI), were able to show that women experienced an increase in memory capacity after being given estrogen replacement preparations. We might conclude that the new millennium will see a phenomenal breakthrough in the treatment of memory weakness and Alzheimer's for both women and men.

Testosterone is the reason men are less likely to get Alzheimer's

Such findings are only possible with modern imaging techniques, which allow for insights into the functioning of the brain. The discovery of X-rays in 1895 was a major medical breakthrough, but those two-dimensional pictures were useless for distinguishing between two organs of the same density.

It was the British scientist Godfrey Hounsfield who revolutionized the diagnostics of brain disease in 1971. He combined X-ray technology with a computer by superimposing several X-ray pictures taken from slightly different angles and thus creating a three-dimensional image. In 1972, Hounsfield tested his prototype for the first time on a female patient, whose neurologist had suspected a brain lesion. Hounsfield found a dark round cyst in her head. He called his new technology "computerized tomography," or CT. This technology exposed the details of head injuries and brain diseases one hundred times more clearly than previously.

Hounsfield invented computer tomography in 1971

In the 1980s, nuclear magnetic resonance technology was developed. Using a gigantic magnet, the protons (or the nuclei of the hydrogen atoms) of an organism are grouped together and aligned according to the north-south polarity of the magnet. A computer "reads" that information and creates an image, using a process known as "magnetic resonance imaging" (MRI). MRI is ideal for the observation and diagnosis of internal organs with fine tissue, like the brain, that have a higher content of water than, say, bones. During an MRI examination, the patient lies in a tube over an extended period of time (15 to 60 minutes).

Magnetic resonance imaging is ideal for brain examinations

These developments in neurology make it possible today to analyze the brain "in action." Using electroencephalograms (EEG), various brain activities such as thinking, speaking, feeling and action can be measured, and the respective regions of the brain and their functions can be identified and displayed as waves. During the normal wakeful state, these waves are so-called beta waves. Whenever you sit at your computer, participate in a conference, read the newspaper or make phone call, you are in a beta state. The state of mental relaxation is called the alpha state. You are not asleep, you can sense the world around you, but your head is pleasantly "empty."

The state of mental relaxation is called the alpha state

Modern neurology also has complex imaging systems at its disposal, such as positron emission tomography (PET), which can display the structures of the human brain and also reveal molecular dimensions. Perhaps this will help answer some of life's banal questions, "Do I know you?" or "Have we met before?" questions that older people invariably ask, although they may have met the person on three separate occasions. In other words, perhaps it will be possible to study memory loss in more detail.

Young people learn faster

As we grow older, does it become more difficult for us to form memories, or is the problem that old memories cannot be retrieved anymore. Modern research findings suggest that older people learn more slowly because they do not have the same capacity to absorb information and to encode it.

As we grow older, we require longer and more frequent phases of learning and repetition in order to form a memory. "Use it or lose it," as they say. So, how does the brain work?

The Structure of the Brain

The cerebrum consists of two symmetrical halves also called hemispheres that are separated by a deep fissure or sulcus. They are connected by way of a thick nerve tract, the corpus callosum, which enables communication between these two hemispheres of the brain. The surface of the cerebrum is the pallium, or the cerebral cortex, which is only about three millimeters thick and consists of convoluted folds, so-called gyri. The cerebral cortex is made up of approximately 14 billion nerve cells and controls highly complex processes like thought and language. It has six different layers, which are known as the gray matter. These layers differ from each other because of their specific cell structure. The white matter, the nerve tissue of the brain composed of neurites, is found towards the interior of the cortex.

Hippocrates was the first to understand how the brain works

Each hemisphere has specific tasks and functions. The Greek scholar Hippocrates was the first to discover the specific workings of the brain hemispheres. He examined people who had been wounded in the Persian wars and found that damage to certain regions of the brain resulted in the loss of particular functions of the body or brain. He concluded that the functions of the body were connected to specific areas of the brain.

The cerebrum is the center of intelligence, the mind, consciousness, learning and memory. The left hemisphere contains the centers of speech as well as of logical and analytical thought. It is the center of abstract thought processes (concepts, words and numbers). It processes these logically, analytically and sequentially. The occipital lobe houses the visual center, and the temporal lobe contains the auditory center. The border area of the parietal and frontal lobes is the motor center controlling the different parts of the body (i.e., controlling the motion of the body). This area of the brain also contains the sensory centers.

The left hemisphere is responsible for speech, vision and hearing

The right hemisphere, on the other hand, specializes in sensory content, (images and patterns holistic and intuitive). Sensory perceptions are processed in the right hemisphere. Intuition and imagination are, it is suspected, located in the right hemisphere.

The right hemisphere processes sensory information

At the command of the hypothalamus, the pituitary gland releases hormones that circulate throughout the body and control the activity of other glands.

The almond-shaped amygdala, in cooperation with the hippocampus, creates feelings and emotional reactions on the basis of perceptions and thoughts. Both the amygdala and the hippocampus are involved in learning processes.

The cerebellum is responsible for coordinating the motions of the body. It also controls the spatial sense of orientation, equilibrium and body posture.

The cerebellum coordinates body movement

The diencephalon comprises the two thalami, which act as relay stations between the cerebrum and the periphery, and the hypothalamus, which contains the superior centers of the autonomic nervous system. It controls such vital bodily functions as the regulation of temperature, water metabolism and energy metabolism. The next area after the diencephalon is the midbrain or mesencephalon. Finally, the brain stem is formed by those parts of the brain that are the oldest in terms of phylogeny. The medulla oblongata contains the control centers for heartbeat, respiration and metabolism. The spinal cord sends the impulses from the brain to other parts of the body and then transmits the information from there back to the respective brain structures.

The first to do research on the differentiated functions of the human brain was the psychologist and zoologist Roger Sperry, who, for many years, worked for the NIH in Bethesda. He arrived at his findings by mere accident in the early 1960s when, together with his colleague Michael Gazzaniga, he examined a severely epileptic patient. That patient's corpus callosum, the direct link between the two brain hemispheres, had been separated. At first, the patient seemed normal, but a series of tests in which he had to name objects or assemble building blocks in

Zoologist Roger Sperry provided the first map of the brain

a certain way showed that he could only perform those tasks when they required the use of only one hemisphere at a time. His left hemisphere had specialized in language processes, and the right one in visual tasks.

The two hemispheres can operate independently of each other

Sperry found that the two hemispheres operated virtually independently of each other. His work contributed to the creation of a kind of map of the brain and thus formed the basis for the treatment of brain diseases. In 1981, Sperry received the Nobel Prize in medicine for his theory of the hemispheres.

How to Keep Your Head Fit

What can we do to stay mentally fit for life, to maximize the power of our brain and to learn the art of concentration so that our thoughts become more efficient and our problem-solving skills are improved?

The functioning of the brain depends just like the rest of the body on our habits. If we consume a lot of alcohol or fatty foods, we impair its performance. But we can also improve its performance through a healthy and balanced lifestyle.

"In what way are individuals different? Each individual, in comparison to others and himself, sometimes retains and reproduces a lot, sometimes only a little. It all depends on the stage of his existence. It will be different in the mornings and evenings, in youth and old age," wrote the German philosopher Hermann Ebbinghausen in his 1885 book "Über das Gedächtnis" (The Memory) on brain capacity.

The memory, just like all other parts of the body, is subject to the aging process. As we grow older, it will happen more often that we do not recognize people we have met before, forget telephone numbers and other everyday things, e.g., where we parked the car the night before. In other words, it is normal for our memory to decline within certain limits.

The Body and Mind as One Unit

Books on Chinese meditation, yoga and other practices from the Far East whose goal it is to increase concentration and memory are becoming more and more popular. And it is top managers who are becoming increasingly interested in those subjects. People want to learn from Asian Zen masters or Indian yogis who, even among screaming kids and surrounded by honking horns and barking dogs on the streets of New York, do not lose their concentration and cannot be roused from their "inner world." These figures have become fixtures of daily street life in big cities of the Western world. American medical scientists have identified "attention deficit disorder" as a disease, and Western civilization has rediscovered Plato's maxim that the body and mind, thought and emotion form an inseparable unit.

The body and mind, thoughts and feelings are inseparable units

What is concentration? People with a low concentration may have some segments of the brain that do not receive enough energy. The neurotransmitter dopamine may also be involved. Most neurologists and neurobiologists are convinced, however, that continuous learning is crucial to the activity and the capacity of the brain. What the brain learned once can be retrieved and processed at any time by supplying the brain with the necessary energy.

Dopamine is the key to concentration

Therefore, it is important that small children start to learn about things in a playful way as early as possible in order to stimulate their intellect. Physical and mental relaxation exercises can stimulate their imagination. Music is also a good method, especially in preschool, kindergarten and during the first two grades of elementary school. It is essential to constantly stimulate children's fantasy and imagination through games that create images in their minds, for mental images are always easier to remember. But in today's world, the influence of television with its rapid succession of images and advertising make it very difficult to foster the ability to create mental images in children.

Brain Jogging

There is a show on German TV featuring people with an extraordinary ability to recall numbers, names and other "crazy" things in a show of "mental acrobatics."

In recent years, computer programmers in the US have shown similar traits. Some of them work about ten times as efficiently as their colleagues, even though tests showed that their intelligence was not above average and they were not harder working, better trained or more capable than the others. The cause of their extraordinary performance lies much deeper. The programmers who were tested all exhibited the same features:

US researchers were surprised by the "super programmers"

● Their attention was significantly less likely to be diverted by external factors.
● They incorporated abstract and spatial models of thought in their work.
● They showed no signs of stress on the job.
● Their performance increased by a factor of ten.

Programming, on the surface, is a matter of logic. But the actual programming process unfolds on a wholly different level. The visual element is very important. These super-programmers employ their visual imagination and spatial models in the development of new software. They often visualize entire lines of programming code and functional units. The software is created as an image in the brain, and all they have to do is simply "copy" these images onto the screen. The programming code is often better structured and more effective in the way they set it up. Frequently, they discover programming errors by just browsing quickly through a program listing, using a kind of pattern-recognition process that can locate errors automatically.

Surgeons exhibit similar high performance

Similar high-performance phenomena have also been found among surgeons. Apart from the fact that some of this may be due to a special talent, one thing has become clear. The brain is like a muscle that must be exercised constantly to keep it fit. Memory exercises cannot guarantee perfection, but they can help increase capacity, especially through memory games that enhance concentration. Why not use these skills everyday, and then put them to the test on concepts, faces, addresses, events or phone numbers? Some progress is fairly assured.

Exercise can sharpen your concentration

If someone gives you thirty words and asks you to repeat them in the right order after 15 minutes, can you do that? Can you memorize the whole agenda of a board meeting? Or the red wines listed on the menu of a restaurant? A good memory is not only a matter of training, but also of the right method.

THE BRAINPOWER CHECKLIST

If you can answer these questions with "yes," you are exercising your brain correctly.

● Do you read books or newspapers regularly?
● Do you enjoy riddles or math problems?
● Are you interested in society and politics?
● Are you learning or practicing foreign languages?
● Do you try to memorize phone numbers?
● Do you watch your alcohol consumption?
● Do you watch your diet and the time spent viewing TV?
● Can you free yourself from the stress of your job?
● Do you practice any sports or, at least, get some exercise outdoors?
● Can you forget or cope with unpleasant events?
● Do you get enough sleep?
● Do find the time to relax every now and then?

The Methods

1. Use the time that you would normally just waste

In the morning, perhaps while in the shower, make a mental list of the things you want to do that day. Mnemonic devices prove quite helpful, especially images that are, for example, related to the shower itself. Let's say you have to fill the tank of your car. Associate that with squeezing the shampoo bottle. Or you want to clean your desk. Think of brushing your teeth (works with any kind of cleaning activity).

2. Test yourself

Whenever you read a newspaper, magazine or book, pretend that you will be expected to summarize the contents later. You will be surprised at how your way of reading changes and how your concentration increases subconsciously. Try to identify the thesis sentences or message on each page or in each article and memorize it. Invent your own subtitles for some of the paragraphs of the article you are reading.

Review in your mind everything you read in a newspaper

3. Review

You probably take the same route to work every day. Try to identify the different features along the way to which you have not paid any attention so far. Memorize street names, as if you had to explain the way to a stranger later on. Such things will help sharpen your concentration. If you get bored driving, there is another little game you could play—memorize license plates.

Memorize license plates

When you are at a restaurant, waiting for your lunch partner, study the faces of the other people there. About 50% of name and face associations can be memorized by exaggerating or generalizing facial features. You could take certain facial features, such as the hair, skin, mouth, or nose, and enlarge, miniaturize or distort them in your mind. You will find it gets easier to remember faces. Similarly, you can memorize names and places using associations.

4. Where is

Every day, walk through a room in your apartment or house and choose ten different objects. When you leave the room, try to remember the ten objects and where they are. Repeat the exercise with different objects in different rooms until you can remember all ten objects and their locations.

5. Name association

This exercise is perfect for the next party you go to. Try to remember at least

Exercise your mind at parties

four names of people you get to know there, as well as their appearance. Then, at each subsequent party, increase the number of names by one. Use mnemonic tricks like "The man who is talking to my wife is Robert." Check your recollection at the end of each party. This exercise at least has practical value.

The storage compartment of our cell phones, laptops and PCs are brimming with information and it is no longer necessary to remember the phone numbers of our favorite restaurants or our lawyer or doctor. We can have the computer or the phone dial their number just by voicing the person's name (voice recognition technology). The risk here is that the capacity of our memory will gradually decline unless we take countermeasures. In the future, try to do without the speed-dialing feature on your phone and retrieve the information you need from memory. Remembering names is very important in the business world, but very difficult for many people.

Do I Have a Healthy Mind?

How do we know whether it is "just a poor memory" or a serious problem? The best way to find out is to take a test at a memory clinic.

Memory tests can tell you more about your memory

The surprising fact is that people who are worried about their memory and learning skills often score high in these tests. On the other hand, people who really have a serious problem, with Alzheimer's for example, do not even think they have a problem.

Again, there is talk of miracle drugs, smart drugs, and vitamin and mineral supplements to enhance our brainpower. Recently, a substance known as NADH has been touted as a miracle remedy. But none of the many substances tested scientifically has been shown to have a real effect on learning and memory, apart from a placebo effect. In the next ten to fifteen years, there will probably be such supplements to support the neurotransmitters in the brain, but at this point none of the products available goes beyond faith healing. Stay away from "brain food" and "memory drugs."

There are no miracle pills for memory

There are studies on the influence of stress and depression on memory and brain capacity. Undoubtedly, they impair the optimal functioning of the brain. But such effects are usually only temporary. Improvement in the person's emotional state automatically results in an improvement in their mental faculties.

WHAT YOU SHOULD KNOW ABOUT BRAINPOWER

Continuous learning is the key to success.
Review everything in your mind when reading a book or newspaper.
Beware of stress. It drastically reduces the brain's capacity.
Stay away from miracle drugs. Most of them are just placebos.
Estrogen helps against Alzheimer's. It can lower the risk of getting the disease.
There is no information overkill of the brain. You can never learn too much.
"Mind machines" are usually ineffective. Some are even dangerous.

The influence of insomnia or other sleep disorders, or a temporary loss of sleep has similar results. Fatigue can drastically reduce memory retention. And then there is the often cited "information overkill" our society thrusts upon us. That is a fallacy. There is no overkill of the brain. We are not even close to using our brain to full capacity. Some people speak six or seven languages fluently and have a number of other skills to boot. Even a thousand computer chips are no match for the human brain.

Loss of sleep drastically reduces your memory capacity

What else can we do to keep our gray cells alert, to enhance our memory, logic and creativity? There are many different approaches. They range from the currently popular "mind maps" to visualization techniques, repetition techniques, verbal mnemonic devices, index card systems, time-lapse learning and increasing creativity.

Other methods are based on thinking techniques, brain-floating methods, affirmation techniques and dream techniques. Relaxation methods using controlled breathing are also very popular. Then there are so-called "mind machines"—biofeedback devices or self-help tapes. Whether mind machines are a type of ecstasy that flows out of a wall outlet, or whether they really have a positive effect on the use of the brain, are questions we will try to answer in this section.

● Neuro Linguistic Programming

Neuro-Linguistic Programming (NLP) is a technique by which behavioral patterns can be modified, communication with oneself and others improved, and mental power maximized.

NLP can maximize your mental power

NLP was created in the late 1970s when two American scientists, Richard Bandler and John Grinder, sought the answer to why some psychotherapists achieved higher healing rates than others. Over an extended period of time, they analyzed the therapeutic work of several top psychiatrists, such as Milton Eriksen, who was a hypnosis specialist, and his colleague Virginia Satir, a family therapist.

From their findings, Bandler and Grinder developed a series of techniques that were supposed to make psychotherapy more effective. Thus, NLP was born. NLP is based on a number of basic assumptions also called axioms:

1. Everyone creates his own model of the world, his personalized "map."

Everyone sees the
world differently

Everyone sees the world differently. NLP is based on the idea that people have different experiences throughout their lives and that, as a result, they all have a different "map" in their minds. Such personalized maps are assessed for their usefulness and adjusted as necessary. We can all improve and expand our map.

2. The body, soul and mind form a unit.

NLP: a change in
posture also
changes your
thoughts

Together they make up a system and influence each other. For example, if we change the posture of our body, our thoughts or feelings may change as a result and vice versa. The immune system and our emotions are linked. The more negative our thoughts, the more susceptible our body becomes to disease.

3. People have all the resources they need.

NLP postulates that we all have the solutions to our problems within ourselves. Experiences, memories, or simply knowledge are all the resources we need to solve any problem.

4. If something does not work, try something else.

The processes of life affect every person differently. If something does not work for you, you must be flexible enough to try something else.

5. The more choices you have, the better.

NLP is based on the assumption that the likelihood of achieving a certain goal is greater the more choices you have in any given situation.

NLP teaches you
how to anchor
feelings

NLP methods must be practiced continuously. A person must constantly improve the power of imagination, visualize things and change them in the mind. NLP also helps a person to deal with problems and feelings, which can be called upon selectively using the "anchoring" method (e.g., motivation, ambition, etc.). According to NLP, anchoring consists of three steps:

1. Relax, take deep breaths. Think about the feeling you would like to anchor. Remember a situation when you experienced that feeling and try to trigger it. Reinforce the feeling. Relive it again. What happened at that time? What was it like? Stop and savor the feeling.
2. When you think that the feeling has become as strong as it will get, trigger the anchor: touch a certain spot on your body, e.g., the lower arm, and associate the touch with the feeling.
3. See if the anchor works. Think of something completely unrelated, then trigger the anchor with the touch. If you experience the feeling again, the anchor works.

Here is another NLP exercise to enhance your visualization:

1. Close your eyes and imagine a strawberry. What does it look like? How big is it? What color is it? Do you see a painting or a photograph of a strawberry? Do you have a three-dimensional image?
2. Now change the image in your mind. Make the strawberry smaller, then larger, make it as big as yourself, push it away and let it rotate on its axis.

In order to sharpen your auditory imagination, do the same exercise with a bell. How does it sound? Is it loud? Change the direction from which you hear the sound.

Feelings, too, can be influenced, as in autogenic training. If you imagine your right leg becoming heavier and heavier over a longer period of time, it will actually become warmer and heavier because your conscious imagination increases the blood circulation to that body part.

Feelings can also be influenced

Imagine you are walking through a desert. What is the sand like? Is it hot? How does it feel on the soles of your feet? Combine all these images into one whole.

Eliminate unpleasant thoughts

NLP also has a solution for unpleasant thoughts. Close your eyes and think of the unpleasant image, even if it triggers negative feelings in you. Continue by imagining a black-and-white TV onto the screen of which you start pushing the image until it is quite small and in black and white. Push the TV far away from you. Do something else, and then repeat this exercise. At some point, you will no longer have a problem when you think of the unpleasant image because it appears to you as a small image in black and white.

Discard thoughts that cause you stress

Motivation through NLP

NLP includes methods for self-motivation. We all like to push unpleasant things away from us—tax returns, car repairs or spring cleaning. The "New Behavior Generator," as Steve Andreas and Charles Faulkner call it, is a method for facing up to unpleasant things.

Create your alter ego

Relax and close your eyes. Think of a person who looks just like you. This is your alter ego. Your alter ego learns to do all the things you hate and are not driven to do with passion and motivation. Observe your imaginary double during these activities. If you are satisfied with the way he solves the problems, you will internalize your alter ego in such a way that you will go about the tasks as motivated as he. Choose a task that you would enjoy doing.

Imagine your alter ego completing the task without any difficulties, being praised for it, receiving recognition for it. If your alter ego performs the tasks the way you would like to, then draw him into your own world. For example, picture yourself giving your alter ego a hug.

Now that you are fully motivated, make a plan for tackling those tasks that so far have been anathema to you. In NLP jargon, this is called the "Future Pace," a point at which you imagine what it would be like if you had already achieved what you wanted to achieve.

There is worldwide boom in NLP. More and more institutions are offering courses. NLP is a legitimate psychological practice we do not hesitate to recommend.

• Biofeedback

Biofeedback increases performance

Biofeedback is a method of mental training in which you are hooked up to a computer through sensors. The computer measures skin conductivity, body temperature, pulse rate and respiratory rate. The computer gives you feedback on your body's reactions to situations and thoughts that can be simulated. You learn techniques for increasing your concentration, your memory and the efficiency of your brain. Biofeedback is used by a number of institutions around the world.

• Superlearning

The processes within the brain can be displayed as waves. Depending on the wavelength of a mental state, a distinction can be made between alpha and beta states. In an alpha state, for example, the brain stores content without checking for meaning, which results in enormous learning capacity. Listening to special CDs with instrumental music and spoken information brings you into an alpha state. When you are fully relaxed, a mix of information and music is fed into your brain through a headset.

Superlearning is quite effective, but it only makes sense when used in conjunction with conventional learning programs because Superlearning does not allow for analytical and meaningful structuring of information.

• Electric stimulation

Electrical stimulation of the brain is conducted with two electrodes attached usually to the earlobes. It is said to be quite effective in drug rehabilitation programs (not scientifically verified), but it is not suitable for increasing brain capacity. The benefit is quite doubtful, and some health risks may be involved.

Electric stimulation of the brain is dangerous

• Optic and acoustic stimulation

Many of the "mind machines" available on the market consist of futuristic pairs of goggles that give off light impulses at certain intervals. These light impulses are intended to stimulate specific areas of the brain. According to the manufacturer's instructions, this setup is supposed to induce an alpha state. In part, it is possible to achieve a meditation-like state of relaxation, but it is highly unlikely that such "mind machines" can train the brain.

"Mind machines" are supposed to induce an alpha state

• Alpha CDs and tapes

The alpha rhythm is in the range of 10 Hz, an inaudible frequency for humans. Companies have developed CDs and tapes with "different" 10 Hz sounds that are supposed to be audible. Again, this method is quite dubious. The benefit to the brain is probably zero.

• Mind Power

An extraordinary method for effectively training the brain was developed by John Kehoe, the pioneer behind "Mind Power." In 1975, he retreated into the wilderness of British Columbia, Canada, for three years, completely cut off from civilization in order to devote himself to researching the power of his thoughts and, by extension, of the human intellect.

Three years in the wilderness gives birth to "Mind Power"

Far away from civilization, he created his program for developing the mental faculties with such success that he later taught it to multinational companies such as Mobil. Here is a closer look at Kehoe's theory.

1. Your consciousness is an enormous power

Strong and concentrated thoughts are strong and concentrated powers. If you want to change your life, you must first have the necessary consciousness. Just hoping for a change is useless. You must change your thinking.

2. Visualize your wishes

Visualization is imagining over and over a situation that has not happened yet. In the process, you see yourself as if you had already completed, or were completing, the task at hand.

There are three steps:

Imagine reality as you want it to be

1. Decide on what it is you want to do.
2. Relax.
3. Imagine for five to ten minutes the reality of your choice as if it were already happening.

Imagine the situation you wish for at least once a day and repeat this again and again.

3. Affirmations

Affirmations are simple sentences that are repeated in a low voice or aloud. Choose a sentence that expresses what you want to do and keep repeating it ("I'll pass the exam," "I'll get the contract," "My plan will be a success," etc.). You do not even have to believe in what you are saying. Just stick with the constant repetition. Always choose positive statements and short sentences (not more than ten words). Avoid affirmations that are directed against you ("I'm jinxed"). Your consciousness creates reality and you are in charge of your consciousness. Whatever you believe in is what you will get.

4. You can do anything you want

Always think that you are unique. You can do anything you want if you put your mind to it: "I can learn any language I want," "No project is too difficult," "I can change my job." Positive and self-confident thoughts create a confident person. Ambitious thoughts create an ambitious person. To the extent to which you change your thinking about other people, other people will change theirs about you.

Positive thoughts make for positive people

5. Problems point you in the right direction

Problems are important and valuable parts of our lives. They point us in the right direction, but we have to be able to interpret them. There are no accidents. Even better, change your attitude so that you no longer see problems as problems, but rather as opportunities.

Whatever you think is possible, whatever you believe in has a strong effect on what actually happens. Men who live in fear of getting sick have a higher risk of actually becoming sick because the body senses the effects of the thoughts. Depressed men are more likely to become sick than happy ones.

How To Beat Stress
Strategies Against the Epidemic of the Third Millennium

For several years, Andreas K. worked for a movie production company specializing in TV commercials. He was very comfortable in his job. One day he was promoted. Totally unexpectedly, he was made assistant to his boss. The company was completely restructured, and Andreas K. even received a new job title, Managing Director. This new position came with a huge office, two secretaries, a lot of employees and a company car. But the promotion also had an unpleasant side effect. From that moment on, Andreas K. felt the entire weight of the company, the sole responsibility for its success or failure, resting on his shoulders. He no longer had time for his hobbies—golf, surfing and tennis—or for regular meals. His laptop computer became his best friend and, thanks to his cell phone, he was available to his clients even past midnight. After six months, Andreas K. experienced heart palpitations and a racing pulse, shaking, numbness in his left hand, pains in the stomach that he had not felt in years, and splitting headaches that he had not experienced since he was a student about to write a big exam. One time during an important meeting, he felt a burning sensation around his heart, which lasted for a few minutes. He recognized it as angina pectoris, the first sign of a heart attack. That same day he went to have it checked out.

After a series of lengthy examinations, the doctor confirmed his suspicions. Other than elevated serum lipid levels and a moderately higher blood pressure, Andreas K. had no physical problems. He was healthy. But he suffered from uncontrolled stress. Andreas K. was a man who had lost his equilibrium.

Stress levels have escalated in the last decade, especially in the Western world. All social classes have been affected, from top managers to taxi drivers. Stress has become an inevitable consequence of modern life.

Mental stress plays a key role in sudden cardiac death

A study published in European Heart Journal in 1999 dealt with the connection between stress on the job and sudden cardiac death in middle-aged employees. The study, which focused on 200,000 Japanese employees over a period of seven years (from 1989 to 1995), is one of the most representative studies of its kind. The findings are alarming. Mental stress, especially the kind that occurs with changes in a person's social and professional life, plays a key role in triggering sudden cardiac death. The mortality rate during the economic recession in Japan in 1995 was twice as high as in 1991 when the economy was booming. The majority of deaths occurred in April, the beginning of the Japanese business year, and in the early morning hours. To doctors, this does not come as a surprise. Coronary spasms usually occur at night or early in the morning.

According to doctors and psychologists at the 10th International Congress on Stress held in Montreux, Switzerland, at the beginning of March 1999, diseases caused by stress will very soon reach epidemic proportions.

Stress is the number one health problem in the US

A study by the American Institute of Stress in New York came to a similar conclusion. Stress and ensuing diseases have already become America's number one health problem.

- Already, 75% of all preventive medical exams are taken for stress-related problems.
- 89% of adult Americans say that have experienced "severe stress" at numerous times in the past.

78% of Americans equate their jobs with stress

- 78% of Americans blame stress on their job. One in two states that the degree of stress has increased significantly in the last ten years. More than a third of Austrian men say that they suffer from chronic stress.
- 60% of industrial accidents in the US have stress-related causes or are the result of a stress-related action.
- The National Safety Council estimates that a million Americans are absent from work for stress reasons on the average working day.
- Because of the increase in stress levels, only 25% of Americans say they are "very satisfied" with their jobs (in 1973, it was 40%).
- Violence in the workplace has risen sharply in the last five years. More than half of those incidents have stress-related causes or are the result of a spontaneous stress-related reaction.

Most of us have experienced stress. People use this trendy term to describe everything that is negative in their lives. But stress involves a lot more than people think. You are at a party until two in the morning, you get into an accident, your dog is sick, you are broke, your new furniture is being delivered, you receive a bonus from your boss—that is all stress. Every change in your life, any move away from your daily routine, be it negative or positive, is stress.

Even long parties cause stress

Types of Stress

Stress can have many causes. The most common are:

• Emotional stress
Conflicts, disagreements, relationship problems, even the baptism of your child can cause emotional stress.

• Stress as a result of overexertion
If you work (or party, for that matter) fifteen hours every day, you shorten your body's regeneration phase. You can do this only up to a certain point and as long as the body still has enough time and energy to repair or replace damaged cells. But the energy metabolism of your body will continuously decline. The body will then mobilize all its reserves to keep the system going and protect your health.

• Stress as a result of disease or accident
This ranges from a common cold to a broken leg.

• Hormone-related stress
During puberty, stress is caused by strong hormonal changes. This is the time when the genitals become functional, the testicles begin producing sperm and new hormones are secreted in large quantities.

Hormonal factors can be the cause of stress

The continuous decline in hormone levels that occurs with age is another stress factor for men.

• Stress as a result of environmental influences
Hot or cold weather, extreme elevations, environmental toxins, etc., can trigger stress.

• Smoking-related stress
The active ingredients in tobacco destroy cells and cause chronic bronchitis, cancer and many other diseases, which makes them stress factors.

• Stress as a result of allergies
Allergic reactions are part of the body's immune system. When your body

Allergies can cause
stress

comes into contact with substances that are toxic or that your body considers toxic, it will attack these and try to neutralize them. If such substances, for example, come into contact with your skin, the body will fight them off by developing acute dermatitis (inflammation of the skin), and if you consume toxic substances, you will vomit. Allergic reactions create stress because your body requires energy to fight the invaders.

Stress is necessary
for survival

Stress is an individual, personal reaction to situations and events that create a physical or psychological strain. Stress is a normal and integral part of life. It is a byproduct of our adapting to ever-changing requirements, a prerequisite for survival for all highly developed life forms, especially humans. The form it takes is called the stress reaction. It is the organism's response to the stressor (stress-triggering event), and its biological function is to readjust the body.

The basic pattern of stress reaction is probably several million years old. In the course of evolution, it became a complex reaction with a specific biological purpose. Since the "fight or flight" phenomenon was first described almost fifty years ago, we have learned a lot about these reactions as well as about the chemical processes in the human body.

Stress From a Medical Point of View

From a medical point of view, two basic types of stressful events can be distinguished. One is intensive, a type of alert, which prepares the body for an emergency situation within a very short time. The other is less intensive and alerts the body to a long-term problem that requires endurance. In spite of the difference in the details, the stress reactions in humans have four distinct phases that always unfold in the same way and in the same order.

Phase 1: The Alert

Stress was a
survival reaction in
prehistoric times

Even for our prehistoric ancestors, stress was a reaction necessary for survival. It was primarily triggered by events on the physical plane, especially through sensory perceptions like vision, hearing, smell or emotions. Stress gave homo sapiens the strength to fight with bears, to run away from a pack of wolves or to avoid falling rocks.

The original purpose of the lightning reaction was to prepare the body for an increase in physical activity, requiring faster energy metabolism. Even if psychological factors are now the predominant triggers of stress, the processes within the body have remained the same.

In stressful circumstances, several bodily functions are affected in different ways. The corticotropin-releasing hormone (CRH) is released in the brain. As a result, the pituitary gland in the brain secretes the adrenocorticotrophic hormone (ACTH). This is the signal for the adrenal gland to produce the classic stress hormone cortisol, and to release the stress hormones adrenaline and noradrenaline from the adrenal medulla. The stronger the stressors, the more hormones are produced. The ratio between the two hormone concentrations (adrenaline and noradrenaline) can vary depending on whether the reaction has been triggered by fear, including a possible flight reaction, or by anger, which would trigger a fight reaction. In the process, the respiratory rate, the contractility of the heart muscle, the heart rate (= pulse rate) and the blood pressure increase. This often results in palpitations and tachycardia.

Under stress, the adrenal gland produces the cortisol hormone

Glucose and fat are mobilized, blood is rerouted to where it is needed, and the blood platelets are activated so that the blood can coagulate faster in case of injury. The digestive tract (including salivation) is largely shut down, which creates a dryness of the mouth. This reaction brings to mind the gesture of spitting on the ground in front of an opponent to show the enemy that one was without fear, which goes back to Greek mythology.

Salivation stops

Phase 2: The Adjustment
Deeper respiration enables the lungs to take in more oxygen, and the heart to increase the blood supply to the muscles, where the nutrients are burned. Overall "production" increases. The resources are consumed as part of the stress reaction, and this leads to phase three.

The heart increases the blood flow to the muscles

Phase 3: Fatigue and Exhaustion
A state of diminished performance occurs, caused by the consumption of the body's resources, especially of glucose, water and salt. The body begins to sweat in order to keep the temperature constant. This is followed by a state of exhaustion, just like in sports.

Muscle spasms serve to protect the organism because it could be life-threatening for it to use up all its resources. Fatigue sets in to slow down or stop the exertion before the situation becomes dangerous. When engaging in longer physical exertion, such as jogging or cycling, it is important to start replacing the lost sugar and water by consuming electrolyte drinks as soon as half an hour into the activity and after each additional half hour.

In the next stage of exhaustion, the body's energy requirements can no longer be met by the biological burning of nutrients. This results in additional biochemical processes that release lactic acid, which cannot be broken down. If the lactic acid accumulates, the muscle fibers cannot work anymore and stop. This reaction is a well-known sight in marathons, where a runner collapses due to exhaustion. Triathletes often experience general fatigue. When taken to an extreme to include sleep deprivation over several days, the stress can actually be life-threatening.

When the body is exhausted, it releases lactic acid

Phase 4: Restoration and Recovery

Flight is one way of reducing stress

In prehistoric times, cavemen survived the first three phases either by fighting or fleeing and then retreating to their caves. Today, we hardly ever fight or flee anymore, so the stress-related tension has no outlet. It builds up because we no longer have time for the phase of recovery. The more intense and longer the exertion, and the higher the level of exhaustion, the longer the body takes to recover. Chronic everyday stress has a negative effect on both the body and the mind.

Chronic everyday stress has negative effects on the body and mind

The Symptoms of Stress

Stress causes physical, psychological and behavioral disorders

The signs and symptoms of stress fall into three groups: physical problems, psychological problems, and mental disorders that affect behavior. Stress usually starts with feelings like listlessness, tightness, irritability, nervousness, hectic fever, impatience or fatigue. Then, the body begins to react to the stress.

Use this stress test to find out if you suffer from the typical symptoms of stress. Some of them might also have a medical cause, which you should clarify with your physician.

Here are the typical physical symptoms related to stress:

Symptom	Yes	No	Sometimes
● Headaches	☐	☐	☐
● Grinding your teeth	☐	☐	☐
● Feeling of tightness or dryness in the throat	☐	☐	☐
● Dizziness	☐	☐	☐
● Tinnitus (ringing in the ear)	☐	☐	☐
● Chest pains	☐	☐	☐
● Shortness of breath	☐	☐	☐
● Difficulty breathing	☐	☐	☐
● Asthma attacks	☐	☐	☐

Symptom	Yes	No	Sometimes
● High blood pressure	☐	☐	☐
● Tense muscles	☐	☐	☐
● Muscle twitches	☐	☐	☐
● Gastritis	☐	☐	☐
● Nausea	☐	☐	☐
● Congestion or indigestion	☐	☐	☐
● Chronic fatigue	☐	☐	☐
● Sleep disorders	☐	☐	☐
● Weakened immune system, frequently sick	☐	☐	☐
● Back pains	☐	☐	☐

Psychological and/or emotional stressors are:

Symptom	Yes	No	Sometimes
● Anxiety	☐	☐	☐
● Irritation	☐	☐	☐
● Feeling of constant threat	☐	☐	☐
● Depression	☐	☐	☐
● Slowed-down thoughts	☐	☐	☐
● Racing thoughts	☐	☐	☐
● Feeling helpless	☐	☐	☐
● Feeling hopeless	☐	☐	☐
● Feeling worthless	☐	☐	☐
● No clear goals	☐	☐	☐
● Feeling insecure	☐	☐	☐
● Sadness	☐	☐	☐
● Apathy	☐	☐	☐
● Over-sensitivity	☐	☐	☐
● Anger	☐	☐	☐

Mental disorders which affect behavior during stress are:

Symptom	Yes	No	Sometimes
● Loss of sex drive	☐	☐	☐
● Impotence	☐	☐	☐
● Premature or delayed ejaculation	☐	☐	☐
● Alcohol abuse	☐	☐	☐
● Smoking	☐	☐	☐
● Drugs	☐	☐	☐
● Increasing isolation from friends and colleagues	☐	☐	☐
● Bad performance on the job	☐	☐	☐
● Burnout syndrome	☐	☐	☐

Each item to which you answered "yes" adds to your stress level score. A high score means that your mind and body will react in a way that is typical of men under a lot of stress.

Men experience stress when their competence is questioned

Timothy Smith of the University of Utah has proven in a study what we have all observed in daily life. Men and women have different stress triggers. Disagreement triggers stress in women, but not in men. But men experience stress when doubt is cast on their performance and competence. Women remain calm in such situations.

Stress as Killer of Relationships

Empirical studies of a group of Swiss psychologists have shown that stress is the number one killer of relationships. One possible reason is that men under stress drastically change their social behavior, even toward their partner. They become more selfish and, depending on their inclinations, more aggressive and reluctant to reconcile with their partners. Stress creates problems of communication within the relationship, and leads to more serious problems that could end in separation or, in the worst case scenario, in violent acts against the partner.

They become more selfish and aggressive under stress

Stress leads to erectile dysfunction

Since men's libido is still very strong even while under stress, they could experience erectile problems if their partner, because of the man's changed behavior, frequently refuse to have sex. If a woman rejects a man's sexual advances one out of two times, or needs to be persuaded first, then the man is almost bound to have erectile problems.

According to a study of the Institute of Sex Research in Hamburg, about 8% of German women, between 1975 and 1977, said they had no real sex drive. Between 1992 and 1994, that percentage was 58%, while the number of men who had lost interest rose from 4% to 16%. At the same time, for the period 1992 to 1994, 63% of men complained of erectile dysfunction.

On-the-job stress can therefore lead to:
- communication problems within the relationship
- lack of trust of the partner
- sexual conflicts
- lack of romance
- lack of tenderness

Job-related stress has also led to a rise in the number of divorces. In Austria, for example, one in three marriages is dissolved, and the numbers are pretty much the same all over the Western world.

What Stress Type Am I?

The Viennese psychologist Brigitte Bösenkopf, who has become Austria's number one expert in stress management. She has conducted stress-management seminars for top male managers of national and international corporations for the last ten years, and she distinguishes four stress types.

1. The workaholic
"Time is money." The workaholic manager or executive typically manifests his stress in relationship problems. He lives almost exclusively for his work, and cannot stand being too close to someone. He prefers to bury himself in his work and excels at it. The workaholic often ignores physical warning signals, and does not pay any attention to his health, a balanced diet or his fitness. As a consequence, he works himself into a wreck, and it is only a matter of time before the burnout syndrome catches up with him.

Workaholics ignore their health and only live for their work

2. The servile sycophant
"I give my time to others." The man who cannot say 'no.' Often, friends and colleagues take advantage of him and he lets it happen because he wants to please everyone. He is willing to do anything others ask him to, even if it comes at a disadvantage to him. The sycophant is desperate for recognition and esteem. He is often sloppy in his behavior, which creates enormous stress for him. This stress type often suffers from psychosomatic diseases, primarily gastrointestinal problems (e.g., ulcers), and tense muscles.

The sycophant has never learned to say 'no'

3. The perfectionist
"Planning is everything." Many executives and men of power fall into this category. The perfectionist always expects 150% performance of himself, and of others around him. He cannot delegate because he can do everything better than others. In his view, they would make too many mistakes or at least would not perform to his full satisfaction. He does not know how to enjoy the moment. He has no inner balance, and his compulsive perfectionism blocks his view of the essential things in life.

Perfectionists demands 150% performance

4. The hedonistic time-waster
"Live for the here and now and enjoy life." This type includes highly creative

men who work in the media or advertising as well as artists. The "time-waster" often has hundreds of ideas at once, but he cannot implement even half of them. With him, stress starts in the head. He wants to do everything at the same time and thus creates a lot of stress for himself as his life turns to chaos. As a rule, he is late for meetings, does not meet deadlines, and his desk is cluttered. This ties in with his supreme motto, "Small minds have to keep order; great minds thrive on chaos."

The stress of being a procrastinator starts in the mind

Try to find out which type you are. Self-assessment is the first step toward change because a number of efficient methods of managing stress exist.

The 15 Most Effective Methods Against Stress

"The only mountains that we need to move are those in our minds."
Austrian mountain climber Reinhold Messner

Stress is not an organic disease

Stress is not a traditional medical disease, but it does have physical consequences. Any successful strategy for dealing with stress starts in the head. You must learn to cope with stressful situations and stress factors and to gradually avoid them. Try to protect your body and mind from stress.

DHEA is the body's anti-stress hormone

Hormones, too, play an important role in fighting stress. The DHEA hormone (dehydroepiandrosterone) is the body's anti-stress hormone. Produced by the adrenal gland, it reduces the activity of the body, which also diminishes the stress factor. DHEA inhibits the production of adenosine triphosphate (ATP) and the stress hormone cortisol.

Many causes of stress are to be found in our lifestyle and our environment. An essential element in stress management is positive thinking. Negative thoughts not only put a strain on the mind, but they also make the body sick. Therefore, change your attitudes about health, relaxation, performance and your behavior toward others. Organize your life and re-prioritize your goals in life.

Reorganize your life

First, it is crucial to find your personal balance in life. Divide your life up into four departments:

● work and performance
● body and health
● social contacts and private relationships
● matters dealing with your purpose in life and your future

Then ask yourself what percentage of your time is spent on each. On average, it would look like this:

- work and performance: 50–70%
- body: 5–20%
- social contacts: 5–20%
- purpose in life: 5–10%

The ideal would be a balanced 25% in each department, but this is unrealistic. Still, it is what we should strive to achieve in the long term.

The following fifteen strategies are currently the best anti-stress methods available from researchers and psychologists who specialize in stress management. If you follow these rules, your life will change completely.

1. Identify the causes of your personal stress
The first step toward stress management is to identify the causes of your stress and the subjective personal stressors. The first question you must ask yourself is what is causing your stress? A new job, the birth of your baby, the wedding of your daughter, the death of your uncle, the divorce from your spouse that you had vowed to love until the end of time, a new apartment? All of these events, whether positive or negative, have one thing in common. They create stress.

Do your own personal stress checkup. You will find included in this section a stress scale, developed by the American stress expert Steve Burns, which shows you whether and to which extent changes in your life have caused you stress. For each of the events that you have experienced in the last twelve months, you should write down the corresponding score from the right-hand side of the scale, and add up all the scores when you are done. Do not be surprised about the long period under consideration (one year). Many events that change your life take some time to show their effects. **Your personal stress checkup**

If you have experienced stress within the last twelve months scoring 250 or more, you may be overstressed even if your stress tolerance is normal. Persons with low stress tolerance may be overstressed at levels as low as 150.

Overstress will make you sick. Carrying too heavy a stress load is like running a nuclear reactor past maximum capacity. Sooner or later, something will melt down.

STRESS SCALE

1. Death of spouse	100
2. Divorce	60
3. Midlife-crisis	60
4. Separation from living partner	60
5. Jail term or probation	60
6. Death of close family member other than spouse	60
7. Serious personal injury or illness	45
8. Marriage or establishing life partnership	45
9. Fired at work	45
10. Marital or relationship reconciliation	40
11. Retirement	40
12. Change in health of immediate family member	40
13. Work more than 40 hours per week	35
14. Pregnancy or causing pregnancy	35
15. Sex difficulties	35
16. Gain of new family member	35
17. Business or work role change	35
18. Change in financial state	35
19. Death of a close friend (not a family member)	30
20. Change in number of arguments with spouse or life partner	30
21. Mortgage or loan for a major purpose	25
22. Foreclosure of mortgage or loan	25
23. Sleep less than 8 hours per night	25
24. Change in responsibilities at work	25
25. Trouble with in-laws, or with children	25
26. Outstanding personal achievement	25
27. Spouse begins or stops work	20
28. Begin or end school	20
29. Change in living conditions (visitors in the home, change in roommates, remodeling house)	20
30. Change in personal habits (diet, exercise, smoking, etc.)	20
31. Chronic allergies	20
32. Trouble with boss	20
33. Change in work hours or conditions	15
34. Moving to new residence	15
35. Change in schools	15
36. Change in religious activities	15
37. Change in social activities (more or less than before)	15
38. Drop in salary	10
39. Change in frequency of family get-togethers	10
40. Vacation	10
41. Minor violation of the law	5

TOTAL SCORE:

2. Analyze your internal and external stress factors

In order to analyze your daily stress events and the symptoms that are triggered by them, you must keep a stress diary over a period of at least one week. Note down all the events that cause you stress. For example:

Keep a stress diary

Day	Time	Feelings/actions	Situation
Monday	8:00 a.m.	muscle twitches headache coming on	traffic jam
	11:30 a.m.	depressed	boss returned report to be rewritten

Analyze the essential causes of your stress and write them on a piece of paper. After a few days, take a look at your diary and separate the stress factors into two groups.

- external stressors (e.g., money problems, health problems, time pressure, pressure to perform)
- internal stressors (e.g., the inability to say no, demanding excessive perfection from oneself, a chaotic attitude toward life, illusory goals, negative feelings, anxiety of failure, low self-esteem).

Medical science distinguishes between internal and external stressors

"Eighty percent of all stress factors are internal stressors," says the psychologist Brigitte Bösenkopf. "They are based on a person's character and his own behavior."

The next step involves identifying your own stressors, which you can note on a piece of paper or on your PC using a table like the following:

External stressors	big problem	medium-sized problem	I can live with it
Internal stressors	big problem	medium-sized problem	I can live with it

You should try to avoid everything that has become a big or a medium-sized problem in your life. It may be a long and difficult road to take, but it is the only chance you have if you want to avoid health problems due to stress.

3. Make sure that you manage your time well

According to Professor Paul Haber, stress management is the conscious and selective control of the ratio of exertion and recovery in favor of recovery. Time management is a lot more than keeping a laptop or palmtop computer schedule. Primarily, it means assessing tasks and setting priorities. Psychological studies have shown that men who do not write down their goals achieve only about a third of them. Always keep track of your time with written schedules. If you need more time, analyze your schedule carefully and revise it. Prepare schedules for each day, week, month and year. Then, try to eliminate anything that is unimportant. Just cancel out that third in your daily plan that you think is least important.

Men who do not write down their goals only achieve a third of them

---

THE 20 MOST COMMON TIME "SINS"

1. The attempt to do too much or everything at once ☐
2. No clear goals and priorities ☐
3. No organized chart of upcoming tasks and activities ☐
4. Personal disorganization / cluttered desk ☐
5. Lack of motivation / indifferent work behavior ☐
6. Lack of teamwork ☐
7. Interruptions by phone calls and other diversions ☐
8. Unpleasant visitors / external interruptions ☐
9. Long unnecessary meetings ☐
10. Putting off unpleasant tasks ☐
11. Inability to say no ☐
12. Incomplete and delayed information ☐
13. Excessive perfectionism ☐
14. Lack of motivation to complete tasks ☐
15. Lack of consistency and self-discipline ☐
16. Insufficientl preparation ☐
17. Lack of communication or imprecise communication ☐
18. Inability to delegate ☐
19. Private conversations with colleagues ☐
20. Too much bureaucracy ☐

Plan 60% of your day

A tip for men in top executive positions: Plan only about 60% of your day and leave yourself enough time for routine tasks, such as making phone calls or going through your mail. Keep 20% of your time as a buffer zone and for unforeseen events (e.g., a client is late, a meeting goes into overtime, you are stuck in a traffic jam, or other events threaten to torpedo your daily planning). The remaining 20% should be reserved for creative activities that allow you to be spontaneous, to retreat from the hustle and bustle or to meditate—for example, going for a walk in the park or jogging. Stress almost never allows for creativity. Set time aside for yourself and your thoughts.

The "Pareto Principle" is a useful tool for proper time management. The Italian economist and sociologist Vilfredo Pareto postulated his "80/20" rule in the 19th century, one of the few reasonable ideas that he had. The rule states that a few elements within a certain set can represent the major part of it. In other words, 20% of a man's performance is responsible for 80% of his success; 20% of a company's customers generate 80% of the volume. Or 20% of a story contains 80% of its informative content. We may conclude from this that you should always limit yourself to what is truly essential. Identify the essential 20% and delegate the remaining 80%. Journalists may have to sift through 20 to 30 newspapers, a dozen magazines and other press material every day. They can only do that by skimming for the essential 20%. Try to do the same.

The Pareto Principle: Only a fifth of things are essential

Another method is the so-called "Eisenhower Principle," which more and more trainers recommend as a viable weapon against stress. It is based on a very simple idea. Everything that we should and must do in our lives gets broken down into four groups:

The Eisenhower Principle can help reduce stress

- tasks that are both important and urgent
- tasks that are important, but not urgent
- tasks that are unimportant, but urgent
- tasks that are both unimportant and not urgent

Here is the solution. The tasks that are both unimportant and not urgent are best discarded and forgotten. If a task is unimportant, but urgent, then delegate it. We take note of the important tasks that are not urgent and make sure that they are executed in time. Tasks that are both important and urgent are those we must attend to immediately.

Bad communication skills—an inability to express your own needs clearly and to delegate tasks— can be another source of stress. Lack of communication can often result in the loss of support of co-workers, which causes you to overreact and experience stress.

Bad communication can be a stressor

4. Your body should be your castle

Stress management starts with your own body. How important is a healthy body to you? Do you eat right? What is it that robs you of your physical strength? Your body should be your number one source of strength. Avoid anything that would deplete your strength.

- Keep your blood sugar level stable

People under stress have a tendency to eat increasing quantities of sweets, for the sudden rise in their blood sugar level gives them a sensation of strength. Eating sweets makes your blood sugar level rise and fall in rapid succession. Avoid such a roller coaster ride. Eat carbohydrates, such as corn, rice, noodles, bread and potatoes. They are digested slowly and the body absorbs them. It is better to eat small meals several times a day rather than one heavy meal.

● Eat lots of vegetables

Vegetables trigger the production of the "happy" hormone serotonin

Vegetables increase the production of the "happy" hormone serotonin in the brain. Serotonin has a very positive effect on the mind and body during periods of stress due to the absorption of the amino acid L-tryptophane. Rather than digging into a steak, you should have some lettuce.

● Take vitamins

When you are under stress, you should supply your body with sufficient vitamins. If your diet does not contain enough vitamins, take vitamin supplements, available at the drugstore. The average daily intake of vitamins your body needs is given in the chapter, "The Proper Diet." One of the most important pieces of advice we can give is to cut out, or reduce, your consumption of sugar, caffeine, tobacco and alcohol.

300 milligrams of vitamin C can give you a lot of strength

5. Set some time aside for yourself

"You cannot fill your life with more days, but you can certainly fill your days with more life."

Conventional wisdom of American managers

Allow your body to regenerate. Enjoy some spare time, even if there is a pile of work sitting on your desk. Relax and try to find the time to completely "switch off." Never take work home with you. Postpone things that could create stress. Remember that change means stress. Put off the renovation of your house, or painting your living room, as long as you are experiencing stress-related problems.

6. Set your internal clock

Deep sleep is the best remedy for stress

The best way to relax is to get enough deep sleep. People under stress often find this difficult. Therefore, set yourself a time for going to bed and waking up. Stick to that schedule because this is how to set your internal clock. This is also Niki Lauda's recipe for success. Lauda, a triple Formula One world champion and owner of a successful airline says, "I listen to my internal clock. I always go to bed at 10 p.m. if I have an early call the next morning. This way, my batteries can never run dry."

Your body may take a few weeks to adjust to the new sleeping and waking rhythms. But what happens if you cannot fall asleep no matter how hard you try? Sleep disorders are among the most common causes of stress and indicate that your internal clock is "broken." If you are still not asleep after one hour of lying down, take a book and start reading. Or switch on the computer and surf the Internet. Sooner or later, you will become tired and find yourself able to fall asleep. Repeat these activities until you have managed to actively control your sleeping and waking.

If your job requires you to work nights or do shift work (for example, doctors or police officers), try to bring some continuity into your life, perhaps by changing shifts every two weeks. If you are a pilot or businessman who frequently has to travel through different time zones, then jetlag will be a problem. Your sleep rhythm will be upset. When you want to go to bed, your body is still wide awake. When you need to work, you feel tired. It can take anywhere from ten days to two weeks for your body to adjust to a new rhythm. If you suffer from very severe stress, you should, for the time being, avoid long trips. If that option is not available, try to stay in bed longer, even if your body is completely awake.

Introduce continuity into your life

One more tip. If you work under artificial light all day, it may happen that your internal clock goes crazy. Fluorescent light does not have the same spectrum as daylight. If you work in a confined space, try to sit by a window or install a special lamp with a daylight spectrum.

Artificial light upsets your internal clock

7. Learn to say 'no'

"The 'no' that I've been meaning to say
have pondered a hundred times, formulated, but never uttered,
it burns my stomach, deprives me of air,
it is ground between my teeth,
and leaves my mouth as a peaceful 'yes.'"

Peter Turrini, Austrian writer

The simplest and most efficient tool of stress management is the little word 'no.' Learn to say no and you will see your stress level drop rapidly. Do not constantly take on new tasks, responsibilities and challenges. Think of yourself and the quality of your life.

8. Balance your life in a healthy way

To avoid stress, you should try to strike an ideal balance between tension and relaxation. This can be achieved in numerous ways:

● Sports

Exercise at least twice a week. See the chapter "Fit for Life."

● Mental training

Autogenic training relaxes the mind and soul

Listen to your body. Do autogenic training, yoga or learn some other relaxation technique. It is no coincidence that more and more people are signing up for courses and seminars in mental development and even spirituality. As a result of the tension between economic success and the pressure to perform, the desire to find new sources of strength and internal peace is growing.

● Biofeedback

Biofeedback is the autogenic training of the 21st century

The latest method for restoring your connection with your body is biofeedback, the autogenic training of the 21st century. More and more men under stress looking for more efficient relaxation techniques have discovered biofeedback. Many people have lost touch with their body, that healthy sensitivity to its physical needs. In biofeedback, the patient is hooked up to a computer through sensors that measure skin conductivity, body temperature, pulse rate and respiration. The patient receives feedback from the computer about how his body reacts to certain situations. Under stress, the heart begins to beat fast, respiration is accelerated, the temperature drops, the conductivity of the skin explodes, the pulse rate rises and the neck muscles become tense. Put in a simulated stress situation while being monitored by the computer, the patient learns efficient relaxation techniques, such as positive thinking, but also how to increase his performance and eliminate stress at the same time. It is mental training for the computer age. The success rates are certainly incredible. Brigitte Bösenkopf, a psychologist at the Institute of Preventive Psychology in Vienna, has even used biofeedback to successfully treat impotence.

9. Rearrange your goals in life

Imagine that you have only three more years to live. Or, to use a more drastic example, only three months. What is important to you all of a sudden? Do your priorities suddenly change overnight? Awareness of the limitations of your earthly existence would suddenly make everything that causes you stress seem trivial.

Nobody on his deathbed ever regrets not working enough

Nobody on his deathbed has ever regretted not working enough. Keep this in mind and reduce your stress by reprioritizing your life's goals and plans. Men often say, "I'll do all those things when I retire." It is not true. Maybe you will not even be around for your retirement because a stress-related heart attack or pancreatic cancer (six cups of coffee a day increase the risk of pancreatic cancer by a factor of eight) has already claimed your life. Or your wife has already left you.

Think about your attitude toward life. Let go of your fantasies of power and your hunger for recognition that you do not need nearly as much as you think.

"We cannot take life to court and sue for lost meaning," wrote Erwin Ringel, an Austrian psychiatrist and university professor, in his book The Austrian Soul, "because it can only have the meaning we attach to it. It is we who are primarily in charge of our lives." He adds, "We do not live in an unbridled performance-driven society, though performance is not such a bad thing for it can lead to self-actualization. Instead, we have a society driven by success. But he who worships success will start a war that pits everyone against everybody else."

Six cups of coffee increases your risk of cancer by a factor of eight

10. Test your ability to deal with success and failure

"It is a skill to say, 'I do not know.'
To know that one does not know anything speaks of wisdom.
To believe that one must know everything speaks of ignorance."

Dalai Lama

Stress is the result of a workload that is so immense that you cannot get it done without overexerting yourself. You have to know your limits, but do not keep pushing yourself to the limit. Many people wrongly believe that it is impossible to admit to their limits.

Avoid pushing yourself to the limit

Set yourself reasonable and realistic tasks; you should be able to complete them without having to push yourself to your physical limit.

11. React calmly to stress

You can plan your day down to the minute, which is important, as we have seen under stress reduction method number three. But inner calm cannot be "scheduled." Try to find inner peace by managing your time properly. That inner peace is a source of enormous strength, a state of contemplation. But more and more people do not have time for introspection anymore. They have forgotten how to deal with inner peace. Hyperactive children are a good example. They behave in abnormal ways because their parents set a negative example by being hectic and nervous all the time. Children internalize such behavior and often become hyperactive themselves, sometimes developing behavioral disorders. Whenever you experience stress, especially if you are going at full steam, just stop for a while.

Inner peace cannot be controlled with your day planner

Stress management also means being gutsy enough to take a break, to do noth-

WHAT TO DO IN A CASE OF ACUTE STRESS

1. Take deep breaths.
2. Relax your posture.
3. Distance yourself mentally from the problem that is weighing you down at the moment.
4. Stand up and leave the room or, at least, open the windows to let in some fresh air.
5. Engage in conversation to take your mind off things.
6. Meditate by "switching off" completely and relaxing.

Take a break every two hours

ing whatsoever. You should take a break of ten to fifteen minutes every two hours and a longer break of about one hour every four hours. Make your breaks more effective by using relaxation techniques that easily fit into your schedule. Also, try to avoid additional stress in your spare time. You should do things that you personally enjoy. It will be invigorating.

12. Learn conflict and communications management

Unresolved conflicts, even the attempt to avoid conflicts, can contribute considerably to your stress. Try to anticipate difficult situations so that you can prepare yourself. State your point of view clearly without assigning blame. Do not say, "You never give me enough time." Rather, you should say, "I need a bit more time for this task." Listen to others. Focus on what the other person says and repeat in your own words what the conflict is all about to show that you have understood correctly.

13. One way to work off stress is by having sex

Men and women differ in their sexual behavior. For men who are always under stress, sex is an ideal way of letting off steam. Sex helps them relax, as confirmed by biofeedback readings.

Women lose their libido when stressed

Women who are stressed, however, are the exact opposite. They lose interest in sex. There are two reasons. On the one hand, their bodies are tense as a result of the stress. And men under stress are irritable at home, which the women in their lives have to put up with. In turn they will often refuse to have sex.

14. Vent your anger

Do not keep your emotions bottled up inside. It is quite normal to vent your anger occasionally, provided that your behavior does not hurt others. At work, the average employee, according to one study, gets angry about fourteen times a day. Often, this cannot be avoided, but it can be managed. The test, created by the Mayo Clinic Health Sources, allows you to determine whether or not your anger has already gotten out of control.

Do not keep your emotions bottled up inside

1. I want to scream or hit someone once a week.
2. I get angry with others when I have to line up for something.
3. When someone cuts me off on the road, I honk, scream at the other driver or make obscene gestures.
4. Anyone who makes me mad will get it.
5. When someone treats me unfairly, I think of ways to take revenge.
6. I do not hold back my feelings when I am treated in a condescending way.
7. I often think that others are out to get me.
8. I strike back whenever someone criticizes me.
9. I just take over when someone takes too long to do a job.
10. I always call customer service and yell at them when I have a problem with a product or service.

If four of these apply to you, then you should quickly look for ways to vent your anger. Try some of the methods listed in this book. Try to accept things that you cannot change, but try to change them whenever possible.

15. Reduce your leisure-time stress

Learn to say 'no' to friends as well. Go out only once a week. Do not spend long nights at bars and nightclubs. Some of your friends might have gotten used to staying at your place and have begun to take your hospitality for granted. Send them a fax with the addresses of a few nice hotels in your area.

Learn to say no to friends

If these fifteen methods for fighting stress do not work for you, consult your physician to find out if your stress has a medical cause.

REDUCE YOUR STRESS

Learn to say no. Think of yourself first and foremost.
Manage your time properly. Try to avoid unimportant things.
Plan your work carefully. Do not overestimate yourself.
Distance yourself. Sometimes a little conversation can shed new light on things.
Be realistic. Do not set yourself unrealistic goals.
Set priorities. Focus on the essential things. Make sure you have enough sleep, exercise and a healthy diet.

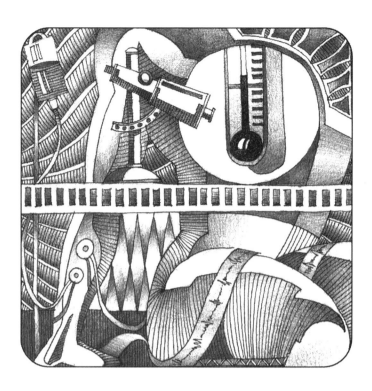

The Pain and Suffering of Men

The Risk Factor Cholesterol

High serum-lipid levels are the main risk factors in heart attack

Eat fatty food. Enjoy your daily servings of ham and eggs as well as lots of bacon for breakfast. Snack on a salami sandwich and at night dig into that steak. And, of course, let us not forget a couple of hamburgers in between. *Bon appétit.*

All of the above are no problem, if we are to believe an article, "The Truth behind Cholesterol," published by a lifestyle magazine in the spring of 1999. According to this article, medical research has already proven that cutting out fatty food does not make you any healthier. Quite the contrary—it will get you closer to a heart attack. The subtitle of the article was "The Monkey Business of 'Bad' Cholesterol." Is the author of that article right? Is it all just scaremongering fueled by industries more interested in the bottom line than in your health and happiness??

Not quite. High serum-lipid levels are among the main risk factors leading to heart attacks in men. Cholesterol is especially dangerous because it does not have any symptoms. Its risk potential should not be underestimated. Cholesterol is sometimes referred to as the "killer of managers." Even though medical science has begun to take a different view of cholesterol, the American Heart Association and the National Heart, Lung and Blood Institute stated unequivocally: "There is clear proof of the benefits to men and women, young and old, high-risk or low-risk, of reducing one's cholesterol level."

What Is Cholesterol?

Cholesterol, as a constituent of body cells and hormones, is vital. Together with phospholipids and triglycerides, it belongs to the group of serum lipids. It is required for synthesis, and the buildup of hormones and cells. It is also responsible for the distribution of fat in the blood vessels, the production of bile acid and vitamin D (calciferol), and the buildup of cell membranes. Most cholesterol originates in the liver, where it is produced from saturated fatty acids. Cholesterol is found exclusively in animal products, especially in meat, sausages, tripe, fish, butter and eggs.

> Cholesterol is necessary for the synthesis of hormones

Men, in particular, tend toward high cholesterol levels because of fatty diets, lack of exercise and excess weight, which often go hand in hand with diabetes, lipid-metabolic disease, nicotine and alcohol. Elevated cholesterol levels are mostly dietary, but hereditary disorders can also lead to higher serum-lipid levels.

Generally, people in Western civilization take in more cholesterol with their food than the body really needs. The daily intake should not exceed 300 milligrams. Austrians, for example, consume an average of 500 milligrams. In addition to this, the body itself produces about 700 to 1,200 milligrams a day.

> Austrians take 500 milligrams a day, instead of 300

The Good, the Bad and the Ugly

There are different kinds of cholesterol. To be soluble in blood, it requires a water-soluble "coating" of fat and protein, the so-called lipoprotein. Sergio

Leone pretty much anticipated the cholesterol story with his Western movie, The Good, The Bad And The Ugly.

There are three types of cholesterol:
- HDL cholesterol (high-density lipoprotein): the good
- VLDL cholesterol (very low-density lipoprotein): the bad
- LDL cholesterol (low-density lipoprotein): the ugly

HDL cholesterol protects the vessels

HDL is called the "good" cholesterol. It serves as a protection against vascular disease because it transports the cholesterol away from the blood vessels to the liver, which is the main organ of lipid metabolism.

LDL cholesterol causes arteriosclerosis

LDL is often referred to as the harmful cholesterol because it is the main culprit behind arteriosclerosis. It deposits on the inner walls of the blood vessels and blocks them, which often results in hypertension, a weak heart, heart attacks, stroke and other problems.

According to the recommendations of the National Cholesterol Education Program (NCEP) and the European Atherosclerosis Society (EAS), the overall cholesterol level should be below 200 mg/dl, preferably below 180 mg/dl, the LDL-cholesterol level should be below 100 mg/dl and the HDL-cholesterol should be at least 35 mg/dl.

THE IDEAL CHOLESTEROL LEVELS IN MEN

- The overall cholesterol level should be below 200 mg/dl (the ideal would be below 180 mg/dl).
- The LDL level should be below 100 mg/dl.
- The HDL level should be higher than 35 mg/dl.
- The quotient of overall cholesterol/HDL cholesterol should be below 5.

75% of Austrians have elevated cholesterol levels

Until recently, the LDL cholesterol level was the main measurement that concerned heart patients. In Austria, 75% of the adult population has an overall cholesterol level of more than 200 mg/dl, and over 25% have an overall level more than 250 mg/dl, which comes with health risks.

But there are more precise ways to determine whether the heart is at risk. Results from a New York study presented at the annual meeting of the American Cardiological Society in 1999 showed that the LDL level is possibly not the best parameter for determining the risk to the heart. These scientists discovered that the two fat proteins, ApoB and ApoA1, as well as their relationship to each other, provide a more sensitive gauge for predicting cardiovascular disease than the LDL level by itself. The year 2000 should see modifications to international guidelines.

Possible Diseases

Cholesterol can cause a series of dangerous conditions:

- The overall cholesterol level and/or the LDL level are elevated or the ratio of HDL and LDL is unfavorable—a condition known as hyperlipemia.
- Hypercholesterolemia, which is hereditary, occurs when the liver cannot absorb and process LDL cholesterol. In order to meet its own requirements, the organ starts to produce more cholesterol. This rapidly raises the overall cholesterol level of the body (especially LDL).
- Some conditions, such as diabetes or hypothyroidism, affect the entire metabolism and thus the cholesterol level. Medication that contains cortisone has similar effects on the body as a whole.

Too much total cholesterol is called hyperlipemia

Hypercholesterolema is hereditary

There is no doubt that arteriosclerosis and thus the risk of coronary sclerosis are triggered by not only one factor (e.g., cholesterol), but by a multitude of factors. Besides elevated serum-lipid levels, other factors include homocystein, genetic predisposition, excess weight, hypertension, lack of exercise, diabetes, inflammations and infections, such as chlamydia, antioxidants and many more.

With the new millennium, there will be a drastic change in methods for predicting heart attacks and arteriosclerosis. A large number of so-called double blind large-scale trials have been done, and the results are conclusive. These studies, known as 4S, CARE and LIPID, are the first to show that a new medication containing so-called "statins" for lowering the serum-lipid level in heart attack patients, can be life-saving in patients with high and average cholesterol levels.

Fewer patients had heart attacks or strokes, and fewer of them required surgery or angioplasty. Based on studies to date, we can conclude that the effective lowering of elevated serum-lipid levels can stop the progress of coronary disease and that, after about five years, some vascular damage may actually be repaired.

Serum-lipid-lowering statins can save your life after a heart attack

One question that is often raised is whether there is any plausible way to identify risk minimization. A formula developed by the University of Zurich (the "Zurich formula") identifies risk potential based on ten years of aging. In this period of time, the body experiences:

● an increase in the LDL level by 36 mg/dl,
● a decrease in the HDL level by 12 mg/dl or
● an increase in the triglyceride level by 90 mg/dl.

Looking at this, it becomes clear that any improvement in the risk scenario leads to an increase in life span. Any positive change to any of the risk factors mentioned, to the extent of the risk potential, thus corresponds to an improvement in the risk scenario by ten years. For example, if a patient reduces his triglyceride level by 90 mg/dl, he will gain ten years. The same is true of a patient who manages to raise his HDL level by 12 mg/dl. If a patient manages both, he can gain twenty years.

Lowering LDL is recommended even after age 70

Another common question refers to the age up to which it is medically sensible to try to lower one's lipid level. There are some indications that the lowering of LDL can be effective even after the age of 70. As a matter of fact, it can be as effective as in younger people. But the important thing is that the reduction does not kick in until two to five years after the start of the treatment. As a result, everyone can do his own calculations and determine when to get actively started.

10% of all men with elevated LDL suffer a second heart attack

The fact that men are often careless when it comes to their health is illustrated by figures from the US. After a heart attack, fewer than 20% of patients have their serum-lipid level checked and consistently take their medication (the proper medication can lower the risk of dying from coronary heart disease by up to 40%). This is alarming given the fact that 10% of all men with elevated serum-lipid levels have a second heart attack within five years of the first.

Exercise and a low-fat diet lower cholesterol

Ideally, the risk of arteriosclerosis and of a heart attack should be minimized beforehand through a combination of low-fat food and exercise. American doctors at Stanford University in Palo Alto confirmed in a 1998 study that a low-cholesterol diet is not enough. Only in combination with physical exercise can a low-fat diet have a real effect. For that study, the researchers divided the 197 patients into four groups. One engaged in sports, one had only the low-fat diet, the third had a combination of both. A fourth group did neither.

HOW TO CONTROL YOUR CHOLESTEROL LEVEL AND
PREVENT A HEART ATTACK

- Reduce your energy input. Overweight people should start by halving their food intake. The reduction of body fat produces an increase in good HDL cholesterol. But do not go on any crash diets.
- Replace animal fat with vegetable fat. For example, use margarine instead of butter.
- Low-fat diet rich in fiber. Eat more fruit, vegetables and legumes. Reduce your intake of carbohydrates and sugar.
- Make sure your diet includes polyunsaturated fatty acids. Polyunsaturated fatty acids, contained in such foods as cold-pressed olive oil and cold water fish oil, should be part of your diet. They lower the LDL level.
- Also take lipid reducers. Doctors often recommend them as an addition to a low-fat diet in order to lower the LDL level. They are available as garlic pills.
- Statins, the new lipid reducers, lower the risk of arteriosclerosis. The statin preparations available from drugstores can minimize the intake of cholesterol contained in your food. Consult your physician about statins.
- Exercise helps. Elevated LDL levels can be effectively lowered by combining exercise with a low-fat diet.
- Avoid alcohol and cigarettes. Try not to drink or smoke. If you do, keep them to a minimum.
- Regularly check your cholesterol level. If you have elevated serum-lipid levels, you should see your doctor at least twice a year to have it checked out. A high cholesterol level that is not diagnosed and treated in time can lead to premature death.

After one year, the result was quite clear. In order to achieve a significant improvement, you must combine a low-fat diet with exercise. The group that combined the two showed a significant reduction in the LDL cholesterol level, and the ratio of good HDL cholesterol had also been improved. The problem is that a low-fat diet also decreases HDL—an unpleasant concomitant effect—but exercise seems to compensate for that.

The Engine of Life

The Heart and Its Peculiarities in Men

Friday, 5 p.m.: The newsroom of a local radio station. A briefing for the weekend anchormen, then a meeting with the producer—the week is over. The election campaign and the war in Kosovo have been covered, the reporting from Belgrade was tough, but objective. Another cigarette, a cup of coffee—the seventh for the day—and then off for the weekend.

8 p.m.: Mario R. arrives at home, sifts through the mail and has dinner with his wife—two glasses of beer, a steak, and potatoes. He feels completely drained, a paralyzing fatigue. There is a feeling of pressure. He blames it on the steak and has a liqueur to help his digestion.

11.45 p.m.: He feels nauseous. There is a slight pressure above his chest, which he attributes to gas and bad digestion. He goes to bed.

1.32 a.m.: Saturday morning. Mario R. wakes up with pressure in his chest like he has never experienced before, and shortness of breath. He wakes up his wife, who gets quite upset. Mario thinks about all the things at the office he has not finished yet. He gets angry with himself for not being able to think of anything else.

2.30 a.m.: He is sweating profusely. A feeling of anxiety takes hold. Mario R.'s wife has already called the ambulance.

2.55 a.m.: Lights flashing, the ambulance takes him to the emergency room.

3.15 a.m.: Saturday morning. Diagnosis: heart attack.

The Engine of Our System

Cardiovascular disease causes 55% of all deaths

Of all deaths in the Western world, 55% can be traced to cardiovascular disease. When the heart stops, so does life. Heart attacks are the number one killer in Europe.

The heart, which weighs between 280 and 310 grams, is nothing but a muscle with a very sophisticated and unique function.

It is the engine of our body. It is the center of our soul, as many cultures have believed in the course of history. It is not much bigger than a fist. The heart contracts 60 to 80 times per minute and pumps about 75 milliliters of blood with each beat depending on sex and body height. Each minute, a total of five liters (over one gallon) of blood is sent through the body—the total amount of blood in an adult man. That biological pump transports 300 liters of blood an hour or 7,200 liters each day. There is no technology that comes even close to that kind of output. The heart beats 41 million times a year and moves over 2.6 million liters of blood. Over a life span of 70 years, this comes to an incredible 2.8 billion heartbeats and 182 million liters of blood.

The heart beats 115,000 times a day

The heart's contraction can best be compared to a shampoo bottle. When you squeeze the bottle and then let go, the plastic will return to its original shape until you squeeze it again. The amount of blood pumped out by the heart is called the ejection fraction. A stroke volume of 60% to 70% means that 75–90 milliliters of blood is ejected with each heartbeat. If you "squeeze the bottle" 60 times, you will achieve 5,400 milliliters or 5.4 liters of blood per minute. This is called the ejection output.

The heart rate, the number of strokes, depends on your age. Newborn babies have an average rate of 140, children 100 to 120 and adults 60 to 90. With increasing age, the maximum heart rate starts to drop. For example, a 25-year-old man has a maximum of 200 beats per minute, a 35-year-old 188, a 45-year-old 176, a 55-year-old 165 and a 65-year-old man has only 155. The heart rate slows not only with age, but also with physical condition. Athletes can increase the pumping output of each beat to such an extent that the heart rate of, say, top cyclists such as the Spanish winner of the Tour-de-France, Miguel Indurain, can drop to a heart rate at rest of 35 beats. For them, this would be normal.

The maximum heart rate decreases with age

She Opened His Chest on the Floor of a Pub

Steven Miland was as good as dead. The 22-year-old man from Britain was out drinking with his buddies almost to the bitter end when someone stabbed him in the chest with a knife. But he was lucky, considering the circumstances. The emergency doctor, Heather Clark, got to the seedy pub in a rundown part of London within a very short time, and she acted quickly. Under the disbelieving stares of Steven's intoxicated friends, the 35-year-old doctor performed open-heart surgery on him right there on the floor of the pub. She cut two holes in the chest to lower the pressure on his lungs. Then, having sedated him, she

She performed open-heart surgery on the floor of a pub

performed a thoracotomy, which means that she opened his chest to raise the thorax and have access to the heart, which had stopped beating because of a blood clot. Clark had learned that technique only two days before, reported the French news agency AFP on April 29, 1999. This open-heart surgery, in the middle of a British pub, without any of the modern tools of an operating theater, clearly shows how vital an organ the heart really is. Steven Miland survived the operation. Without it, he would have died.

The heart, the capacity of the heart, heart disease and, in particular, heart attacks have many similarities in men and women, but also many differences. The most recent studies on male and female heart attacks show that they can be almost like two different conditions, with different symptoms.

Women are usually seven to ten years older than men by the time they suffer a heart attack

Women who suffer heart attacks are usually seven to ten years older, often have diabetes, hypertension and not enough red blood cells (anemia). But they also manifest substantial psychological and psychosocial differences compared to men.

Even the symptoms may be different. An American study of 810 men and 550 women who had heart attacks, published in the American Heart Journal, has proven that men complain of neck pains, back pains, pains in the jaw and nausea less frequently than do women. But men complain more often of sweating. More than 80% of the men and 70% of the women mentioned chest pains, but 15% of the men and 25% of the women did not experience these at all. While 90% of all cases do feel some kind of pain in the upper body, it can be said that symptoms like pain in the left shoulder, upper abdominal pain, nausea, respiratory distress and weakness may lead to a wrong or delayed diagnosis. Regardless of these factors, it is a fact that women suffer more severe heart attacks and they are more likely to die with the first heart attack than are men.

Men are less likely to die of a heart attack than women

On the other hand, women's risk of sudden cardiac death is not even half that of men. However, it is a threat that should not be underestimated at a more advanced age. There are no doubt extenuating factors that protect the female heart, but scientists are still in the dark about them. For now, the only recommendation is to avoid the risks.

Women do not use bicycle ergometers as often as men

The January 1999 issue of Women's Health Source of the Mayo Clinic features a discussion of the differences between the sexes. Women are less likely than men to have a cardiac-stress test (bicycle ergometer), a cardiac probe or a bypass operation. Their treatment is less aggressive than that of men, and they seem to have a higher mortality rate from heart attacks. Based on this evidence, the Women's Health Initiative was founded.

The Women's Health Initiative (WHI) is a multimillion-dollar project that was created in 1991 by the National Institutes of Health in Bethesda, Maryland. As part of this initiative, more than 167,000 women, who participate in one or several studies, are examined and cared for. Some of the studies deal with the influence of hormone replacement therapy on the prevention of heart disease and osteoporosis. Others focus on the significance of changes in people's diets and eating habits to prevent breast cancer, colon cancer and heart disease. The usefulness of calcium and vitamin D-replacement therapies for the prevention of osteoporosis and colon cancer is also being researched. The program also involves longitudinal studies, which are meant to shed light on the connection between lifestyle, health and risk factors related to specific women's diseases.

This American initiative clearly shows the way. But there should also be a Men's Health Initiative, which is long overdue. This makes sense because there are not only hormonal differences between men and women: the size of the brain is different and so is the risk of cardiovascular disease. Even the life cycle of a cell differs in men and women. Only longitudinal studies can provide the answers we need to identify the risk factors as well as to decide on preventive and specific treatment.

The Birthplace of Modern Cardiology

Framingham, a small suburb of Boston, has been the mecca for cardiology for the last fifty years. During the late 1940s, more patients between the ages of 50 and 60 died than ever before in the United States. Most Americans at the time were not familiar with cholesterol levels, hypertension and the connections between smoking, diet and health.

The Framingham Heart Study is the biggest of its kind

In the fall of 1948, therefore, the American Public Health Service commissioned an unprecedented study. In the small town of Framingham, they persuaded 5,000 people, out of a population of 25,000, to participate in a lifelong health study that involved regular, complete, physical checkups. The so-called Framingham Heart Study, which has been conducted by the National Heart, Lung and Blood Institute and Boston University for more than 50 years, is the longest epidemiological study of all time. So far, thousands of scientific discoveries and findings have been made. Much of it was pioneering work in the fields of prophylaxis and the fighting of heart disease. The scientific discoveries made thanks to Framingham include:

- 1960: smoking increases the risk of heart disease
- 1961: the cholesterol level, blood pressure and irregularities in the electrocardiogram are correlated to a heightened risk of suffering a heart attack
- 1967: physical activities, such as sports, can lower the risk of a heart attack
- 1970: high blood pressure increases the risk of having a stroke
- 1988: a high HDL-cholesterol level (high-density lipoprotein) provides protection against heart disease and lowers the mortality rate
- 1996: scientists find out why high blood pressure can lead to heart failure

Diabetes is one of the main causes of cardiac disease

So far, more than 10,000 inhabitants of Framingham have participated in regular biennial physical checkups. The findings of the Framingham Heart Study have been beneficial for medical science around the world. For example, it was found that heart attacks can occur without any pain whatsoever and leave scar tissue without any symptoms. Among other findings, high blood pressure can trigger a heart attack, smoking is generally bad for the heart, and diabetes is the most fundamental cause of heart disease.

That may all sound banal to us these days, but those findings have changed the world and will continue to do so well into the new millennium. Before Framingham, people assumed that a heart attack or stroke was merely a twist of fate, a matter of good luck or bad luck. It was these studies that provided incontrovertible evidence of the dangerous effects of certain lifestyles.

The future of cardiology has already reached Framingham. An article published in the scientific journal Lancet on January 9, 1999, shows that the risk of a healthy man's developing a coronary disease is one in two after the age of 40. For women, it is one in three. This, too, was unknown before.

Arteriosclerosis: Strokes Are Caused by Inflammations

Arteriosclerosis has different causes than once thought

The causes of arteriosclerosis are different from what we have come to expect. So are some of the risk factors of coronary disease or a heart attack.

Arteriosclerosis is now seen as an inflammatory process that leads to the destabilization of the calcific deposits along the walls of the blood vessels. The progression is usually as follows:

Unhealthy lifestyle ➤ accumulation of harmful serum lipids ➤ deposition on the walls of arteries ➤ activation of the delicate inner cell layer (the endothelium) ➤ inflammatory cells enter ➤ activation of inflammatory cells, destruction of muscle cells and tissue ➤ rupture of calcific deposits with disastrous consequences ➤ stroke, heart attack, intermittent claudication.

The role that inflammatory changes and markers play is becoming clearer and clearer. Several factors, besides the harmful LDL cholesterol, are of prognostic importance when it comes to arteriosclerosis. In particular, they are the serum-lipid components apolipoprotein A, apolipoprotein B, the ratio of apolipoproteins A and B as well as inflammation-related blood parameters such as the blood-clotting factor fibrinogen and the inflammation parameter C-reactive protein (CRP). If elevated, all represent a higher risk factor.

Elevated apolipoprotein-A/B levels increase the risk to the heart

For two years, there have been rumors of another "killer": homocystein. Homocystein is an amino acid, a constituent of protein that is normally present in the body. It is taken in with one's food. The body needs homocystein to produce protein and thus sustain tissue. Problems occur whenever we have too much homocystein. In a study published in 1999, Dutch doctors have discovered that an elevated homocystein level in the plasma increases the risk of a heart attack by a factor of 2.4 and the risk of a stroke by a factor of 2.5.

According to the scientists, the high homocystein levels could be caused by a deficiency of vitamins B6, B12 and folic acid. Currently, nobody is recommending that we all undergo a homocystein screening. But members of families with a history of arteriosclerosis (narrowing of arteries of the brain, legs or heart) at a young age or coronary disease should be screened. The normal level is between 14 and 17 micromoles or, ideally, even lower. A level over 18 micromoles carries a drastically higher risk. If your level is higher, you should take vitamin-B complexes (B6, B12 and folic acid) to lower them.

The amino acid homocystein increases stroke risk

Early Warning Signs

Symptoms are the only early warning signs. A symptom tells us how our body feels and allows us to draw our own conclusions as to our condition. Every symptom differs from person to person. The following symptoms and warning signs point to a heart attack. Keep in mind that not all of them have to occur and that some disappear as quickly as they appear:

THE SYMPTOMS OF A HEART ATTACK
- Sense of fullness or constrictive pain in the center of your chest, which lasts a couple of minutes
- Pain that extends to your shoulder, neck or arms
- Sense of pressure in your head
- Dizziness, sweating, feeling faint
- Nausea
- Shortness of breath

The more symptoms there are, the higher the probability of a heart attack. Call 911 for an ambulance immediately.

Other signs and symptoms usually connected to heart disease are general weakness, edemas (excessive accumulation of fluid in tissue), syncope (fainting), presyncope (feeling faint), dyspnea (labored breathing), tachycardia, arrhythmia, abnormal complexion, dry skin, shock, and sudden changes in vision, strength, coordination, speech or feeling. Typical of angina pectoris are chest pain, feeling of impending doom, constriction, retching feeling, pressure, feeling heavy, feeling of fullness, feeling of a heavy weight on one's chest, burning sensation, pain, burping, coughing, feeling cold while sweating, weakness. In these cases you should call a doctor.

The first few hours decide between life and death

The first few minutes after a heart attack determine whether the patient lives or dies. The first few hours determine what your future life is going to be like. Do not hesitate. If you detect the typical symptoms, call 911 for an ambulance immediately, and sit or lie down if you feel dizzy. Breathe slowly and deeply. Chew an aspirin unless you are allergic to aspirin. Aspirin thins your blood and can increase your chance of survival.

High blood pressure, excess weight and stress are risk factors

How high is your risk of developing heart disease in the next few years? Smoking, high blood pressure and high cholesterol levels are among the main risk factors in coronary disease. The probability of having a heart attack or dying from heart disease within the next eight years increases with each additional risk factor that you are exposed to. Calculate your risk by adding up the points for the questions contained in the following risk chart of the Mayo Clinic:

HOW HIGH IS YOUR RISK OF HEART DISEASE?

1. Do you smoke?   No = 0   Yes = 3
2. Look for your systolic blood pressure (always the first level to be measured) in the chart below and take the score underneath as your assessment:

100	110	120	130	140	150	160	170	180	190	200
1	2	4	5	6	7	8	9	10	12	13

3. Take the score at which your age and cholesterol level intersect (use the level from your most recent checkup):

Total Cholesterol	Age 40	50	60	70
165	4	12	18	21
180	5	13	19	21
195	7	14	19	21
210	8	15	20	21
225	9	16	20	22
240	11	17	21	22
255	12	18	22	22
270	13	19	22	23
285	15	20	23	23
300	16	21	24	23
315	17	22	24	23

4. Now add up your points

Smoking	
High blood pressure (systolic)	
Age/blood cholesterol level	
Sex, male	5

TOTAL SCORE

Your Risk

Locate your total score in the following chart. Next to it, you will see the probability in percent of your having a heart attack in the next eight years or of your suffering from some other form of heart disease.

Total score	Probability	Total score	Probability
Up to 10	<1	25–26	6
11–13	1	27	7
14–17	2	28	8

18–21	3	29	9
22–23	4	30	10
24	5	31	11
32	13	41	31
33	14	42	34
34	16	43	36
35	17	44	39
36	19	45	42
37	21	46	46
38	24	47	49
39	26	48	52
40	28	49	55

For your information, the cholesterol level in this chart refers to the total cholesterol level. If you have a very low HDL level (the good one), you will be even more at risk. Men suffering from diabetes should add three points to their score.

A Matter of Probability

Imagine that you travel 10,000 km by car every year. The probability of your having a car accident would be higher than if you traveled only 500 km. Still, it is possible for someone traveling 10,000 km never to have an accident, while the other driver, who covers fewer kilometers, gets into a head-on collision with a truck.

Cardiac diseases can have different causes

The same is true of the probabilities and risk factors in this case. The risk factors of developing coronary heart disease are hypertension, high cholesterol levels, smoking, excess weight, stress, behavioral disorders, certain drugs (cocaine), a family history of coronary heart disease, age, and just being male. But it is all just a matter of probability because someone without risk factors such as homocystein may suffer a fatal heart attack out of the blue. Some of the risk factors, such as heredity, age and sex cannot be influenced directly. But others we can control.

Is prevention really worth it? Maybe you do not want to live forever, but certainly you will want to keep your health as you grow older. Therefore, you should take every step you can to reduce the risk.

Risk Factor: Smoking

Did you know that…
- in Austria, for example, 26 people die everyday as a direct consequence of smoking, but only three die in car accidents?
- smokers, on average, have seven years less to live?
- one in three fatal cases of cardiovascular disease is due to smoking?
- ten in a thousand non-smokers suffer a heart attack, but 131 in a thousand smokers?

Every day, 26 Austrians die from smoking

"Do something for your heart before your heart stops doing things for you," is the slogan of the Austrian Cardiological Society, the Austrian Heart Foundation and the Austrian Medical Association.

More than 500,000 people die from smoking every year in the US. One third of these, 150,000 deaths, get cardiovascular disease. Smoking kills more people every year than AIDS, alcohol, cocaine and all accidents put together. According to the US Surgeon General, 20% of all deaths are related to smoking. Tobacco smoke contains more than 4,000 substances (counting only the ones that have been identified), including nicotine, nitrosamine, polycyclic aromatic hydrocarbons, and other products that may have severe side effects.

Smoking kills more people than AIDS, alcohol, cocaine and accidents taken together

Tobacco affects mainly the vessels and can cause arteriosclerosis. Nicotine reduces the good HDL cholesterol and increases the harmful LDL, thus making the blood more viscous and clogging the vessels. It also damages the inner layer of the blood vessels, the endothelium.

The inhalation of smoke also has short-term side effects on the heart and vessels, which may provoke a heart attack. Nicotine raises the blood pressure and the heart rate, and carbon monoxide—the same gas that is found in car exhaust—enters the bloodstream and reduces the blood's oxygen content. Smoke can also constrict the coronary vessels. All of this also applies to those breathing second hand smoke.

Nicotine increases blood pressure and heart rate

Non-smokers have fewer problems breathing, they are in better physical shape, and their sense of taste has not been distorted. They also do not suffer from smoker's cough, their teeth do not turn yellow, they experience less heartburn, and they have a considerably lower risk of cardiovascular disease, lung emphysema, lung cancer and esophageal cancer. In short, non-smokers have a higher life expectancy.

Other substantial factors in heart disease, such as cholesterol, hypertension, stress, body fat and blood sugar are explained in the corresponding chapters of this book.

Fats—Harmful Doping of the Heart

Change your diet if you love your heart

Your diet can also have a substantial effect on the likelihood of heart disease. You should follow these recommendations for a heart-friendly diet:

- Cut down on meat, poultry and fish
- Use oils that have a large content of polyunsaturated fatty acids, such as sunflower or corn oils.
- Avoid hidden fat, such as the fat in sausages, cheese, dairy products, mayonnaise and nuts.
- Use a low-fat way of preparing your food (e.g., barbecuing, stewing or braising).
- Eat fruit and vegetables five times a day.
- In restaurants, do not have meat as your main course. Remember that red meat, poultry and seafood should be the "side orders" to fruit, vegetables and whole grain products (natural rice, whole wheat pasta, whole wheat meal, whole wheat bread and buns).
- Use low-fat dairy products. Dairy products provide the body with essential calcium and protein, but they can also have high contents of saturated fat and cholesterol. Instead of the usual dairy products, buy one-percent low-fat milk, low-fat yogurt, low-fat or fat-free ice cream and low-fat or fat-free cheese and sour cream.
- Prepare your food with little or no salt. Eliminate salt and replace it with herbs and other spices such as onions, garlic, mustard, fresh lemon and vinegar.
- Use sugar, as well as honey and syrup, sparingly.
- It is better to have small meals several times a day. Eating five small meals is better than eating three big ones.

Omega-3 Fatty Acids Can Protect Your Heart

How often do you eat fish? This is one of the most important questions to ask yourself if you are interested in a heart-friendly diet. Fish is not the only source of protein, but it has one advantage for your cardiovascular system in that it contains omega-3 fatty acids.

These are found primarily in fish. Some fish, especially cold water species like salmon, mackerel and herring, contain relatively high quantities of these acids. Omega-3 fatty acids, to a lesser degree, are also contained in soybeans, nuts, and green vegetables.

Omega-3 fatty acids have a positive effect on the heart in many ways. They can reduce certain serum-lipid levels, especially triglycerides. Triglycerides are a type of fat that the body uses as a source of energy. If there is an excess of triglycerides, they are stored in the body as fat. A permanently elevated triglyceride level raises the risk of arteriosclerosis. If the triglyceride level is especially high, and conventional drugs do not work, your physician will prescribe fish oil supplements in addition to the drugs. The use of fish oil capsules is the only recommendation of the American Heart Association. *Omega-3 fatty acids protect the heart muscle*

Omega-3 fatty acids also reduce the risk of thrombosis, the coagulation of blood in a blood vessel. They function as natural anticoagulants by preventing the blood platelets from clotting. The blood platelets, or thrombocytes, are then less likely to stick together. Some studies have even shown that omega-3 can reduce blood pressure. In America, therefore, the motto is "fish on your dish." Fresh fish, or frozen unprocessed fish, is best. Stay away from breaded fish like fish fingers. Cold water fish such as mackerel, Atlantic salmon, halibut and herring have an especially high content of omega-3 fatty acids. *Reduce your risk of thrombosis*

Antioxidants Prevent Heart Disease

The three vitamins C, E and beta carotene are antioxidants (see our chapter on the proper diet). They protect the body cells by neutralizing various toxins in the body. The toxins known as free radicals destroy part of the protective layer that surrounds the cells. The American Nurses Health Study showed that people that had been taking at least 100 units of vitamin E per day over a period of more than two years were 41% less likely to suffer from cardiovascular disease than the control group. Another study showed that people who had suffered a heart attack or stroke had considerably lower levels of vitamin C and beta carotene than those of a control group. *Vitamins C, E and beta carotene are antioxidants*

Aspirin—Should We Take It Everyday?

Aspirin has been the focus of media reports for decades, and many of these reports say the same thing. Taking aspirin regularly can prevent a heart attack, lower the risk of colon cancer and diminish the frequency of migraines. But is *Aspirin protects against heart attack and colon cancer* it really necessary to take aspirin everyday or every other day, even as a prophylaxis to be on the safe side? The answer is a qualified 'no.'

Before you start taking aspirin, you should consult your doctor. Aspirin is not good for everyone. Your doctor will be able to weigh the benefits of aspirin against specific health problems.

Aspirin is a non-steroid anti-rheumatic Aspirin is actually acetylsalicylic acid. Its natural precursor is salicylic acid, which is found in the bark of the willow tree. Both salicylic acid and acetylsalicylic acid, which after synthesis is known as aspirin, can reduce pain, fever and inflammation.

Medically speaking, aspirin is an analgesic or non-steroid anti-rheumatic (NSAR). In the last few decades, scientists have discovered that aspirin interacts with the coagulation of the blood and prevents the thrombocytes from sticking together. Aspirin can therefore reduce or even prevent the formation of blood clots (so-called thrombi), which results from constricted sclerotic vessels, or arteriosclerosis. Heart attacks result when coronary vessels are blocked by just such a blood clot.

Men who have already suffered a heart attack can reduce their risk of a second attack by 30% if they regularly take aspirin. Aspirin also reduces the risks of a second stroke, a short-term blood-circulation disorder of the brain, a so-called transitory ischemic attack, a heart attack as part of an angina-pectoris attack, and complications during a heart attack.

The benefits of aspirin are not completely clear So, does this mean that aspirin can actually prevent heart disease? If you do not suffer from heart disease, then the benefits of aspirin are less clear. A study involving 22,000 male doctors in the US, the Physicians' Health Study, had one half of the doctors take aspirin every day, while the other half received a placebo (an inactive substance without any effects). After five years, it was shown that aspirin did, in fact, reduce the frequency of heart attacks by 44%, but not the total mortality rate due to cardiovascular disease. And those taking aspirin exhibited a higher rate of gastrointestinal bleeding and strokes.

Although it is very likely that aspirin can lower the risk of a first heart attack, most experts agree that the benefits of aspirin do not outweigh the risks for everyone. However, another study that looked at 600,000 adults and their frequency of gastrointestinal cancer found that those who were taking aspirin had a significantly lower incidence of colon cancer, rectal cancer and esophageal cancer. Those subjects who took 16 or more aspirin tablets per month over a period of at least one year had a 40% lower frequency of gastrointestinal cancer than those not taking aspirin. How is that so? Aspirin contains a hormone-like substance—so-called prostaglandin—which scientists assume inhibits the growth of tumors.

Aspirin contains prostaglandin, a hormone-like substance

Another tip: If you take aspirin regularly and you are about to undergo surgery, you should tell your doctor. Aspirin increases the risk of severe bleeding after a surgical intervention.

How to Reduce the Risk of a Heart Attack During Exercise

The probability of having a heart attack during cardiovascular exercise is very low. Still, if you are older, out of shape, or suffer from heart disease, you should consult your doctor before embarking on any exercise program. Here are some further recommendations:

- Exercise regularly. The cardiovascular risk rises if intensive workouts are alternated with weeks or months of inactivity.

Exercise regularly

- Avoid stop-and-start activities. It is better to take up continuous exercises such as cycling, swimming or walking.
- Do not be competitive. Avoid the physical and emotional intensity of competitive sports.
- After a large meal, wait two to three hours before starting your workout. The digestive processes draw blood away from the heart and into the gastrointestinal tract.
- Do the speech test. If you can speak without any difficulty during the exercise, then there is no risk of overexertion.
- Adapt your activities to the weather. Reduce your speed and distance when it is hot and humid.
- Do not forget those warm-up and cool-down exercises. They relieve stress, both for the heart and the muscles.
- Listen to your body. If you feel dizzy, weak or nauseous, or if you feel pressure in your chest or become short of breath, stop immediately and see your doctor.

Heart Attack During Sex—Myth or Real Danger?

Anger, over-excitement or just getting out of bed in the morning can trigger a heart attack, but the chance of this happening is very slim, so do not bother worrying about it.

There is a correlation between sex and heart attacks

But what about sex? There are plenty of tales of well-known personalities who passed away while engaging in sex.

For a long time, nothing was known about the correlation between sex and heart attacks in men.

But a study published in the Journal of the American Medical Association in 1996 shed some light on the notion that sexual intercourse could trigger a heart attack. "There was enough anecdotal evidence that made men believe that sex could be a substantial potential trigger of heart attacks," said Dr. Mittelman, "and some of it seems to be true."

The heart-attack risk is twice as high up to two hours after sexual intercourse

The scientists interviewed 850 men and women who had been sexually active during the year before their heart attack. The results were amazing. Scientists found that the risk of having a heart attack is twice as high within the two hours following intercourse. But as is the case with all statistics, some perspective must be maintained. If a very low risk level is doubled, it will remain a low risk. Statistically speaking, this means that a 50-year-old man who has had no previous heart attacks has a probability of one in a million of suffering a heart attack. After intercourse, this risk doubles to two in a million. A 50-year-old man suffering from heart disease has a risk of ten in a million before intercourse, and about twenty in a million after.

During sex, the stress hormone epinephrine is secreted

The most likely cause of these heart attacks is stress hormones like epinephrine that are secreted during sexual intercourse. Mourning can also be an important trigger, but for completely different reasons. The risk of having a heart attack the day after a close friend or family member dies increases 14-fold. Then it drops off with each day that passes.

The Monday Factor

Heart attacks occur on Mondays and in the mornings

We know that the human body has an internal clock and, therefore, its own specific rhythm, the circadian rhythm. A disproportionate number of heart attacks occur in the morning hours, especially on Mondays. The frequency of life-threatening arrhythmia is also higher on Mondays than during the rest of the week, even among people who do not have to go to work. It may be that these people are automatically associating Monday with stress.

The Miracle Drug Viagra

About 10% of men cannot achieve an erection sufficient for sexual activity. Of these cases, 80% have a physical reason.

Among the physical causes, cardiovascular disease ranks first, followed by diabetes. Many cases of erectile dysfunction are caused by drugs, especially beta blockers (used to lower high blood pressure), the heart drug digoxin, antidepressants, other hypotensive drugs and diuretics such as thiazides, as well as muscle-building anabolic steroids. Other risk factors include alcohol and nicotine, which also play a role in heart disease.

Therefore, it comes as no surprise that coronary heart disease and erectile dysfunction often occur together. A large percentage of men with coronary heart disease, who develop angina-pectoris-like problems during sexual activity, took Viagra in combination with nitroglycerine or another vasodilative drug. This led to a series of complications, from heart attacks to cardiac death. About 40% of coronary patients show angina-pectoris symptoms during intercourse after taking Viagra. Following a number of lawsuits against the manufacturer in the United States, the media jumped on the story. As the German edition of this book was going to press, the American Heart Foundation was about to publish information on this subject.

Careful: do not mix Viagra with nitroglycerine

Sexual activity for men demands energy output of about 75 watts—the same as for climbing a staircase quickly—and increases the heart rate to about 110 to 175 beats per minute during sexual activity lasting between ten and fifteen minutes.

Men's output during sex is 75 watts

Intracoital coronary death, or cardiac death during sex, has long been familiar to us. Risk factors that could trigger it include fatigue, excessive eating and drinking as well as a high emotional state.

By the end of November 1998, the American Food and Drug Administration (FDA) had reported 128 deaths related to Viagra. Three patients had suffered strokes and 77 had had cardiovascular complications; 41 of the latter group were definitive heart attacks, with 27 cardiac arrests. In another 48 cases, the cause of death is unknown. The average age at the time of death was 64, and the majority of men had taken 50 mg of sildenafil (Viagra). Sixteen men had also taken nitroglycerine or a similar vasodilative drug.

50 million tablets sold

Still, there is no end in sight to the Viagra boom. Up to the time of printing this book, there had been six million prescriptions for about 50 million tablets issued worldwide. Given these figures, the number of deaths and complications is relatively low. The FDA did not revise its benefit-risk analysis, but recommended that there be closer scrutiny.

RECOMMENDATIONS ON HOW TO USE VIAGRA

Be careful. Heart patients who regularly take nitrates must not use Viagra under any circumstances. The same goes for patients taking nitrates for a short time only. Nitrate sprays and similar substances, such as molsidomine, fall into this category as well.

Viagra is strictly prohibited if you suffer from very low blood pressure (below 90/50) and had a heart attack or stroke within the last three to six months. The same is true of:
● liver disorders
● patients suffering from heart insufficiency
● severe hypertension

You should also be careful when it comes to mixing Viagra with other medication that lowers the serum lipid level: statins, cimetidin (gastric-acid blocker) or the antibiotic erythromycin.

Too Much Coffee and Its Effect on the Body

Men (or women) who work in stressful jobs tend to consume a lot of coffee. Is there a connection between coffee and heart disease?

Four cups of coffee per day is the maximum

There have been numerous scientific studies, but with no clear results. The problem is that heavy coffee drinkers are often in high risk categories for other reasons as well. They may smoke, eat fatty food and not exercise. The final word is not out on this matter, but there is enough scientific proof of the side effects of coffee that we can safely recommend that you not drink more than three to four cups of coffee a day. Caffeinated coffee, as well as of other caffeinated drinks like tea, cola and certain soft drinks, can trigger arrhythmia and tachycardia.

Alcohol and the French Paradox

That alcoholic beverages can have any beneficial effect on your health sounds almost too good to be true. But a series of studies conducted in France and elsewhere seem to point in this direction. Epidemiological studies have shown that people who consume a moderate amount of alcohol have a 40% to 50% lower risk of developing coronary heart disease.

French men have a significantly lower rate of coronary heart disease than American men, even though they consume more fat and alcohol than the average American. The most common explanation is that the French drink more red wine. Red wine increases the good HDL cholesterol level and probably lowers the harmful LDL cholesterol. Scientists have come to the conclusion that red wine, in moderation, is not bad for the health. However, we must not forget the disadvantages that come with the regular consumption of alcohol: alcoholism, alcoholic gastritis and alcoholic cirrhosis.

1/8 of a liter of red wine a day is good for the heart

The All-Important Question: Do You Treat Your Heart Right?

By now, you know the risk factors in heart disease. The following test will tell if your lifestyle is good for your heart or if you have to make some adjustments.

	YES	NO
Do you eat a lot of red meat?	☐	☐
Do you like to eat sweets?	☐	☐
Are vegetables only rarely part of your diet?	☐	☐
Do you eat fresh fruit only rarely?	☐	☐
Do you have an elevated cholesterol level?	☐	☐
Do you know your cholesterol level?	☐	☐
Does your family have a history of cardiovascular disease?	☐	☐
Are you permanently under stress?	☐	☐
Do you have high blood pressure?	☐	☐
Are you overweight?	☐	☐
Do you suffer from diabetes?	☐	☐

Do you drink a lot of alcohol every day (more than half a liter)?	☐	☐
Do you never have a physical?	☐	☐
Has it been a long time since your last EKG?	☐	☐
Do you exercise only rarely?	☐	☐
Are you engaged in sedentary activities?	☐	☐
Do everyday affairs weigh you down?	☐	☐
Do you often have problems at work?	☐	☐
Do you take everything personally?	☐	☐
Do you smoke more than five cigarettes a day?	☐	☐

Up to 7 affirmative answers:

Your lifestyle is such that you deliberately or subconsciously are trying to do the best for your heart. Still, be careful with the known risk factors.

8 to 14 affirmative answers:

You are on your way to doing long-term damage to your heart. Try to follow the recommendations in this book and live a healthier life. Avoid risk factors, and consult your physician.

15 and more affirmative answers:

You lead a dangerous lifestyle. The heart is the engine of life. You should not forget this, and change your ways quickly if you want to grow old in good health. Discuss this with your doctor and have your cardiac condition and EKG checked.

The Virtual Heart

In the future, it will be easier to explore the male heart and its peculiarities. The heart as generated by computer software has become a reality.

The virtual heart has become a reality

Scientists have managed to simulate the human heart and all its workings on a computer. The simulated heart is surprisingly real, as if it had just been lifted from a person's chest cavity. The virtual heart is a three-dimensional image of the human heart, with all the properties and all the inherent and potential weaknesses of a real heart.

Using just such a "cyberheart," scientists at Oxford University and the Johns Hopkins University in Baltimore are trying simulate the function of individual heart cells, the effects of hormones and metabolic products, as well as the effects of drugs. Using a computer program, they are able to play out scenarios such as arteriosclerosis or angina pectoris on a screen. By 2010, this method will possibly have become a tool in the everyday treatment of heart disease.

THE HEART AS THE ENGINE OF LIFE

- The heart beats about 41 million times a year.
- Each year, it pumps 2.6 million liters of blood through the body.
- 55% of all deaths are due to heart disease.
- Up to two hours after sexual intercourse, the risk, though low, of a heart attack is doubled.
- Taking aspirin regularly can lower the risk of a heart attack by 44%.
- The amino acid homocystein increases the risk of a heart attack by a factor of 2.4.
- Omega-3 fatty acid (in fish, for example) minimizes the risk of thrombosis and has a positive effect on a number of cardiac factors.

Under Pressure

High Blood Pressure–The Enemy Within

The two friends just wanted to have fun. Ever since their schooldays, they have shared a passion for cars, betting on horses, smoking, long nights at bars and clubs, and just plain having fun.

Both are successful real estate brokers. One used to race motorcycles, while the other has always been the classic couch potato.

They are now advanced in years and have gained some extra pounds. Both are under immense stress in their work. One always had a very red complexion and frequent pressure in the chest. So, just for the heck of it, the two decided at a health fair to have their blood pressure taken.

Following standard procedure, a paramedic applied a cuff to the upper arm and started pumping. In moments the results were ready. Baffled at first, the paramedic repeated the process to the concern of his patients. What numbers did he come up with? The results read: 205/115 for the non-athlete, and 190/110 for the sports-loving broker. At first, they refused to believe the readings, and the paramedic suggested that it might have resulted from the excitement and stress of the test.

With the warning that high blood pressure, if left untreated, could lead to cardiac insufficiency, arteriosclerosis, heart attacks or strokes, he advised them to see their physicians. When they hesitated, he added mental debility and impotence to the list, and the two friends immediately booked appointments for a checkup.

One in two men fails to check his blood pressure

Do you know your blood pressure level? If not, then you are just like the 50% of Austrians who have not had their blood pressure taken in years and prefer not to worry about it. In fact, one in four adults in Austria suffers from high blood pressure, but about 800,000 of those affected are not even aware of their condition. How is this possible?

The problem is that high blood pressure (or hypertension) has no symptoms for a long time. Hypertension is the most common disease in Western countries and the most prominent risk factor in strokes and heart attacks. Hypertension, if not treated, can shorten a person's life span considerably. For example, a 35-year-old man with a constantly elevated blood pressure of more than 150/100 will probably die at 60, or 16 years younger than the average life expectancy of 76. By normalizing the blood pressure level, life expectancy can be restored to the normal range provided there are no other risk factors involved. It is interesting to note that more men than pre-menopausal women suffer from hypertension. However, with the onset of the climacteric, hypertension occurs more frequently among women. It would appear that the male and female sex hormones provide protection not only against cardiovascular disease, but also against hypertension.

If untreated, a man with high blood pressure dies 16 years sooner

A Reading of 130/85 mm/Hg is the New Norm for Adults

The World Health Organization (WHO) and the International Society of Hypertension recently published new guidelines for the diagnosis and treatment of hypertension.

Normal blood pressure for younger and middle-aged people is set at below 130/85 mm/Hg (mercury). Optimal blood pressure for younger people would be below 120/80 mm/Hg. These levels are based on recent studies that have shown that the risk of cardiovascular disease increases continuously as the blood pressure rises above them. What are considered to be normal levels are, thus, much lower than originally thought. The old rule of thumb of 100 + your age has been discredited.

The optimal blood pressure is 120/80 mm/Hg for young men

When Do You Require Treatment?

According to the new guidelines, blood pressure can be optimal (120/80), normal (130/85) or high-to-normal (130-139/85-89). High blood pressure is broken down into three stages:

- Stage 1:   140-159/90-99 mm/Hg
- Stage 2:   160-179/100-109 mm/Hg
- Stage 3:   higher than or equal to 180/110 mm/Hg

Blood pressure is measured at two different points. The higher blood pressure reading, or systolic pressure, is measured when the heart ventricles are contracting. The second reading, the diastolic pressure, is taken when the ventricles are relaxed and refilling (between heartbeats).

The systolic pressure is the blood pressure as the heart strikes a beat

In order to avoid a faulty measurement, you should sit comfortably and keep your arms at heart level. In the thirty minutes before the readings are taken, you should not have any caffeinated food or drinks and you should not smoke. The blood pressure should be taken after you have been sitting still for at least five minutes. With upper arm sphygmomanometers, it is important to adjust the cuff to the arm's circumference. In the case of self-test kits that are applied to the wrist, you should ensure that the cuff is not too tight, as this may distort the readings. Just to be sure, you should take two or more sets of readings, each two minutes apart. Your blood pressure level would be the average of all the readings.

Do not drink coffee before checking your blood pressure

If the first two numbers deviate from each other by more than 5 mm/Hg, you should take additional measurements and compute the average. Blood pressure varies quite a bit. The systolic pressure may fluctuate by 60 mm/Hg, and the diastolic pressure by 40 mm/Hg. For comparison's sake, therefore, you should always take your blood pressure at the same time of day.

Blood pressure is subject to enormous fluctuation in the course of a day. It is at its highest during mid-morning hours. At night, it drops 10% to 15%. It should also be pointed out that self-measured blood pressure levels are usually lower than those measured by a doctor, since people are usually calmer at home.

The blood pressure drops by 15% during the night

Doctors call this phenomenon "white-coat hypertension." The reason for this is a reaction of the vegetative nervous system. Nervousness and anxiety lead to an increase in blood pressure.

The Biorhythm of Blood Pressure

As already mentioned, blood pressure varies with the time of day. But it also depends on the type of physical activity as well as on psychological and emotional factors. Over a period of 24 hours, blood pressure has a typical progression. After a person wakes up, the blood pressure rises sharply and continues to do so for the rest of the morning. After lunch, the blood pressure drops for about an hour, only to rise again throughout the afternoon. In the evening, there is a slight peak, and at night it drops significantly. It is at its lowest level during sleep.

A flushed complexion is often a sign of hypertension

What are the usual symptoms of hypertension? Often, they are atypical complaints such as sleep disorders, excessive sweating, diminished performance or a flushed complexion. More typical symptoms are dizziness, pressure in the head, frequent headaches, an oppressive feeling and shortness of breath. But all these symptoms usually occur at a more advanced stage, when the blood pressure is already significantly elevated. By then, the hypertension, having been untreated for years, has already caused considerable harm to the blood vessels.

Men who suffer from hypertension often suffer from impotence as well. Only rarely is this caused by medication taken for the hypertension.

In 95% of Cases, the Cause Is Unknown

Secondary high blood pressure often has organic causes

There are two types of hypertension—primary and secondary. Secondary means that hypertension is caused by a physical problem. But this is only the case for 5% of people suffering from hypertension. Typical of such physical problems would be kidney disease or an adrenal condition, hyperthyroidism or the constriction of a renal artery.

About 95% of hypertensive patients have primary or essential high blood pressure, the actual cause of which is unknown to this day. There is some speculation about hereditary or environmental factors, excessive salt intake, excess body weight and stress.

THE KNOWN RISK FACTORS IN HYPERTENSION

● Genetic (in about 50% of patients)
● Overweight
● Stress
● Alcohol
● Too much salt

In 50% of hypertensive patients, the condition is caused by genetic factors. In other words, it is hereditary. This is of special importance, because men with this genetic predisposition usually exhibit symptoms much sooner, usually between the ages of 35 and 55. Therefore, if the parents suffer from hypertension, it is crucial to have the children regularly checked out.

Other significant factors leading to high blood pressure are excess body weight and the excessive intake of salt (sodium chloride).

We consume about five times as much salt as the body needs. Usually, we excrete the surplus salt with the urine. But people whose ability to excrete salt is defective react to increased salt consumption with an increase in blood pressure. A large-scale international study called Intersalt, involving 10,000 people, showed a clear connection in salt-sensitive people between the intake of salt through food and their blood pressure level.

We consume five times as much salt as we really need

American scientists have come up with a possible explanation for the various degrees of salt-sensitivity. They found that salt-sensitive people have a mutated gene for the messenger substance angiotensin. Only an extreme low-salt diet is effective for such people. In about two to three years, this genetic test will probably have become routine, and people will be able to know in advance whether or not to go on a low-salt diet.

A modified gene for angiotensin affects sensitivity

Other triggers of hypertension are bad diets, too much alcohol, lack of exercise, lack of minerals and, as recently claimed, second-hand smoke and cell phone signals. It has long been a common belief that coffee leads to high blood pressure, but there is no scientific proof of this as yet. However, the consumption of alcohol, especially when taken regularly in larger quantities, has been roundly condemned. As with salt, some people are more sensitive to alcohol than others. Men and women also differ as to the amount of alcohol they can

A poor diet can cause high blood pressure

consume without endangering their health, and there are individual differences among men in their threshold for alcohol.

Impatient and ambitious men are more prone to high blood pressure

One question has always been debated. Is there is something along the lines of a "hypertension personality profile." Psychological studies have shown that the alpha-type male is the more likely to suffer from hypertension. The alpha-male is characterized by his fierce competitiveness, impatience, ambition, need for recognition, suppressed aggressiveness and sense of time pressure.

Many Hypertensive Patients Snore

Snorers have a higher heart-attack risk

Another characteristic of hypertensive patients, almost exclusively among men, is a tendency to snore. Snorers are also more likely to be overweight and to have a higher risk of heart attack or stroke. Snoring is often attributed to abnormal daytime fatigue. Snorers frequently feel more irritable during the day, and can be drowsy or moody. If you detect any of these symptoms in your own behavior, have your blood pressure checked several times and consult your physician.

It is established fact that blood pressure is closely connected with weight, the amount of fluid intake, and the consumption of salt—the higher those factors, the higher the blood pressure.

HYPERTENSION IS A DEATH TRAP

A number of studies on men have shown that there is a direct correlation between high blood pressure, strokes, heart disease and kidney failure. Hypertensive men are:
- three times more likely to suffer from coronary disease,
- six times more likely to suffer from myocardial insufficiency and
- seven times more likely to suffer a stroke than men with normal, controlled blood pressure.

Hypertension causes the heart muscle to become thicker

The body can be compared with a refinery, with its miles of tubes and pipelines. As the body's main 'boiler,' the heart has to work harder in event of high blood pressure. In order to transport the blood through the pipes at the elevated level of pressure, the heart must increase its own level of performance. The result is that the heart muscle—like any other muscle under increased strain—becomes thicker and thicker.

But this leads to a number of complications. Once the heart muscle becomes too thick, it cannot perform at its most efficient anymore. High blood pressure in the 'pipelines' also accelerates the onset of arteriosclerosis, which affects all the blood vessels, from the largest to the smallest. This increases the probability of a stroke or a heart attack. It may also result in the development of aneurysms. Even in the case of mild hypertension, the ongoing damage that is being done to the blood vessels can harm the kidneys and result in kidney failure if left untreated over several years.

A 24-hour blood pressure check will provide answers

For a better understanding of high blood pressure and its consequences, take part in a public blood pressure program. You will have to wear a cuff with a blood pressure recorder around the clock. This will monitor your blood pressure on a typical workday. The doctor will be able to follow the fluctuations by day and by night.

A blood pressure profile makes it possible to identify certain rare secondary forms of hypertension. These secondary forms may be due to kidney disease, hyperthyroidism, the constriction of a renal artery or the secretion of the adrenal hormone. After identifying a secondary form of hypertension, a further search for the underlying causes is necessary. Generally, hypertensive men should also have an eye test to determine if there is any micro-damage to the vessels of the fundus of the eye, as well as an ultrasound of the heart muscle and both kidneys.

Have your eyes checked if you suffer from hypertension

I Have High Blood Pressure—What Do I Do Now?

The answer is as easy as ABC—lead a healthy lifestyle. But most people do not want to hear that.

A healthy lifestyle is the best remedy for high blood pressure

Alcohol has been proven to be one of the main causes of hypertension in men. Numerous scientific studies have shown that by reducing the consumption of alcohol, or by staying away from it all together, the blood pressure can drop and sometimes even return to normal levels. In most cases, a reduction is sufficient. There is no need to become a teetotaler.

Recent genetic research has shown that, as with salt, men have different degrees of sensitivity when it comes to alcohol tolerance and a tendency toward high blood pressure. In other words, not all men react the same way. But alcohol often leads to another very different, though just as serious, result. It supplies the body with a lot of calories, which can lead to excess weight.

Half of all men
with hypertension
are overweight

Body weight has a very strong influence on blood pressure. About half of all men suffering from hypertension are overweight. This probably makes it the factor most commonly leading to hypertension. Losing ten pounds can lower the blood pressure by one percent. In some cases, cutting back on salt may also reduce blood pressure.

There are many non-medicated treatments for high blood pressure. As an example, 30 to 45 minutes a week of any kind of moderate endurance exercise can reduce the blood pressure by 10 mm/Hg.

A Healthy Diet Can Take Off Some of That Pressure

A diet rich in fiber
minimizes blood
pressure by about
11.5 mm/Hg

A recently published study has shown that a diet low in fat and rich in fiber (vegetables, fruit) can lower the blood pressure by an average of 11.5 mm/Hg (systolic) and 5.5 mm/Hg (diastolic). Forty percent of the hypertensive patients in the study were able to stop taking their medication after going on such a diet.

Another study, at Harvard University, called Dash, has shown that a low-fat, fiber-rich diet—eight to nine portions of fruit and vegetables, less meat, more poultry, fish and low-fat dairy products—has the same effect after two to four weeks as mild hypotensive medication, but without the side effects. For breakfast, the experimental subjects had muesli, orange juice, low-fat milk and bread with low-fat margarine. For lunch, they had turkey schnitzel with raw vegetables and a plate of fruit. Dinner consisted of fish, broccoli, tomato salad and a plate of strawberries.

Nicotine damages
the arteries

It is important to reduce the stress in your life and stay away from cigarettes. Not only does nicotine have a direct or indirect influence on blood pressure, but, like high cholesterol and blood sugar levels, it damages the arteries and speeds up the process of arteriosclerosis, thereby increasing your risk of suffering a heart attack or a stroke.

Other effective remedies include old fashioned R & R—relaxation, sleep, vacationing, or staying at a health resort—and stress management. By following this advice, you can prevent a catastrophe like a heart attack or stroke while still in your prime.

HOT—Hypertension Optimal Treatment—is the name of the largest study of the disease ever conducted anywhere in the world. It involved 19,000 patients and proved that reducing the blood pressure could drastically lower the risk that patients would develop a secondary disease. Check your blood pressure level regularly, and remember that high blood pressure is reversible if caught in time. The treatment of high blood pressure is hindered by problems arising from a lack of detailed knowledge of hypertensive conditions. New treatments that work differently and have fewer side effects are in the development stages. In future, ever smaller groups of patients with more precisely identified types of hypertension will be diagnosed using completely new microbiological methods. In some cases, it will be possible to predict the effectiveness of treatments before they are administered.

Check your blood pressure regularly

Warning: If you are taking any of the following medications or substances, your blood pressure may be difficult to control.
- Nose drops
- Asthma medication, sympathomimetic drugs
- Appetite suppressants
- Cocaine or hallucinogens
- Excessive caffeine
- Adrenal steroids
- Antidepressants
- Non-cortisone antirheumatics
- Erythropoietin

Panic attacks and chronic pain can also lead to high blood pressure.

Panic attacks can cause high blood pressure

The most common drugs now available are primarily diuretics and, for younger patients, beta blockers or the next generation of ACE inhibitors, as well as angiotensin-II blockers. There are also alpha blockers and calcium antagonists, and scientists at large pharmaceutical companies are working on totally new forms of treatment. At this point, it is not possible to say whether these new substances (dopamine antagonists, rennin inhibitors, potassium channel openers, inhibitors of neutral endopeptidase) will prove effective.

It's a Man's Business

No Need to Be Ashamed of Prostate and Testicular Problems

The Safe Deposit Box for Sperm—The Prostate

It is a never-ending story, one that drives a man to despair. You feel the urge to go to the washroom, but when it comes to the moment of expected relief, nothing happens. And if it does, it is just a few droplets. This phenomenon comes and goes and normally you would not give it a second thought.

Every man suffers from prostate problems at some point in his life

The urge to urinate, which goes away at the moment of relief, is triggered by a gland that most men do not know anything about. Yet, it is one that affects their lives in a big way—the prostate. Almost every man in the Western world, according to estimates of the WHO, has prostate problems at least once in his life. One in three men has to undergo surgery at some point.

The prostate weighs only 15 to 20 grams

The prostate is of vital importance to human life. It is responsible for the liquefaction and activation of semen leading to the production of sperm. A healthy prostate weighs only about 15 to 20 grams, and its size and form are similar to a ripe chestnut. It is made up of millions of small glands as well as muscle and fiber cells. The glandular tissue is surrounded by a layer of connective tissue. The center contains the upper part of the urethra. The prostate gland itself is situated below the bladder on the pelvic floor muscles. In the back, the gland touches the front surface of the rectum.

Its growth is controlled by testosterone

The prostate gland belongs to the sex organs. It already exists at birth, but it does not reach its full size until the end of puberty. Its growth is controlled by the sex hormones, especially testosterone. But it has one design flaw. With age, it becomes enlarged, and that is where the trouble begins.

How the Prostate Protects the Sperm

Not all of the functions of the prostate gland are fully known. The most important, however, is the production of the whitish secretion that makes up about 30% to 40% of the male ejaculation. This secretion supplies the sperm with nutrients such as amino acids and sugar. It also activates the mobility of the sperm. The characteristic smell of seminal fluid is caused by the prostatic fluid.

The prostate secretion protects sperm in the vagina

Another function of the secretion is to protect the sperm in the female vagina from the acidic environment there, which itself protects the vagina from bacteria. In addition, the prostate gland is responsible for the ejaculation of sperm. It prevents urine from flowing back into the seminal duct and the testicles. It also produces enzymes such as acidic phosphatase and the prostate-specific antigen (PSA), which keep the semen liquid so that the sperm can move around more easily. These two enzymes are very important in the diagnosis of prostatitis and prostate cancer, as you will see in the chapter on "The Silent Killer."

An analysis of prostate conditions requires a urine sample and the palpation of the prostate by inserting the finger through the rectum. By doing this, the doctor can feel the size and shape of the prostrate and the existence of any abnormalities, such as nodules or swelling. A blood test or an ultrasound, through the abdominal wall or transrectally, may be required as well. For this purpose, a tiny ultrasonic device is inserted into the rectum, and the structure of the entire prostate gland in all its depth is displayed on a screen.

The most common condition that occurs is the enlargement of the prostate in older men (benign prostate hypertrophy/BPH). This is completely normal and, in general, benign. But one in three men may experience more serious problems with it over the course of time.

Rectal ultrasound: the probe is inserted through the rectum

Usually, BPH starts with difficulty in urinating. The emptying of the bladder is delayed, the urinary stream takes a couple of seconds. Sometimes, the urinary stream may suddenly stop in the middle of urination and not resume until many seconds later. The force of the stream is diminished, and after urination, "terminal dribbling" may occur.

Other symptoms are an ability to urinate only under strain, incontinence, an unpleasant feeling during urination, increased urinary urgency and nocturia. Often, there are also sensations of incomplete emptying.

Warning sign: the urinary stream stops abruptly during urination

The causes of benign prostate hypertrophy have not been fully exposed yet. But there is agreement that the onset of this condition is based on a change in the ratio of male and female sex hormones. Testosterone, which is transformed into dihydrotestosterone (DHT) by the 5-alpha reductase enzyme in the prostate gland, almost certainly plays a huge part in it. This enzyme is of great importance because some drugs inhibit 5-alpha reductase production as a treatment for prostate enlargement.

5-alpha reductase inhibits prostate enlargement

The enlargement of the prostate gland brings with it many changes to a man's lifestyle. Most men reduce their intake of fluids (a male bladder can hold about half a liter of urine), especially before going to bed. They may feel depressed about their condition, with their need to know at all times where the nearest washroom is as a constant reminder. In the case of severe prostate enlarge-

An average bladder holds half a liter of urine

ment, they also experience a diminished libido and difficulty maintaining an erection.

An increase in the size of the prostate gland and the narrowing of the urethra can also cause bladder problems. Because the bladder has to void against resistance, the bladder muscles are overexerted. Another consequence may be the thickening and deformation of the bladder muscles. If the urethra constricts any further, the bladder will not be able to empty completely. This is referred to as residual urine. The bladder muscles may also become stretched as a result of the constant strain. This produces a sudden urge to urinate and the permanent feeling of incomplete emptying. The danger here is that there could be reflux of urine in the draining urinary tract. This creates a veritable hotbed for germs, which cause inflammation of the bladder, urethra and even of the renal pelvis and the kidneys, with potentially disastrous consequences.

Urine reflux often causes bladder inflammation

How Dangerous Is an Enlarged Prostate?

If the symptoms are weak, it suffices just to keep an eye on them. If the problems get worse, you should have your prostate checked regularly at short intervals. When it comes to treatment, discuss with your urologist the different options: herbal remedies, drugs or surgery.

The urologic examination may be performed using the following methods:

1. Palpation
Even when performed by a highly experienced urologist, palpation of the prostate (i.e., examination by touch through the rectum) does not guarantee that small cancerous growths will be detected.

2. Urine sample
Urine is tested for sugar, protein and PSA

The urine sample is used to analyze the sugar and protein content in the urine. It includes the so-called three-glass test, which helps determine if there are any pathogens in the urine (bacteria, red blood cells, micro-organisms, etc.).

3. Measurement of urinary outflow
Uroflowmetry: measuring the urinary stream

Uroflowmetry is a modern method that measures the rate of the urinary stream to assess the severity of the obstruction. This examination is completely painless. The man has to urinate into a special toilet using a tube that is connected to an electronic measuring device. The results are printed out as a diagram. In the case of normal voiding, the urinary curve at first rises sharply, only to drop just as quickly. This method allows for a painless diagnosis of any obstruction of the urinary stream (e.g., in the case of BPH) as well as of constricted urethras and impaired coordination of the bladder and sphincter muscles.

4. The prostate-specific antigen (PSA)

Another examination involves measuring the prostate-specific antigen (PSA). This is a protein that is produced almost exclusively by prostate cells. The analysis is done on the basis of a simple blood sample. If your PSA level is shown to be elevated, you should definitely see a specialist for further tests. PSA is also a tumor marker (see the chapter, "The Silent Killer"). The serum level of this protein is elevated in the case of almost all benign conditions of the gland, but it is extremely high in the presence of a malignant disease. Higher concentration levels, therefore, may indicate cancer even five years or more before a tumor is palpable or shows any symptoms whatsoever.

An elevated PSA level is a warning sign

Although an elevated PSA level does not signify a diagnosis of prostate cancer in all cases, it certainly requires a closer urologic examination. It must also be noted that normal levels change with age as the prostate gland grows in size.

- Up to the age of 50   max. 2.5 nanograms/ml
- Between 51 and 60   max. 3.5 nanograms/ml
- Between 61 and 70   max. 4.5 nanograms/ml
- Over 70   max. 6.5 nanograms/ml

In the last two years of the 20th century, the American Cancer Society and the American Association of Urologists published a number of recommendations. In one of the studies on which they based their recommendations, 1,000 men older than 50 with a PSA level between 2.6 and 4.0 were given a checkup. A finger examination did not reveal anything unusual, yet it turned out that one in five suffered from prostate cancer. This was discovered after conducting a trial biopsy. Perhaps we can conclude that a man should not feel completely safe just because he has a normal PSA level and positive results from a finger examination. Follow-up exams and observations are very important.

A harmless PSA level does not provide 100% protection

X-rays are sometimes taken as well. In such cases, the doctor looks for signs of sclerosis in the abdominal region. The patient is injected with a contrast medium, which concentrates in the kidneys and is excreted through the draining urinary tract and the bladder.

New methods of examination include computer tomography and nuclear magnetic resonance tomography. By means of layered x-ray images or a strong magnetic field, the minor pelvis is examined, without any exposure to radiation. Both methods employ the latest technology, but they do not yet provide reliable and conclusive information about the prostate gland.

Bladder stones are crushed during urethroscopy

Essential diagnostic methods for detecting changes to the urethra or the bladder are urethroscopy and cystoscopy. A five-millimeter instrument is inserted into the urethra and then into the bladder. The examining doctor can see any irregularities in the urethra or the bladder on a monitor. During such an exam, the doctor can also crush small bladder stones or take tissue samples. Formerly, these would have required extensive abdominal surgery. The examination is usually done on an outpatient basis, is painless and is carried out with the patient under local anesthesia.

Another valuable examination, which allows benign irregularities to be distinguished from malignant ones, is the biopsy. For this test, the doctor takes tissue samples by going in through the rectum. By means of an aspiration biopsy, prostate cells are siphoned off through a hollow needle. These cells are then sent to a laboratory to be analyzed under a microscope. In rare cases, a punch biopsy may be employed.

Phytopharmaceutic as help against prostate problems

If the samples are negative, yet the prostate is causing problems such as a frequent urge to urinate, then the benign enlargement of the gland can be treated with drugs. There are many herbal medications, or phytopharmaceuticals, available in different formats, such as tablets or tea. The best known are stinging nettle, pumpkin seed, umbrella dwarf palm, South African star grass, goldenrod, pygeum africanum, serenoa repens and rye-pollen extract.

Exercise can protect against prostate conditions

An American study carried out by the Harvard School of Public Health found that physical activity (e.g., walking, running, rowing, or swimming) provides protection against prostate problems. Since the muscle tone of the nonstriated prostatic muscles is diminished during exercise, active men have a lower risk of developing a benign enlargement of the prostate. Men who engage in several hours of regular exercise each week, it was shown, can lower their risk by up to 25%.

Moderate symptoms can be treated only with drugs. Drugs can reduce the cramping of the bladder (spasmolytics).

There are two categories of drugs:
- One group consists of alpha blockers that reduce muscle tension in the bladder neck and the prostate gland. These treatments can provide relief from

problems such as the frequent urge to urinate and delayed urination. But these drugs do not address the problem of enlargement.

- The latest remedies actually reduce the size of the enlarged prostate gland. Such drugs (e.g., Finasterid®) inhibit the 5-alpha reductase enzyme, which converts the male sex hormone testosterone into dihydrotestosterone. The drugs in this group can result in a 20% reduction in the size of an enlarged prostate.

Alpha blockers lower the muscle tension of the bladder neck

If the drugs do not take effect, surgery is the only other option. Prostate surgery is inevitable:

- if the condition is so severe that drugs are ineffective,
- if the kidneys or the bladder could potentially be harmed,
- in the case of overflow incontinence and urine reflux, and
- in case of cancer

Before opting for surgery, you should discuss it thoroughly with your urologist (including all the possible risks and consequences).

In contrast to surgery for malignant growths, the entire prostate gland is not removed in the case of benign irregularities. Only the proliferative gland tissue is removed.

The transurethral resection of the prostate (TURP) involves the removal of proliferative tissue by means of an electric wire sling through the urethra. This type of surgery is a lot less risky than open surgery, which involves the removal of the prostate gland through an abdominal incision. Because of the high risk associated with open prostate surgery, it is hardly ever performed on older patients. Other methods include cryosurgery and laser surgery.

TURP: surgery through the urethra

What About Sex After Prostate Surgery?

Since, in most cases, the entire prostate gland is not removed, surgery—especially transurethral surgery—does not necessarily have a negative effect on potency, erectility or libido. Occasionally, men complain of a less intense orgasm. This may stem from the fact that in one-third of the men who have undergone surgery, some of the sperm flows back to the bladder during ejaculation, which would indeed cause some reduction in the intensity. From a medical point of view, this is completely harmless, for the sperm is washed out of the bladder the next time the man urinates. Fertility may be reduced somewhat, but potency is not affected.

Prostate surgery has no effect on libido or potency

A major worry for men who face the decision of whether to have their prostate removed is the question of impotence and the urethra's inability to close. Apart from the psychological problems that come with a diagnosis of cancer, it can indeed happen that nerves get severed during the operation, rendering the patient incapable of having an erection. Recent surgical practice involves leaving the nerve bundles running along the prostate intact rather than removing them, which lowers the risk of impotence and incontinence. In the event of impotence, a sufficient erection can be achieved using drugs (Viagra), or by means of penile prostheses or penile injections of a substance that will act on the blood vessels. For more information on the diagnosis and treatment of prostate cancer, see the chapter titled "The Silent Killer."

Viagra helps with impotence

The Pathology of the Prostate Gland

• Acute prostatitis

Careful: acute prostatitis can affect other organs

Acute prostatitis is a sudden infection of the prostate gland that results in the inflammation of part of the gland. Frequently, acute prostatitis may lead to an inflammation of the bladder (cystitis). This will require immediate treatment to prevent it from infecting adjacent organs. It is possible that the tissue of the prostate may become purulent and form abscesses. In extreme cases, the urethra may be blocked. The signs and symptoms of acute prostatitis are the sudden onset of moderate to high fever, chills, pain during urination with a burning sensation in the urethra, urinary urgency (resulting in small amounts of urine) only a short time after the last urination. Typically, a man would also experience pain in the back and lumbar vertebrae as well as in the lower abdomen (between the rectum and testicles). In extreme cases, there may be blood or pus in the urine, and even bowel movements could be painful. The most common triggers are intestinal bacteria and bacteria that are sexually transmitted (e.g., chlamydia, gonococci or fungi). Treatment of acute prostatitis is with antibiotics. The sexual partners must also be notified because they may have been infected as well.

• Chronic prostatitis

Back pains may point to chronic prostatitis

Chronic prostatitis is an infection of the glandular tissue. In some cases, it may be the result of acute prostatitis. The symptoms are usually less severe than those of the acute kind. It may possibly be linked to other inflammations of the urinary tract. Chronic prostatitis is partly triggered by bacteria, but also by anatomical changes such as the narrowing of the bladder neck or of the urethra; by external mechanical irritation of the prostate due, for example, to cycling or sitting down too long; or by reducing the temperature of the abdomen.

The problems and the symptoms are manifold. The key symptom is a painful and unpleasant sensation in the lower abdomen, which may sometimes radiate into the groin and testicles. Many men tend to confuse this feeling with backache. Other symptoms are increased urinary frequency and a burning sensation during urination, painful ejaculation, a watery outflow from the urethra or premature ejaculation. If the seminal vesicles become infected as well, the ejaculate will in most cases contain traces of blood, which can be quite a shock to the man. In addition, if the seminal tract and seminal vesicles are infected, he may experience pain during sexual intercourse.

Inflammations lead to blood in ejaculate

An infection caused by bacteria or other pathogens is treated with antibiotics as well as anti-inflammatory drugs or analgesics. Other possible treatments are a warm half-hour bath and a prostate massage. Also possible are microwave-hyperthermia, acupuncture, laser treatment, relaxation techniques and, in serious cases, sedatives and spasmolytics. For chronic non-bacterial prostatitis or chronic prostate problems, it is advisable to stick to a low-fat diet that is rich in vegetables and fiber, to avoid congestion and to drastically reduce alcohol, caffeine and nicotine (these can have a direct negative effect) intake.

Warm baths and massages

The Testicles—The Center of Masculinity

The testicles are the male sex glands, two oval-shaped organs with a length of about four centimeters and a diameter of approximately two centimeters. Located in the scrotum, they are positioned slightly raised to protect against any external pressure. The scrotum consists of an outer, almost hairless, skin and an inner layer of muscle tissue. Each testicle is made up of chambers that contain the convoluted seminiferous tubules. They are surrounded by a protective capsule.

The testicles have two main functions. They produce spermatozoa that are required for procreation, and they produce hormones, testosterone in particular, in the Leydig cells that are key to the development of the male body. The testicles lie surrounded by a firm fibrous capsule in the scrotum at the end of a spermatic cord outside the abdominal cavity. The reason for this is that the production of semen/sperm requires a lower temperature than is found in the interior of the body.

The testicles are the main producer of hormones

Sperm requires a lower temperature to survive

Sperm as a Source of Energy

Results of recent studies have raised a few eyebrows. In Denmark, older men have more sperm than younger ones. In the US, the sperm count has been constant for 60 years, while the population of Hamburg saw its sperm count drop by half between 1956 and 1995.

Now, for the first time, scientists at the university hospital in Kiel, Germany, seem to have discovered a possible cause. They found that, among 22 infants between the ages of one and twelve months, those that had plastic diapers had a higher testicular temperature than those with cotton diapers. "There may be a link to infertility later in life, and it is being explored further," says Prof. Wolfgang Sippel, who is in charge of the study.

Seminal tubes are six meters long

The seminiferous tubules in the testicles continue into the epididymis. The epididymis is a network of tubes for storing sperm. If these tubes were laid out in a line one by one, the line would be five to six meters (16 to 18 feet) long.

When the sperm moves from the testicles to the epididymis, it has usually not yet fully matured. It is in the epididymis that the sperm becomes fully capable of fertilization.

Sperm contains sugar, protein and prostaglandin

During an orgasm, the sperm leaves the epididymis and goes, through the seminal duct, to the penis. Before it reaches the penis, it comes into contact with the prostate and the seminal vesicles, which are located between the bladder and the rectum. The seminal vesicles give off a fluid rich in a protein that gives it a viscous quality. This seminal fluid contains a number of substances, especially sugar, that provide the sperm with energy. But it also contains other essential substances such as prostaglandin. The most important function of prostaglandin is to stimulate the cervix of the uterus so that it opens more widely, making it easier for the sperm, headed for the ovum, to enter the uterus.

The Color Codes of the Ejaculate

If the sperm is not white, it may indicate a number of conditions. There are four typical color variations: crystal-clear, brownish, red-brown or yellow.

It is completely normal for a clear fluid, the prostate secretion, to trickle out before ejaculation.

Red sperm points to ruptured vessel

If the sperm is brownish or yellowish and cloudy, an inflammation of the prostate gland and/or seminal vesicle is likely. If the sperm is clearly red or red-brown, it is likely that blood has gotten into the sperm. The most common cause would be the rupture of a small blood vessel in the prostate, which occurs mostly after the age of 45, when the prostate starts to enlarge significantly. If there is blood in the sperm on a regular basis, a urologist should be consulted. Apart from an inflammation or high blood pressure, the reason could be a malignant growth of the prostate gland.

Sperm or ejaculate that is yellow is usually due to the insufficiency of the constrictor muscle of the bladder. Normally, the bladder is closed during ejaculation. But if the muscle does not function properly, urine may become mixed with the sperm. By itself, this is not a cause for concern. If the problem persists, however, a urologist should be consulted to have the bladder muscle checked out.

Yellow sperm means the sphincter of your bladder does not work

The Pathology of the Testicles

● Strangulation of the testicles (testicular torsion)

The characteristic complaints are sudden acute pains in one testicle along with swelling and redness of the scrotum, sensitivity to touch, nausea, vomiting, tendency to vascular collapse, sometimes even fever. The pain usually radiates into the groin.

If you experience sudden acute pain in the testicles, treat it as a true emergency situation. It may happen while you sleep or during exercise. Testicular torsion is, by and large, a rare complication. But it can happen at any age, especially between early childhood and puberty. It is very rare, however, in babies. The strangulation of the blood vessels is dangerous as the testicles may necrotize within hours. Therefore, you should see a doctor at once. Usually, the condition requires immediate surgery to reposition the testes. In some cases, the doctor may be able, through skillful manipulation, to reposition the testes without surgery. But even that does not mean that surgery can ultimately be prevented, because the testicle tends to twist around again. So, surgery may be required after all in order to anchor the testicle in its normal position.

Strangulating the vessels kills the testicles

● Epididymitis

The characteristic symptoms of epididymitis are hardened and painful epididymides and testicles. In addition, the skin of the scrotum is red, there is fever and a burning sensation during urination, as well as pain that starts gradually and continues for hours and days. The pain radiates into the groin. The most common cause of epididymitis is an infection brought on by bacteria or viruses, almost exclusively transmitted through sexual intercourse. In some cases,

In the event of epididymitis, the sex partner needs to be treated as well

epididymitis may be the consequence of an inflammation of the urethra below the prostate. Usually, only one side is affected. The condition can be controlled pretty well by drugs, and it usually leaves the sexual organs undamaged. In very rare cases, it may evolve into chronic epididymitis, which may require surgery (again, in exceptional cases). Generally, antibiotics and drugs that reduce swelling are used. It is important, however, to inform your sexual partners of the condition. It does not matter whether they have symptoms or not, they have to be told and treated prophylactically. Recovery can be helped along by staying in bed, by putting ice on the scrotum and, if the pain is severe, by taking analgesics.

● Testicular pain

Testicular pain is often connected to fever

The testicles are highly sensitive. Even medium pressure or a blow of medium force can result in terrible pain. Injuries during football or falling off a bike can result in severe testicular pain—some men may even faint from the pain. Testitis, an inflammation of the testicles, is accompanied by pain that radiates into the groin, along the sides and to the back as well as into the area of the spermatic cord. In most cases, there is fever as well as swelling on one side of the testicles and the scrotum. As well, the testicular region starts to feel very heavy. This is generally triggered by bacterial infection or the mumps virus. Sometimes, testitis coincides with prostatitis. In some rare cases, other conditions or infections have been known to inflame the testicles. Doctors do not always find it easy to distinguish between testitis and epididymitis. The tests in this case are similar to those for the epididymis—palpation by the urologist, ultrasound, blood and urine samples. Testitis can cause lasting damage to both testicles, resulting in shrinking of the testicles and even infertility. In cases of a bacterial infection, the patient is treated with antibiotics.

● Hydrocele (dropsy of the testicular membranes)

In the case of hydrocele, the swelling may be as big as a tennis ball

The term hydrocele is derived from the Greek "hydro" meaning 'water' and "cele" meaning 'tumor.' Testicular hydrocele is the accumulation of fluid between the testicles and their membrane that may be watery or amber. This produces a painless enlargement. The swelling may even reach the size of a tennis ball. The causes are not always clearly identifiable. Sometimes, this dropsy may be the result of an injury, an inflammation or a dysfunction. Less serious cases of hydrocele are usually left untreated. In more severe cases, the fluid needs to be suctioned off. Because the fluid may re-accumulate, a liquid is injected into the gap between the testicles and their membrane to serve as a kind of glue. With the man's fertility at stake, massive recurring cases of hydrocele are treated with surgery.

● Varicocele

A varicocele is the accumulation of swollen veins and varicose veins in the area around the spermatic cord surrounding the testicles. Varicocele is a fairly common condition that affects one in ten men and, in 90% of these cases, it occurs specifically in the left testicle. The testicle is often smaller, softer, and hangs lower. There is a kind of pulling sensation that stops once you lie down. This condition is caused by missing venous valves, which leads to an enlargement of the veins and an increase in their number. The diagnosis is relatively easy for an experienced urologist. After carefully gauging the swelling, the doctor holds a light source up from behind the testicles. In the case of varicocele, the testicles are translucent. A painless ultrasound test is then done to confirm any suspicion. In general, varicocele is not a dangerous condition. The pain can be relieved by means of a suspensory bandage or strap supporting the scrotum similar to the one used in many sports. If the swelling becomes troublesome and if fertility is at risk, the patient will undergo surgery to remove the varicocele. After six months, the diminished fertility will normalize again.

One in ten men has varicose veins in this testicles

● Testicular cancer

Testicular cancer usually starts in the cells that produce sperm. The tumor manifests itself as a firm lump or nodule in the testicles. It is usually not painful to the touch. The early stage is symptom-free. Most men discover the tumor themselves by palpation. The tumor usually occurs on only one side (enlargement and swelling). Subsequently, the weight of the cancerous testicle may increase. There may be pain and a pulling sensation. The sooner it is diagnosed, the better.

The tumor is often a hard lump

Testicular cancer is the most common tumor among younger men between the ages of 15 and 35 and the third most common cause of death in that age group. In recent years there has been an unfortunate increase in the incidence of this type of cancer. It may be linked to a genetic disposition. For example, if your brother has had testicular cancer, your risk of getting it will be five to ten times greater. Another risk factor is an undescended testicle (it had not descended into the scrotum at birth and remained in the abdomen). If diagnosed and treated in time, testicular cancer can be cured in most cases.

There are three types of testicular tumor—seminoma, teratoma and choriocarcinoma. Teratoma mostly affects men between the ages of 15 and 25; seminoma usually occurs between 25 and 30.

Testicular cancer has a 90% recovery rate if detected early

Self-examination of the testicles is absolutely necessary if you want to catch the condition in its early stages. If diagnosed in time and if there are no metastases, 90% of all cases are curable. Therefore, it is immensely important to check the testicles regularly. This is something that even young men in puberty need to be made aware of. It should become a routine, just as women examine their breasts regularly.

A simple two-minute self-examination every month is sufficient. Do it after taking a shower or a bath, when the skin of the scrotum is soft and relaxed. Always check one testicle after the other. Softly roll it between your thumb and index finger and feel for nodules below the surface of the testicle. You should also try to see if there is any enlargement, hardening or any other change to the testicles since the last exam. Exert slight pressure and repeat the procedure several times.

Nodes in the testicles: see a doctor immediately

Each testicle should feel soft and smooth or, as urologists would say, "like a hard-boiled egg." If you feel something strange, do not be alarmed. It does not have to be cancer. But you should definitely consult a specialist. Do not be shocked to feel a small firm shape with a cord leading to your testicles. These are the epididymis and the spermatic cord.

The urologist will do a urinalysis and an ultrasound, and also take a blood sample. The blood sample will be tested for tumor markers, i.e., alpha-fetoprotein and beta-human chorionic gonadotropin. These substances are given off into the blood by 80% of testicular tumors. Almost all testicular tumors are malignant, and in this case, removal of the testicle, possibly even of the lymph nodes, will be absolutely necessary.

Almost every testicular tumor is malignant

The most common type of testicular tumor, the seminoma, can be cured in almost all cases if caught in time. All types of testicular tumor taken together have incurred an average survival rate for the patient of more than 90%, even in the worst cases where the tumor was left untreated for as long as five years.

Removal of testicles does not entail loss of masculinity

But it will be necessary to remove the testicle. This does not result in the loss of masculinity or sexual functions. The remaining testicle can perform all the necessary hormonal functions. If both testicles have to be removed, which is very rare, the man will be rendered infertile. But normal sexual functions can be maintained by way of a regular hormone-replacement therapy every three weeks. In advanced stages of cancer, chemotherapy may also be required.

If you examine your testicles regularly and see a urologist if you feel a lump, you will have a very good chance of a full recovery.

The Last Puff

The Risks of Alcohol and Nicotine

Alcohol "A Mean Spirit?"

Patrick K., a 38-year-old university graduate, achieved his life's goal. At 36, he was named deputy director of a major bank. His resume says all the right things, and the new job is exactly what he had been wishing for all his life—demanding, involving a limited amount of publicity, paying a wonderful salary and including business trips overseas.

Shortly after accepting the position, the introverted manager realized that he had grossly underestimated the new challenge. Suddenly Patrick K. could not shake off the feeling of being overworked. He became increasingly nervous, and suffered recurring fear of failure. Gradually, he developed sleep disorders, for which he started taking pills on the advice of a friend.
More and more often, he would drink alcohol at night, especially when his loneliness was its worst and his head was full of gloomy thoughts. Alcohol to relieve the daily stress and help him fall asleep at night became Patrick K's refuge.

He began to drink a bottle of red wine by himself every night. At first, he would drink expensive vintages, but then he made do with the cheaper stuff. All he wanted was to be able to forget everything and to relax. Sometimes he would even drink until he passed out. Under the influence of alcohol, Patrick K. would calm down and even relax, and he fell asleep more easily. His alcohol consumption became greater and greater. During the day, he would get restless and begin to sweat, so he would start drinking hard liquor even at business meetings while the others were having tea. It came as a shock when his friends started talking to him about his alcohol problem. In full denial, he told them that he was fine. But his fear of being found out and of losing his prestigious job drove him to the doctor's office.

Patrick K. is not alone. One in five men and one in ten women drink too much.

One in five men and one in ten women drinks too much

Even the Bible Contains References to Alcohol

Even in prehistoric times, people in various cultures knew about alcohol and its disinhibiting, relaxing and intoxicating effects. Fermentation was probably discovered by accident, but people probably learned very quickly to produce alcoholic beverages, mostly from fruit juices and corn and, in some rare cases, from honey and milk. And so wine and beer were born.

Noah cultivated vineyards and got drunk

The Bible reports an increase in the consumption of wine for the first time after the Flood. Supposedly, Noah cultivated vineyards and regularly got drunk.

In the Western world, a Scottish doctor named Trotter (1780) was probably the first to understand that the urge to get drunk could be a disease triggered by the chemical nature of alcoholic beverages.

Health risk: 40 grams of alcohol is the limit

Today's definition of alcoholism distinguishes between alcohol abuse and alcohol addiction. The World Health Organization has issued a recommended limit on alcohol consumption—20 grams for women and 40 grams for men. This is equal to a liter (1fl pints) of beer, three quarters of a liter of wine or a glass of whiskey.

THE ALCOHOL CONTENT OF VARIOUS BEVERAGES

- 0.33 liters beer   13 grams
- 0.21 liters wine   16 grams
- 0.1 liters sherry   16 grams
- 0.02 liters liqueur   5 grams
- 0.02 liters whiskey   7 grams

If you prefer not to do without alcohol, you can assume that, provided your liver is healthy, drinking a liter of beer two to three days per week will not harm your internal organs.

Alcohol dampens the central nervous system

The alcohol found in beverages is ethyl alcohol (ethanol), a colorless liquid with a burning taste if consumed in a pure concentration. Ethanol is the fermentation product of sugar, which occurs naturally in corn and fruit. Alcohol subdues the central nervous system in the same way that a sedative does. Alcohol has a stimulating effect on many people when they take the first drink or the first few drinks. It is only if they continue drinking that it will have its sedative effect. With the impairment of the central controls in the brain, the mind relaxes and we loosen up. The more we drink, the more sedated we are.

Anyone who has ever spent a night "out on the town" drinking will know what it is like when alcohol first affects the thoughts and emotions and, finally, the judgment.

Larger quantities of alcohol lead to an impairment of speech and muscle coordination as well as to fatigue. The critical point for men suffering massive intoxication is a blood alcohol level of 2. This degree of intoxication results in nausea, vomiting, stomachaches, indigestion, headaches, dizziness and a racing pulse. Higher concentrations may lead to alcohol poisoning with blackouts and respiratory paralysis that can be fatal.

The critical limit is a blood alcohol level of 2

The blood alcohol level is expressed in parts per thousand. The concentration in men depends on the amount of alcohol consumed, on the quantity of food eaten while drinking, as well as on bodyweight. Another important factor is the speed with which the body excretes the alcohol.

Although the blood alcohol level is subject to much individual variation, the following rule generally applies: A man weighing about 70 kilograms (155 pounds) reaches a blood alcohol level of about 0.5 parts per thousand after one liter of beer or half a liter of wine. With this much alcohol in his system, he starts to loosen up and shed his inhibitions. Also, his rational thinking becomes significantly impaired. At this level, he is not allowed to drive in Germany or Austria.

One liter of beer corresponds to a blood alcohol level of 0.5

Beer and Schnapps Increase the Risk of Cancer

A large-scale study was recently undertaken in Denmark to determine the connection between the occurrence of malignant tumors in the upper digestive tract and the consumption of beer, wine and schnapps, as well as smoking . More than 15,000 men and 13,000 women between the ages of 20 and 98 participated in the study. The surprising result is that the moderate consumption of wine does not markedly raise the risk of cancer, while the moderate consumption of beer and schnapps (7 to 21 glasses of beer or schnapps per week) does raise the risk significantly. People who drink 21 glasses of beer or schnapps, but no wine, have an even higher risk.

Wine does not increase colon-cancer risk

Alcohol can cause changes in the brain

Heavy alcohol consumption triggers a series of changes in the cells as well as in the metabolism of the body. Since alcohol is mostly consumed in the form of spirits, wine, beer or aperitifs, a distinction must be made between the effects of the non-alcoholic ingredients and the pure alcohol in these drinks. Alcohol may result in acute alcohol poisoning (intoxication), alcohol-withdrawal syndrome, alcoholic delirium, changes in the brain and polyneuropathy (a disorder of certain nerves resulting in movement disorder and malaise). Chronic alcohol abuse incurs a significantly higher incidence of malignant growths in the oral cavity, larynx, throat and esophagus, of damage to the gastric mucosa, chronic pancreatitis and alcohol-related liver disease ranging from fatty liver and hepatitis to cirrhosis, or shrinking, of the liver.

Alcohol often causes heart-muscle disease

The most serious alcohol-related heart disease is cardiomyopathy that results in enlargement of the heart, insufficient cardiac output and increased heart rate. Chronic alcohol abuse of at least 60 to 80 grams (more than 3 pints of beer) per day also causes high blood pressure.

The effects of alcohol depend on various factors:

● It depends on whether you drink regularly and your body has become accustomed to it, or whether you drink only occasionally.

If you do not drink regularly, even an amount of 100 milligrams of alcohol per deciliter of blood will be enough to produce changes in line with alcohol poisoning. Characteristic signs are speech impairment, slowing of thought processes and staggering. At a higher blood alcohol level, you will experience confusion and dizziness, and in extreme cases, you may lapse into a coma.

Regular consumption of alcohol leads to alcohol tolerance

People who drink regularly have a higher alcohol tolerance and are better at compensating for the outer effects.

● It depends also on whether or not you eat and how much food you consume before and during drinking. If you have not eaten, alcohol enters the bloodstream from the stomach that much faster. Coffee, too, accelerates the absorption of alcohol.

● Your height and bodyweight are also factors, for they influence the distribution of alcohol in the body. In addition, drinking the same amount of alcohol on a regular basis has fewer effects on men than on women.

- Alcohol is converted into acetic acid in the liver. The rate in men per kilogram (2.2 pounds) of bodyweight and per hour is 0.1 grams of alcohol. So, if you drink very fast, you will accumulate a high concentration in your blood.

  0.1 grams of alcohol are metabolized every hour

- Cocktails and alcoholic beverages that contain sugar (mulled wine, etc.) accelerate the absorption of alcohol. Fatty food, however, slows it down.

Am I an Alcoholic?

The transition from having a drinking problem to being an alcoholic is slow and gradual. There is no strict medical classification for drinkers but, in general, four types can be distinguished.

1. The problem drinker

The problem drinker frequently drinks by himself in order to cope with psychological conflicts and disagreements. He is often mentally dependent on alcohol, but he never loses control.

The problem drinker wants to flee from mental conflict

2. The social drinker

The social drinker only drinks with other people around. He is not dependent on alcohol and he does not lose control.

3. The regular and the periodic drinker

The regular drinker has to have alcohol all day long, and always in the same amount. But he does not lose control. Still, he is clearly addicted to alcohol.

The regular drinker consumes alcohol everyday

By contrast, the periodic drinker alternates phases of excessive consumption with phases of complete abstinence.

4. The real alcoholic

The real alcoholic is physically dependent on alcohol. People who consume large quantities of alcohol over a period of one year and lose control over their condition cause severe damage to themselves physically, mentally and socially. Long-term physical damage includes chronic inflammation of the stomach and pancreas, liver cirrhosis, psychoses, changes to their blood count, eye disease, nervous disorders, sleep disorders and impotence.

The alcoholic has a mental and physical dependence

Alcoholism is generally a chronic condition that is progressive and ends in disaster. Those affected keep on drinking even if they are well aware of the effects and the side effects.

It is also characteristic of alcoholics to deny that they have a problem. To hide it, they drink by themselves, or "in the closet." They often forget appointments and ritualize the idea of having a drink before, during and after dinner. And they get angry if that ritual is in any way compromised. They become irritable if they cannot drink; they keep secret stashes of alcohol in the strangest places at home, at work and even in the car; they regularly order double shots of schnapps or whiskey, and they intend to get intoxicated because they want to feel good or normal.

Alcoholics often deny they have a problem

THE ALCOHOL SELF-TEST

There are a number of tests for alcoholism. Here is the short version of the Alcoholism Screening Test (SAAST) of the Mayo Clinic in the US. This test can identify alcoholics in 95% of cases.
1. Do you like to drink a glass occasionally?
2. Do you feel that you are a normal drinker (no more than average)?
3. Have you ever woken up in the morning after a night out drinking and found that you had gaps in your memory about the night before?
4. Has your drinking ever created problems between you and your spouse, parent or other near relative?
5. Are you able to stop after a drink or two?
6. Have you ever had a guilty conscience after drinking?
7. Do your friends and relatives consider your consumption of alcohol normal?
8. Are you always able to stop drinking when you want to?
9. Do you feel tense and restless if you do not drink?
10. Have you ever been arrested, even for a few hours, because of driving while intoxicated?
The following answers indicate a risk of alcoholism:
1. Yes 2. No 3. Yes 4. Yes 5. No 6. Yes 7. No 8. No 9. Yes 10. Yes.

If you want to try this test on another person, keep in mind that a true alcoholic will often lie. If three or more answers match those given above, the person in question will, at the very least, be at risk.

Most alcoholics refuse to undergo treatment because they tend to deny they have a problem. Very often, they have to be forced into treatment. If you suspect that someone you know has an alcohol problem, try to collect proof before you approach him or her about it. This will save you the embarrassment of being wrong and it is a prerequisite for a discreet and very difficult personal conversation.

Observe how much alcohol that person really consumes and try to find friends and relatives of that person who are willing to discuss the problem. Having an understanding of the disease is a crucial first step toward getting real help.

Wait for the right moment, usually the day after a bout of drinking, when the person is recovering from drinking. But do not talk to them when they are drinking again. Other people from their social circle who are also worried about the person should be invited to participate in the confrontation.

You must have a clear plan for helping that person. The best thing to do is to contact a self-help group or a doctor who could act as a confidant. Some people are more likely to accept professional help than advice from friends. Since alcoholism is a disease, the best solution, apart from taking medical therapeutic measures, is self-help groups such as Alcoholics Anonymous and special walk-in clinics.

Self-help groups can aid in bringing about a solution

Patrick K. has also started in outpatient therapy. First, he contacted Alcoholics Anonymous, but he was afraid of running into someone he knew and jeopardizing his position, so he opted for an individualized outpatient program with a specialist on alcoholism.

The beginning was tough and painful, with many minor and major setbacks and anxieties. But after a short time, he was able to go without drinking for a couple of days. Now, at the time of recording his story, Patrick K. has been sober for two months.

FIRST AID FOR HANGOVERS

● **Drink lots of fluids**
Drink at least one to two liters of fluid within a short space of time (water but never alcohol). Popular remedies, such as fighting a hangover with more alcohol, can only lead to further deterioration in your condition.

● **Get fresh air**
Leave the house and get some fresh air. A little exercise can get your circulation going.

● **Hot and cold shower**
Take a shower and alternate the temperature between hot and cold.

● **Do not go out in the sun**
Avoid heat and physical exertion. Let your body rest.

● **Remedies for a hyperacid stomach**
If you have a splitting headache, take medication with an analgesic effect that also works to soothe a hyperacid stomach (e.g., Alka-Seltzer®). These are available at every drugstore.

The Last Puff—The Dangers of Nicotine

Are you among the countless millions of men who smoke cigarettes, cigarillos, cigars or pipes everyday?

1.3 million Austrian men smoke

In Austria, as an example, one in every four men is addicted to nicotine. Each year 15 billion cigarettes are sold and smoked in Austria. Unfortunately, more and more young people are picking up the habit despite vigorous international anti-smoking campaigns.

One in three between 30 and 39 smokes

The average age at which an Austrian starts smoking these days is twelve. The age group 15 to 19 has a 28% share of smokers. Among people aged 30 to 39, the percentage of smokers is even higher, at 38%. That number declines somewhat for the group of over-60-year-olds.

Whenever we inhale the smoke of a cigarette directly, or indirectly as second-hand smoke, we are inhaling not only nicotine. About 4,000 active ingredients in tobacco travel through the body to the vital organs (the brain, lungs, heart and blood vessels). By smoking, we expose our body to chemical substances that can cause cancer and lead to addiction. The nicotine toll in Austria each year as a direct consequence of nicotine is 10,000 cardiac deaths (of a total of 30,000 cardiac deaths per year), 10,000 strokes (out of a total of 20,000), approximately 3,000 lung cancer deaths, and a third of all leg amputations.

Nicotine stimulates adrenal glands

Take nicotine, the most widely known ingredient in cigarettes, as an example. Nicotine stimulates the adrenal glands, which produce hormones (stress hormones) that, in turn, increase the heart rate and blood pressure. The carbon monoxide we inhale from tobacco smoke reduces the supply of oxygen to our blood cells. As a result, vital organs such as the brain and the heart are under-nourished.

It has been shown that, of those 4,000 superfine ingredients, 40 can cause cancer even in small quantities. But the worst offender is without doubt nicotine, for it creates an addiction just like that of cocaine. Nicotine releases neuro-transmitters in the brain, especially dopamine, that create a feeling of bliss in the mind of the smoker. This "dopamine intoxication" is part of the addiction.

Nicotine causes the same addiction as cocaine

Smokers and ex-smokers like to say that smoking starts in the head. Two-thirds of all smokers claim to smoke to relieve stress. Only one-third say they do it for the mere pleasure of it. Two-thirds have tried to quit at least once.

The benefits of quitting are quite clear. Recent studies by the Vienna Institute for Social Medicine have shown that blood pressure and pulse return to normal levels twenty minutes after the last cigarette. Twenty-four hours after the last cigarette, the risk of a heart attack recedes. After nine months, the energy reserves of the body start to build again. And after six to nine months, the damaged mucous epithelium of the lungs begins to be restored and the bronchia start to become clean again. This reduces the risk of pneumonia and infections considerably. It also explains why many ex-smokers report more mucus and coughing during the transition.

The blood pressure normalizes 20 minutes after a cigarette

The real, positive, consequence is that the risk of lung cancer is cut in half. Five to fifteen years after quitting, the risk of a heart attack is similar to that of a non-smoker. After ten years, an ex-smoker can have the same risk of lung cancer as a non-smoker. These are all quite convincing arguments but have little influence over the power of craving and habit.

After ten years without smoking, the cancer risk returns to previous levels

Stop Smoking

Many smokers want to quit, but they find it very difficult to beat their addiction. Some people require more than just willpower to quit. Here are a few recommendations:

● Create your own personalized program by obtaining free literature from some of the many organizations (e.g., cancer-aid organizations or insurance companies) who distribute it. You should also talk to former smokers to find out what helped them quit.

Stop smoking in stages

● Take small steps. Limit yourself to smoking in only one room at home or even leave your house or apartment when you want to smoke. Start by not smoking in the car.

● Start a gradual fitness program.

● Watch your smoking habits. When do you smoke? Where? With whom? What are the typical triggers (coffee, alcohol, food, stress, tension, TV, etc.)? Think of how you would deal with these situations if you no longer smoked.

● Motivate yourself. The key to success is true commitment to quitting. Studies by the Mayo Clinic have shown that smokers, with the right amount of motivation, are twice as likely to quit in the end than those less motivated. This may sound trivial, but it is a key to success. Only try to quit when you are convinced and motivated to do so.

Set yourself a date for your last cigarette

● Set a date for the last cigarette you are going to have. That day should be stress-free. Tell your friends, your spouse, your family and your co-workers of your intention. They can support you, and it will strengthen your motivation.

● Seek help. More and more people are trying to cope with the symptoms of withdrawal by using nicotine-replacement substances.

Chewing gum helps

These substances include Nicorette® chewing gum, produced by Pharmacia & Upjohn, as well as Nicorette® inhalator, plastic cigarettes that contain a nicotine capsule and, the latest addition to the line, Nicorette® tablets. You place a tablet under the tongue. It gives off two milligrams of nicotine while dissolving in your mouth. All of these substances are said to reduce not only the craving for cigarettes but also withdrawal symptoms such as anxiety, increased appetite and sleep disorders.

New Ways

Buproprion blocks dopamine in the brain

Recently, a new "miracle" remedy hit the market. Zyban® is an antidepressant containing buproprion. Zyban blocks the neurotransmitters (dopamine) in the brain and thereby kills the craving for a cigarette. Initial studies in the US have shown that Zyban, when taken together with nicotine-replacement products, is so effective that 38% of people managed to quit after one year, as compared to 18% who quit after receiving only a placebo during the studies. This is certainly an impressive result. But buproprion, like any drug, has side effects, such as headaches and dryness of the mouth. If you have a history of dizziness or fainting, you should definitely stay away from this drug.

Only 5% of smokers can stop smoking on their own. The more support you receive, the more likely you will be to kick the habit. Men who take nicotine-replacement products and receive counseling have a 30% to 40% probability of eventually quitting.

TIPS AND TRICKS FOR COPING WITH NICOTINE WITHDRAWAL

- Try to think of something else when you feel nervous or have a craving to smoke. Take deep breaths.
- Drink a lot of fluids, especially low-calorie beverages, in order to counter any increase in appetite. Eat a lot of fresh fruit and vegetables, and stay away from sweets.
- In the event of loss of concentration, drink a lot of water, go for a walk, try to simplify your daily routine and take more breaks.
- In the event of fatigue, do more exercise to counter your lethargy. Make sure you get enough sleep. Take a nap after lunch at times.
- In the event of sleep disorders, go for a walk before bedtime or drink warm milk. Avoid caffeine late at night.
- In the event of congestion, drink a lot of fluids and eat a lot of fruit, raw vegetables and fiber. Gradually change your diet.

While you are trying to quit, keep in mind that smoking is one of the main causes of heart attacks and cancer, two diseases that will define a man's life in the 21st century.

If you stop smoking, you will reduce your risk of cancer

The Silent Killer

Cancer and Early Detection in Men

His name was Wayne McLaren. He was a stuntman and rodeo cowboy, but his worldwide fame came by way of an odd job. The giant tobacco company Philip Morris was looking for a man to embody the classic adventurer type for a new advertising campaign for Marlboro cigarettes. McLaren, the clear favorite of the Philip Morris executives, became the "Marlboro Man."

The Marlboro Man died of lung cancer

In commercials and billboards, he was the easy-going yet daring outdoorsman who rode through the rugged wilderness of the Grand Canyon, alone but for his horse and his best friend, a Marlboro cigarette that always dangled from the corner of his mouth. McLaren's message was one of freedom, "Everything is possible if you put your mind to it."

Today, Wayne McLaren is dead. A chain smoker, the great outdoorsman died ironically of lung cancer. His death was long and painful, and he had a camera team document it all. In his last interview, McLaren, clearly marked by a series of chemotherapy sessions, without hair and unable to breathe on his own, said, "I'm paying the price for my addiction. My life is ending under an oxygen tent. I'm telling you, 'Smoking isn't worth it.'"

62% of Austrians are afraid of cancer

According to a survey for Forum Healthy Austria, Austrians fear no disease more than cancer. They know little about actual survival rates and possible treatments, and they have a terrible fear of being confronted with a fatal diagnosis. Cancer is the second most common cause of death after heart attacks, according to statistics. Although 62% of Austrians are most afraid of cancer, the actual mortality rate from cancer is "only" 23%.

We Will Already Know at 20 if We Are Going to Die at 50

DNA chips reveal information about personal risks

We are at the beginning of a new century—one that will see the complete reinvention of medical science. The successful treatment of cancer, and of many other diseases for which there is no conventional cure, will soon be a reality thanks to rapid developments in microbiology. Many conditions will become treatable because of what we are learning about human genetics. In a few years, doctors will be able to go straight into the cells and fight disease from there. Even now, scientists are developing DNA chips that will feed us comprehensive information on our personal predisposition and our risks.

The consequences of looking into our genetic structure are unpredictable and not all positive. It will be possible to identify many diseases in the genome even before they express themselves physically or psychologically. But that kind of treatment is still out of reach, except in some rare cases. In the not-too-distant future, twenty-year-olds, for example, may find out from genetic tests if they are likely to die from a disease of the nervous system (Huntington Chorea) by the time they are fifty. Pregnant women, if diagnosed with "damaged chromosomes," will have to decide whether they want an abortion or whether they want to carry a severely disabled child to term. Many women may have to learn to live with the knowledge that, based on genetic predisposition, they have an 80% probability of developing breast cancer. The psychological and psychosomatic consequences for the patient are very difficult to predict.

So far, about 800 of almost 5,000 genetic diseases can be identified, but only a fifth of them can be detected directly using DNA tests. Such tests only make sense at present if knowing about the condition can in some way alter its progression. The next decade may see a major change. No longer will we feel helpless when confronted with a disease that has been identified genetically but cannot be treated. Within the next five years, the complete decoding of the human genome, which contains the complete genetic information about a person, will provide new opportunities for treating diseases.

Only 800 of 5,000 genetic diseases can be identified

Even your wildest dreams could become reality. Overweight men may look forward to having their fat simply melt away, top managers will undergo testosterone therapy, "sunshine pills" will lift depression, and fitness and health food, together with anti-aging products, will produce more attractive people and enhance the quality of life.

Your fantasies will come true

In order to increase life expectancy in the long term, however, men will still have to change their ways. "They should stop believing they are invincible. Men must follow the example of women and learn to listen to the signals from their own bodies. They have to treat their bodies with more respect. Some scientists complain about deteriorating medical services, and they blame many premature deaths on that fact. They say there are no 'andrologists' that men can turn to, as women go to their gynecologists," concludes the magazine Der Spiegel about "the weaker strong sex."

The Future of Diagnostics: Genetic Analysis on Palmtop Computers

Revolutionary diagnostic methods will drastically simplify prophylaxis for men in the next century. Professor David Burgh at the University of Michigan predicts that, in a matter of three to five years, we will have small handheld computers (palmtops) that can do a complete genetic analysis of a patient after decoding the human genetic sequence. The University of Michigan in Ann Arbor is already using an "instant test" to identify criminals in one to two hours on the basis of specific genetic analyses.

DNA profiles on hand-held computers

This explosion of knowledge will not only affect therapy and diagnostics, but also preventive medicine, especially with respect to cancer. In the next few years, molecular-biological diagnostics will help identify families with hereditary cancer, which account for about 10% of all malignant tumors. But early detection of cancer by means of an oncogene test—an oncogene is a gene that causes, or is conducive to, cancer—will also be more efficient and lead to much faster identification. Thus, it will be possible to analyze tumors in terms of their molecular-biological and genetic properties, which would allow for an individualization of the therapy in terms of intensity and vulnerability to side effects.

Soon, genes will be inserted into tumor cells

Soon, it will be possible to introduce genes into tumors in order to activate killer cells that destroy the cancer cells. It may also be possible to introduce defective genes that can bring about the death of the malignant cells. Scientists have already found ways to use harmful viruses in the fight against cancer.

As valuable as this genetic knowledge may be in battling disease, scientists have found that more than a third of all cancer cases could be avoided through changes to a person's lifestyle, and many more cases could be healed through proper early-detection measures.

Cancer in Men and Its Complications

One in three gets cancer; one in four dies of cancer

One in three European men develop cancer at some point, while one in four actually dies of cancer. In 1990 alone (the most recent statistics available), there were 1,351,083 new cancer cases in the European Union. Of these, 706,870 were men. In the same year, 497,464 men died of cancer.

In 1996, 17,428 Austrian men developed cancer. The most common types were:
1. prostate cancer (21.2%, 3,690 cases),
2. lung cancer (15.6%, 2,718 cases) and
3. colon cancer (15%, 2,626 cases).

These were followed by: 4. bladder cancer (7%, 1,215 cases), 5. stomach cancer (5.9%, 1,021 cases), 6. cancer of the kidneys and other urinary organs (4.5%, 778 cases), 7. pancreatic cancer (3.4%, 585 cases), 8. liver cancer (2.9%, 512 cases), 9. skin melanoma (2.6%, 451 cases) and 10. leukemia (2.2%, 390 cases).

This means that, among men, half of all newly diagnosed cancer cases affect only three organs. "Prostate cancer has increased excessively among the number of new cases," says university professor Wolfgang Höll, who works for Austrian Cancer Aid and heads a campaign called "Men and Cancer."

In 1996, 9,614 men died of cancer in Austria. Here are the mortality rates for the three main types of cancer:
1. lung cancer (24.7%, 2,373 deaths)
2. colon cancer (14.1%, 1,356 deaths)
3. prostate cancer (12.2%, 1,170 deaths).

The good news is that the risk of developing cancer can be substantially lowered with a healthy lifestyle. This includes nicotine abstinence, maintaining an ideal weight, adopting a balanced diet, eating more fiber such as whole grain products, reducing fat intake, consuming alcohol only in moderation, reducing consumption of salted and smoked foods, and reducing exposure to UV radiation.

The bad news is that, at this point, one in seven cancer cases seems to be hereditary, so nothing can be done about it. People with a family history of cancer belong to a high-risk group. These so-called "cancer families" have had

15% of all cancers are hereditary

EARLY DETECTION: WHAT CAN YOU DO?

1. Regular self-examination
Palpate your genitals once a month after a warm bath to look for nodules.

2. Prostate prophylaxis
Men past the age of 45 should see a urologist at least once a year. If your family has a history of prostate cancer, you should have regular checkups after the age of 40. Make sure that your doctor analyzes your PSA level.

3. Bladder and kidney prophylaxis
After the age of 35, you should have a urinalysis once a year.

4. Watch out for moles
Men with a lot of moles on their body and those with a family history of melanoma should check their skin once a month for changes in appearance. In addition, you should see a specialist twice a year.

a certain type of cancer in their family over generations. The probability that the next generation will also be affected is as high as 15%.

Other high-risk groups involve people who smoke, drink or have an unhealthy diet.

Unfortunately, "I feel good" does not provide any protection against cancer. Only 30% to 50% of cancer patients suffer from any pains at the time they are diagnosed. At a more advanced stage, it is 60% to 90%. Therefore, the primary objective has to be early detection. But this is a decided weakness in men.

Men do not care about prevention

A representative EU survey in January 1998 showed that 80% of European doctors had the impression that women were more concerned with cancer prophylaxis than men. They reported that men were more introverted when it came to discussing medical problems. In a Eurobarometer survey, 32.5% of the women interviewed stated that they had seen a doctor within the last two weeks. Of the men, however, only 21.1% had consulted a doctor within the same period of time.

Diagnosis: Cancer

"When I was diagnosed with cancer, I made a solemn vow to myself. No, this is not going to get me. I summoned all my strength to fight the disease. I said to the cancer, 'I'm gonna show you.' It is all right to despair sometimes, but you must not hide it. No matter how down you are, don't keep it inside. Despair of the world—it is part of the therapy."

Hans Peter Heinzl, Austrian satirist and comedian

The sooner diagnosed, the better the chance of recovery

All tumors are subject to the same principle: the sooner cancer is diagnosed, the greater the chance of being cured. Some carcinomas have a better prognosis (e.g., testicular tumor), others are worse (e.g., lung cancer).

Since the 1990s, it has been taken for granted that, apart from the medical treatment employed, it is the patient's mental attitude that determines whether he can be cured or not. "Patients who are willing to fight the disease and determined to get better again definitely have a better chance to be cured than those who, upon hearing the diagnosis, become lethargic and entrust their lives to fate," says Christoph Zielinski, an oncologist from Vienna, who treated Leonard Bernstein and the comedian Hans Peter Heinzl. Heinzl, who had pancreatic cancer, is a textbook example of what willpower can achieve. Normally, the life expectancy in the case of this highly aggressive type of cancer is six to nine months, but Heinzl lived another four years before he died.

Those with an iron will have a better prognosis

WARNING SIGNS FOR MEN

If you think that you detect one of these warning signs, consult a doctor immediately:
1. I have difficulties swallowing. I am always hoarse.
2. I cough quite frequently.
3. I do not have any real appetite and I have been losing weight.
4. I have traces of blood in my urine.
5. I have difficulty urinating.
6. My testicles have hardened.
7. My bowel movements have changed.
8. I have found a strange, new mark on my skin.

Source: Austrian Cancer Aid

Do not panic. None of these signs automatically means you have cancer. But you should see your physician.
Pay attention to the following:
● enlarged lymph nodes (neck, armpit or groin)
● chronic fever or febrile attacks without any clear cause
● blood in the stool
● brownish spots ("moles" or "liver spots") on your skin that are getting bigger in size, change color and itch or bleed
● sudden enlargement of a goiter that you have had for some time

---

The most common types of cancer among men are:

1. Lung cancer

Lung cancer (bronchial carcinoma), among men in Austria and Germany, is the type of cancer with the highest mortality rate. About 28,900 men—more than three times as many men as women—get this cancer every year in Germany alone. Of these, 85% to 90% die of it.

Since bronchial carcinoma tends to be detected at a relatively late stage, the prognosis is usually bad. The survival rate is only 10% to 15%. The average age

Lung cancer is often detected too late

of the male lung cancer patient is 62. Recent years, however, have also seen a significant increase in its occurrence among younger people.

LUNG CANCER: SMOKING IS DANGEROUS	
Non-smoker	Risk factor 1.0
1 to 10 cigarettes a day	Risk factor 5.5
11 to 19 cigarettes a day	Risk factor 11.2
20 cigarettes a day	Risk factor 14.2
21 to 31 cigarettes a day	Risk factor 20.4
More than 31 cigarettes a day	Risk factor 22.0

Source: Dr. Peter Drings, Medical Director of the Thorax Clinic Heidelberg-Rohrbach.
(Information he provided to German Cancer Aid)

There are two types of lung cancer:

Small-cell bronchial carcinomas metastasize quickly

● non-small-cell bronchogenic carcinomas, divided into:
squamous-cell carcinoma (40–50% of all lung cancer cases)
adenocarcinoma (10–15%)—the most common type of cancer among non-smokers
large-cell bronchogenic carcinoma (5–10%)
● small-cell bronchogenic carcinomas (25–30%). Because of their rapid growth and the early formation of metastases, the prognosis is bad. At first diagnosis, 80% of patients show metastases mostly in the brain. That is why they complain of headaches, nausea, paralysis and impaired vision.

The etiology

Smoking causes 85% of all lung cancer

In 85% of all cases, lung cancer is caused by smoking and the combustion products of tobacco. So far, more than 4,000 different chemical constituents have been identified in cigarette smoke. Many of these active ingredients are toxic, carcinogenic and change the genetic structure. Since the lungs are the organs primarily exposed to cigarette smoke, it is here that most malignant tumors form. But smoking is also responsible for 90% of carcinomas in the oral cavity, 80% of esophageal tumors and 80% of laryngeal tumors in men. Smokers also show a high incidence of tumors affecting the pancreas, kidneys, stomach and bladder.

Only 5% to 15% of lung cancer cases among men are related to occupation-al agents. These primarily affect people exposed to toxic substances such as asbestos, arsenic compounds, chromium-VI compounds, nickel (e.g., costume jewelry) or radioactive substances such as uranium (e.g., miners), as well as people constantly exposed to benzene or exhaust from diesel engines (shipyard or factory workers, etc.). Exposure to such substances for many years often results in lung cancer.

Secondhand smoke is another risk factor. This is borne out by two studies of the Institute for Medical Computer Science, Biometry and Epidemiology at the uni-versity hospital in Essen, Germany, and the Institute for Epidemiology of the GSF Research Center for Environment and Health in Germany. These studies were carried out over seven years and involved 5,307 lung cancer patients and 5,455 persons from the general population. Of these, 375 were included in the study of secondhand smoke—they had never smoked themselves, but, as chil-dren, they had been exposed to smoking parents or siblings' smoking and, later on, to a spouse who smoked or to a smoke-filled working environment. Their risk of getting lung cancer was one-and-a-half times higher than for people who had never been exposed to smoke. The risk was significantly higher in cases where people had had to work in a heavily smoke-filled environment over a period of ten to fifteen years. It was actually twice as high as for non-smokers without any exposure to secondhand smoke.

Secondhand smoke increases cancer risk

Another significant risk factor has to do with genetics. If the parents had lung cancer, then the child will have a risk level three times as high.

Currently, other factors are also being looked into. A discovery made in February of 1999 caused a furor in the medical scientific community. Janet Butel, a researcher at the Baylor College for Medicine in Texas, published an article in the British scientific magazine Journal of the National Cancer Institute, in which she claimed that there were indications that the polio vac-cine would cause cancer later in life. It led to a special form of lung cancer called mesotheliom. According to Butel, it affected only people born between 1941 and 1961, when the Salk vaccine was still used. It was later replaced with the harmless Sabin oral vaccine. The cultures used to produce the Salk vaccine consisted of kidney cells from monkeys that had the SV 40 virus. The virus was almost certainly spread to people. It also appears that children vaccinated between 1941 and 1961 passed the virus on to the next generation, for SV 40 is found in about 10% of the blood samples of people who have never been vaccinated against polio. The London oncologist and researcher Gordon

The virus spread in people

McVie even believes that SV 40 is the cause of certain types of bone cancer, prostate cancer and brain tumors. Several studies are now looking at the cancer risk from SV 40, but definitive results are not expected until 2001.

The diagnosis

Early symptoms of lung cancer are rare. Coughing, difficulty in breathing and chest pains may, but do not have to, occur, and they are not always characteristic of a tumor. Men over 40 who experience breathing problems and frequent inflammation of the respiratory tract that last more than three weeks should see a pulmonologist.

At an advanced stage of the cancer, the patient shows clearer symptoms: spitting blood, weight loss, massive breathing problems or fever. By this stage, a cure is often impossible.

A bone scintigram detects metastases

The diagnostic methods currently employed are x-ray and computer tomography of the lungs. These allow a tumor to be localized and "staged." That is, the extent of the cancer and the effect on the lymph nodes can be ascertained. In order to show possible metastases, a sonogram of the abdomen, a bone scintigram (a nuclear-medical test involving radioactive substances) or a CT of the head may be done.

A reliable diagnosis, however, can only be made with a bronchoscopy, by which means lung tissue is taken and examined histologically.

There are four stages of cancer:
1. Stage G1: well differentiated (prognosis not that bad)
2. Stage G2: moderately differentiated
3. Stage G3: poorly differentiated
4. Stage G4: undifferentiated (very bad prognosis)

Small tumors (T1 and T2) without an invasion of the lymph nodes (N0) and without metastases (M0) have a more favorable prognosis.

The treatment

Non-small cell carcinomas are inoperable

The tumor should be completely removed surgically. In order to be a candidate for surgery, patients must have small, non-small-cell bronchogenic carcinomas without any effusion (T1 to T3, N0 to N1, M0). Only 20% of lung cancer patients meet these requirements. Of those who have surgery, between 30% and 50% survive the first five years. The patients also receive radiation therapy.

But of those who receive only radiation therapy, only 20% to 30% survive the first five years. For men, the prognosis looks even worse. According to statistics of the Robert Koch Institute in Berlin, Germany, only 9% of male patients survive the first five years.

Only 9% of men survive the first five years

In the case of small-cell tumors (the very malignant ones), patients first undergo chemotherapy, which also attacks certain metastases. But the disease can only be slowed for a few months. Radiation therapy is unavoidable. The average survival rate for small-cell bronchogenic carcinoma is between four and twelve months.

The future

It is very difficult to detect lung cancer early on. Several international clinics are currently testing new procedures for detecting malignant changes as early as possible:

1. Automated sputum cytometry

A sample of sputum (mucus expectorated from the lungs) is taken for analysis of the density of the DNA, the structure and form of the cell nuclei in saliva. Based on the results, it can be determined whether the cell accumulations are normal or cancerous. Due to automation of the procedure, the saliva of large numbers of people can be tested routinely in future. This will increase the odds of identifying possible candidates for the disease early on and to order additional testing. If the findings of the cytometry reveal any irregularities in the mucous membrane, the saliva will be further analyzed under an electron microscope. If any deviations are found there, additional tests, i.e., computer tomography and bronchoscopy, will be ordered.

DNA analysis of sputum can provide more answers

2. Autofluorescent bronchoscopy

This test is based on the principle that light of a certain wavelength is reflected by the mucous membrane of the bronchia. The autofluorescence of healthy tissue is at least ten times more intensive than that of cancerous tissue. This new method, which is being tested at several clinics across the US and Germany, can detect twice as many bronchogenic carcinomas as can conventional bronchoscopy.

The cancer cell that "committed suicide" with the p53 gene

The treatment of lung cancer will see breakthroughs at the beginning of the new millennium. Research teams worldwide are working hard to develop genetically based treatments for patients for whom chemotherapy or radiation therapy would not be effective. The goal is to restore the limited willingness of cancer cells to die off after their conventional treatment by manipulating their DNA. For this purpose, a so-called gene-transfer system is developed that can distinguish between healthy cells and cancer cells. In many cases of lung cancer, genetic mutations result in an overproduction of the Bcl-2 protein. This is the reason that cancer cells do not die off even after being severely damaged by radiation.

The p53 gene causes cancer cells to self-destruct

Other clinical tests that use genetic therapy to treat lung cancer focus on adenoviruses to transfer the tumor-suppressor gene p53. This gene functions like a guard that orders dysfunctional cells to self-destruct. If the gene itself is damaged, this order will never be given. The result is that the cancer cells grow and spread. Since damaged p53 genes have been found in more than half of all cancer types, the objective now is to introduce fully functional p53 genes into the cancer cells to make them "commit suicide." The first findings at the University of Texas in Houston are promising. But the tumor-suppressing gene works only with certain types of lung cancer, i.e., the non-small-cell bronchogenic carcinomas. The Vienna General Hospital is currently participating in an international study on p53 and its role in preventing tumors of the nose, throat and ears.

The BEC-2 antibody vaccine stimulates the immune system

Since April 1998, a study has been conducted at 80 clinics worldwide that deals with preventing a relapse of small-cell bronchogenic carcinomas by using a new vaccine called BEC 2. This vaccine is produced by injecting mice with human cancer cells. The monoclonal antibodies—genetically engineered, highly specific antibodies that stimulate the immune system—formed by the mice are processed and given to the patient.

2. Prostate cancer

70% of prostate cancer patients survive the first five years

Dependent on hormones, the prostate gland is an organ the size of a chestnut. It is located below the bladder, wrapped around the urethra. It consists of many individual glands that drain into the urethra and produce the prostate secretion, the fluid that feeds and moves the sperm. During ejaculation, the secretion is mixed into the semen. As revealed in laboratory tests, active agents such as the prostate-specific antigen (PSA) are also given off into the bloodstream. The production of the secretion is triggered by the testosterone hormone.

The incidence of prostate cancer increases with age. Among 55-year-olds, 20 men out of 100,000 have prostate cancer. Among 70 to 80-year-olds, the number with cancer increases to 500 to 600 per 100,000. In Germany, for example, this translates into 25,000 new cases every year. The chances of being cured are quite good, with 70% of patients surviving the first five years.

The etiology

Changes in the tissue of the prostate gland that occur in half of all men over 50 are quite normal. In most cases, these changes are benign and not dangerous. But, next to the benign growth, a malignant one may be forming. Genetic factors can play an important role here, especially in families that have had cases of prostate cancer before the age of 60. The risk of prostate cancer is two to three times higher if, for example, the father or a brother have already had the disease. Unfortunately, there is no way of actively preventing the formation of prostate cancer.

Risk factors include age and fatty diets. So far, no connection has been established between prostate cancer and lifestyle or sexual activity.

Age and fatty diets are risk factors

The diagnosis

The early stage is practically free of symptoms because this cancer usually occurs in regions far away from the urethra. In some rare cases, there may be blood in the seminal fluid. At a more advanced stage, the patient has problems voiding the bladder because the cancerous growth constricts the urethra. In many instances, prostate cancer is not detected until the patient experiences pain in the bones as a result of metastases.

Traces of blood in semen are warning signals

The urologist checks on the prostate gland rectally, i.e., he palpates it through the anus. In Austria only 22% of men have had a prostate exam.

If the urologist finds the gland to be enlarged or hardened, he will order a blood test. The purpose of the blood test is to detect changes to the prostate-specific antigen (PSA), a tumor marker, and to draw conclusions about possible prostate diagnoses. Cancerous cells can produce ten times as much PSA as normal prostate cells. With a PSA level of more than 10 ng/ml, the probability of cancer is 50%. In order to confirm the diagnosis, the level of free PSA is determined as well, because the probability can be computed more reliably from the ratio of these two levels.

A PSA level over 10 mg/ml translates into 50% cancer risk

In the event of suspected prostate cancer, six tissue samples are tested with an ultrasonic probe, which is inserted into the anus. Samples are taken from the gland (biopsy) and examined under a microscope. Ultrasound examinations can detect certain conditions of the prostate.

The treatment

If the cancer is still limited to the prostate gland, it can be surgically removed. Radiation therapy is also an option. If prostate cancer is detected in time, the chances of its being cured are very good.

Testosterone feeds the prostate carcinoma

If the cancer has already gone beyond the gland, it is surgically removed, but the patient is also given drugs that suppress the testosterone hormone, which otherwise would feed the malignant tumor.

LH-RH suppresses testosterone production

Drug therapy using so-called LH-RH analogs (previously, estrogens were used, but these have side effects) inhibits the production of hormones in the pituitary gland. The pituitary gland normally controls hormone production in the testicles, but because of the drugs, testosterone production in the testicles is suppressed. The drugs, so-called depot treatments, are injected intramuscularly, and they remain below the skin for one to three months. The carcinoma often reacts quickly to the withdrawal of hormones and goes into permanent remission.

Chemical castration and impotence are inevitable

But an unpleasant side effect like a chemical castration takes place. The therapy results in temporary impotence and the loss of sex drive. The patient may also experience hot flushes and excessive sweating.

It is possible to avoid this side effect. The testicular tissue that produces testosterone may be surgically removed.

PROSTATE CHECKLIST

1. Do you often have to go to the washroom during the night?
2. Do you often have to "push" during urination?
3. Is the urine stream sometimes interrupted during urination?
4. Has your urine stream become weaker?
5. Do you often feel a sudden urge to urinate?

If you have one or several of these symptoms, you should have yourself checked out by your urologist just to be on the safe side.

---

3. Intestinal cancer

Too much beer may cause rectal cancer

Drinking too much beer can have fatal consequences. Not only does it make for an unsightly belly, but it can also cause cancer. In the Upper Palatinate in Germany, beer consumption is 40% over the national average of 150 liters (over 250 pints) per person per year. This results in the region's having the highest percentage of rectal cancer in the country. Intestinal cancer is a cultural disease that is closely linked to our eating habits.

About 23,000 German men are diagnosed every year with a malignant colon tumor. Rectal and colon carcinomas are among the most hideous types of cancer because there are no symptoms. Colon carcinomas usually go undetected for years, and the patient suffers no symptoms and no pain. Of those afflicted with colon cancer, 49% survive the first five years.

The etiology
One of the main causes of colon cancer is an unhealthy diet—too much meat and animal fat, and not enough vitamin E and beta carotene.

But there are also genetic factors. Defective genetic information for the intestinal mucosa, which may be passed on by a parent but may also result from the regeneration of the mucous membrane lining the intestines, is another cause of intestinal cancer. The tissue-forming cells of the mucous membrane regenerate very quickly, generally within five to seven days, by way of cell division. In this process, it may happen that the "copy" contains an error, passed on to the daughter cell from the original cell. If repair enzymes do not correct the erroneous information, the defective cell will start a "self-destruct" sequence, leaving only cell remnants to be eliminated by the immune system. But if larger quantities of potentially carcinogenic substances enter the colon frequently and stay there for a longer period of time, the repair enzymes may fail and damaged cells of the intestinal mucosa are not automatically destroyed. Instead, they gradually evolve into malignant cancer cells. In the case of polypoid intestinal cancer, hundreds of small polyps grow in the intestines, and they can quickly take a turn for the worse.

Repair enzymes fail because of carcinogenic substances

Approximately 10% to 15% of intestinal cancer cases have genetic links. The defectiveness of the repair enzymes may also be hereditary. Oncologists often speak of familial non-polypoid colon carcinoma.

There are four stages (Dukes Scale):
1. Dukes A: the mucous membrane and the outer layers of the intestinal wall are attacked by cancer.
2. Dukes B: the carcinoma has gone deeper into the intestinal wall and has reached the surrounding tissue.
3. Dukes C: there are metastases in the adjacent lymph nodes.
4. Dukes D: metastases occur in more distant organs.

The diagnosis

Blood, mucus or other unusual excretions in the stool should be seen as warning signs of colon cancer. Do not panic, for these symptoms may also have other, less dramatic, causes. Still, Susanne Takats, manager of Austrian Cancer Aid, cautions, "Blood in the stool must be assumed to be cancer until it has been proven otherwise." With a special test (hemocult test), which you can also do at home, you can tell very quickly if there is blood in the stool. A bit of stool is applied to a test strip, with any resulting discoloration an invisible sign of blood.

The hemocult test can be done at home

A coloscopy, using a tube with a tiny optical camera that is inserted into the intestines through the anus, provides ultimate certainty. After all, the problem may also be due to a harmless intestinal polyp (although this is often a precursor of tumors). The doctor examines the intestinal mucosa and takes tissue samples, using a tiny tool in the tube. The examination is unpleasant, but is the best way to detect cancer.

You should always consult a doctor in the event of frequently occurring flatulence, congestion or indigestion over a longer period of time, as well as in the event of any hardening in the abdominal region.

The treatment

With hereditary colon cancer, the only effective treatment in most cases is surgery. Usually, the entire colon has to be removed.

Surgery is often the only alternative with other forms of intestinal cancer as well. The affected part of the intestine is removed together with the lymph nodes, and the ends of the remaining intestine are sewn together. Many patients have tumors close to the anus, so the anus has to be removed too and replaced with an artificial outlet.

Cytostatic drugs block cell division

If the tumor has already reached the Dukes-C stage, the risk of metastases' spreading to the lungs and liver is high. Chemotherapy is then the only viable option. This may take two forms—cytostatic drugs that block the cell division and immunotherapeutic drugs. These drugs have a series of side effects because they also block the division of other cells in the body.

Radiation therapy is recommended for cancer cells that have a high rate of cell division.

The future

In the new millennium, the treatment of intestinal cancer will be massively improved. New surgical procedures are being developed, as are more effective forms of chemotherapy.

The latest treatment for colon cancer is to mark tumor cells with monoclonal antibodies (MAB). These protein molecules, which the immune system produces using certain blood cells, can be produced artificially outside the body in a cell culture. They are Y-shaped. The two short ends of the antibody molecule, where the antigen is bound, fit perfectly to a specific chemical structure on the cancerous cell. The longer end, however, is considered an invader by the immune system.

New therapies involve marking tumor cells

If an antibody with the two short Y-ends "docks" onto the surface of the cancer cell, this cell, too, will be interpreted as a foreign body by the killer cells of the immune system and destroyed. In effect, the killer cells "gang up" on the cancer cells and destroy them. These antibodies do not work with larger cancerous growths because they cannot get deep enough into the carcinoma, but their effectiveness on metastases has been confirmed. Cancer researchers all over the world are working feverishly to improve the effect of the MAB even further.

Monoclonal antibodies have one major advantage over cytostatic drugs—they also destroy cancer cells that are not in the process of cell division. These dormant cancer cells have up until now posed a considerable risk. In many cases, it was believed that the cancer was in remission, but one or two years later, the "dormant" cancer cells suddenly woke up.

Monoclonal antibodies dock onto cancer cells

Here is a list of other types of cancer that may affect men:

● Cystic carcinoma

Risk factors: smoking, unhealthy working conditions (especially in chemical factories that produce dyes and rubber), long-term abuse of painkillers, chronic inflammation of the bladder.

Symptoms: hematuria (mostly painless), burning sensation during urination, increased urinary urgency, stinging sensation after voiding.

Diagnosis: testing urine for tumor cells, ultrasound and x-ray, cystoscopy and tissue sample.

Treatment: with a carcinoma of the inner layer of the bladder, endoscopic removal through the urethra, injection of drugs (a type of local chemothera-

Cystic cancer is treated with local chemotherapy

py); with extensive spreading, complete or partial surgical removal of the bladder. In some cases, a replacement bladder can be made from intestinal parts.

Chance of recovery: bladder tumors tend to occur repeatedly. The deeper the cancer has eaten into the bladder wall, the smaller the chance of recovery.

• Renal carcinoma

Ultrasound is a sufficient exam in 95% of renal cancer cases

Risk factors: long-term abuse of painkillers, smoking.
Symptoms: upper abdominal pain, high blood sedimentation rate, red blood cells in urine, colic-like pain, febrile attacks.
Diagnosis: ultrasound test (sufficient in 95% of cases).
Treatment: surgical removal of affected kidney; in some cases, post-op treatment with drugs.
Chance of recovery: high, provided there are no metastases.

• Testicular carcinoma

Please refer to the chapter entitled "It's A Man's Business."

New Forms of Cancer Prophylaxis

In recent years, a number of new substances have been tested for their effectiveness against cancer. Here are some examples:

• Ginseng

Ginseng cuts cancer risk in half

The Chinese have known about its life-prolonging qualities for centuries. Ginseng is a medicinal plant that in the past was available only to the emperor. It is said that the Chinese populace was forbidden to use it on penalty of death. Marco Polo brought the root, which has curative and potency-enhancing properties, to Europe. Ginseng increases performance and relieves stress as well as exhaustion. Taken regularly, it can also lower the cancer risk, especially gastric and lung carcinomas, by more than half. Two scientists, T.K. Yun and S.Y. Choi, at the Korea Cancer Hospital in Seoul, South Korea, reached the same conclusion in their ten-year study that involved more than 4,000 subjects. The study analyzed the cancer-inhibiting effect of the plant. The survey showed that taking ginseng regularly, i.e., every month, was most effective. The scientists also discovered that even taking ginseng only two to three times a year could reduce the risk of cancer by a third. Fresh ginseng is more effective than extracts or powder. However, the effectiveness of ginseng in cancer prevention has not yet been reliably confirmed.

● Selenium

Scientists at Harvard University, in a study with 33,000 Americans, found that selenium, a trace element that is an important constituent of many enzymes, can slow or stop the development of prostate cancer. Those with the highest blood selenium level—they took 159 nicrograms a day—were about two-thirds less likely to be suffering from advanced prostate cancer.

Selenium can help stop prostate cancer

Selenium's proven effect may be based on its role in binding and neutralizing free radicals. Small traces of selenium are found in fish, whole grain products, dairy products and vegetables grown on soil containing selenium. Earlier research at the University of Arizona found that by taking a selenium pill every day, a person's risk of prostate cancer could be reduced by 63%, intestinal cancer by 58% and lung cancer by 45%. Selenium also helps in the supply of oxygen to the heart and makes tissue more elastic.

● Beta carotene

The vitamin beta carotene is said to lower the risk of prostate cancer and, probably, of other types of cancer. This is the conclusion of Prof. Meir J. Stampfer of the Harvard Medical School, following a study of 22,071 men that were treated with beta carotene and/or placebos. The group that took the vitamin contained a significantly lower number of cancer cases.

Heated Debate Over Alternative Cancer Treatments

Olivia Pilhar was only six years old and the Wilms' tumor in her stomach was as big as a football, when her parents fled with her from conventional medicine in the province of Lower Austria to Malaga in Spain. Shocked by pictures of children who had been treated with chemotherapy, they entrusted their daughter to the self-proclaimed faith healer Geerd Ryke Hamer. Chased by Interpol and hounded by the media, Hamer explained his alternative treatment to the parents. He told them that cancer is triggered by an "acute personal conflict," and that "it will go away by itself."

Olivia Pilhar: alternative treatment almost turned deadly

That Olivia survived Hamer's therapeutic nonsense is due to the fact that her parents lost custody of her for a short time. The authorities were able to fly her back to Vienna General Hospital, where doctors removed the tumor and a kidney. Chemotherapy killed off the remaining cancer cells in Olivia's tiny, weakened body. Today, she is a healthy and happy girl.

Hamer's bizarre theories—he was sentenced to jail for 19 months for other "therapies"—have discredited alternative methods of cancer treatment.

Many alternative methods are considered dubious and often rightly so. Others can have a positive effect in retarding the progression of the disease, but only as concomitant measures. Their effectiveness has either not been scientifically proven or at least not established beyond any doubt. Still, it may be useful to discuss alternative methods of treatment openly with your oncologist. Such therapies may never replace conventional treatment, but they can provide additional support.

The best known alternative cancer treatments are:
- **Immunological therapies**
- cytoplasmatic therapy: using a protein remedy derived from the organs of cows and pigs, which is supposed to correct the congenital predisposition for cancer and to strengthen the body's immune system
- factor AF2 therapy: using an organic extract from the livers and spleens of newborn sheep to strengthen the body's defense against cancer
- thymus preparations: from the thymus glands of sheep and calves
- active-specific immunotherapy ASI: three immuno-stimulating measures are employed at the same time—interleukin-2 and interferon-alpha, as well as virus-modified vaccines

Interleukin-2 and interferon are used against cancer

- autologous tumor therapy according to Klehr: the patient is given cytokines grown in cell cultures
- immuno-augmentative therapy IAT: cancer patients are injected with processed blood from their own body several times a day
- Cancer diets
- Homeopathy
- Vegetable products
- Other methods

Strange oxygen therapies, dubious petroleum treatments

- oxygen therapies: in addition to oxygen inhalation and hyperthermia, the patient is given drugs
- petroleum preparations: this method goes back to Paula Ganner, an Austrian butcher's wife, who is said to have defeated cancer that way; these treatments are supposed to kill viruses that cause cancer and strengthen the body's defense mechanisms
- oral vaccination against cancer: using furfurol, which is to increase the acid level of the cancer cells and destroy them by way of hyperacidity
- earth rays and water veins: according to this theory, patients who develop cancer are exposed to water veins, especially intersecting veins; the first thing to do is move your bed

These alternative forms of treatment are seen as a last resort for many desperate patients or their families, but the German Cancer Society recommends that patients ask themselves the following questions before deciding on such a treatment:

1. Has the method been practiced for a long time? If it has not been recognized officially, it is very likely that it is ineffective.
2. Is the method cryptic and mysterious, tied to certain people or places? The more mysterious it sounds, the higher the probability that the method is bogus.
3. Is the number of successful cases higher than that of failures? If the method promises 100% success, it is probably too good to be true.
4. Are there any side effects? Usually, if there are no side effects, the method will not be effective either.
5. Does it require a strict diet? A healthy diet is important, but any exaggeration in this regard should set off your alarm bells.
6. Do the proponents of this method condemn conventional medicine? If so, stay away. Verbal assaults and exaggerations do not make up for lack of evidence.

TEN RULES FOR PREVENTING CANCER

1. Do not smoke.
2. Reduce your alcohol intake.
3. Often eat fresh fruit, vegetables and cereal products with a lot of fiber.
4. Avoid excess weight.
5. Avoid exposure to intensive sunlight.
6. See a doctor whenever you detect inexplicable symptoms.
7. Have an annual checkup.
8. Avoid unnecessary X-rays.
9. Avoid contact with carcinogenic substances (asbestos, gasoline, etc.)
10. Regularly examine your genitals.

Men Under Attack

Osteoporosis–The Male Affliction of the 21st Century

She is the embodiment of children's nightmares. Whenever there was a full moon, the old witch would roam the area and look for children to devour. She especially liked little children. She would be waiting for her victims in a dark forest, with her hump aching and leaning on her cane. Even today, the wicked old witch frightens children more than Stanley Kubrick's movie, "The Shining."

Fairytale witch: perfect example of osteoporosis

Jacob and Wilhelm Grimm, who created Hansel and Gretel at a time when Louis XVI was executed and French troops were retreating to the Rhine, were true visionaries. Grimm's witch lived an isolated life on the margin of society. Her ill will was the result of her ailments and constant pain. The Grimm brothers, in their description of the witch, captured one of the most fundamental ailments of modern women—osteoporosis.

Witch's hump = osteoporosis

What Jacob Grimm could not know in 1860, three days before his death when he wrote his "Discourse on Aging," was that in the 21st century, osteoporosis, which became the mark of the witch in fairytale land, would threaten the well-being of the modern man.

Estrogen—The Bone Density Hormone

Femoral neck fractures are more and more common among men

Discussion of this problem is so new that the Herald Tribune, in April 1999, called the discovery revolutionary. In the next ten years, femoral neck fractures caused by osteoporosis will be as common among men as among women. This holds true for any age group, but especially for those between 40 and 50. The ratio in this age group is still about three women to one man, but among older age groups, that ratio has already been reduced to two to one. So, man in the 21st century will be confronted head-on with a new disease.

Until recently, osteoporosis experts focused exclusively on women. Only five years ago, at a scientific conference, the speakers claimed they did not really know anything about male osteoporosis. It is quite clear why. Men do not develop osteoporosis until they reach a more advanced age, but men's life expectancy has always been below that of women. Therefore, it has never been an issue in the past.

13% of men suffer from osteoporosis, and their number is growing

While we can assume that 25% of women will develop osteoporosis in the second half of their lives, the corresponding percentage for men is currently 13%. Although men are usually at risk of bone fracture, especially femoral neck fractures, about five to ten years later than women, osteoporosis in men will become a bigger problem in the next few decades, both in terms of health policy and health economics.

Recent statistics from the American health sector show that annual costs related to osteoporosis account for about $14 billion. Even now, three billion of it is spent on osteoporosis-related bone fractures in men. No American health economist doubts that this will increase further. The problem is that even a slight decrease in bone density puts men at risk of bone fracture. Men also have a higher rate of morbidity and mortality in the case of femoral neck fractures than women.

According to the Journal of Endocrinology, which published a new study from the Mayo Clinic, male osteoporosis has so far been attributable to an unhealthy lifestyle or as a secondary disease brought on by the use of certain drugs. However, hardly anyone has established a link between osteoporosis and hormonal changes. The most recent findings of the Mayo Clinic show a clear correlation between low bone density and a low level of estrogen (estradiol). Finally, there is scientific proof that the bones of men are also heavily dependent on sex hormones—steroids, in particular.

Too little estrogen reduces your bone density

Production of the estrogen hormone, the main ingredient in bone density, declines more significantly in women in midlife than in men. Therefore, osteoporosis in men is, statistically speaking, still of lesser importance.

But one thing is sure. The book on osteoporosis needs to be rewritten, especially the part about how male bones become brittle.

The Male Skeleton

Men usually have no problems with their bones. That is why we do not really appreciate how important they are. We do not think about our bones unless they are being destroyed by disease or broken in an accident.

Bones primarily provide support by bearing the weight of the body. The weight that rests on the bones of the feet becomes even more of a strain when we run or jump. A single bone may have to absorb several hundred kilograms of pressure. Apart from their function as part of the locomotor system, bones also provide protection to organs such as the brain or the heart. A lot of people do not know that bones also store calcium. Life is not possible without calcium. It is responsible for a number of bodily functions, and it controls processes in our cells as well as, in the form of lime salts, for the stability of our bones.

The bones withstand the force of hundreds of kilograms

Calcium is necessary for bone stability

The Eiffel Tower in Paris is a symbol of human achievement, of proving the impossible possible, but also of firmness, inner stability, support and enormous endurance. In a way, it is a perfect representation of long tubular bones. Our bones contain concrete-like, compressed lime salts, connected to tensile fibers. This allows for a combination of high stability and elasticity. That is why we can lift heavy weights and exert great force. This ingenious "Eiffel Tower" of a skeleton could be called the work of a consortium of three different task forces:

- bone-forming cells (osteoblasts)
- cells resorbing calcified bones (osteoclasts), and
- osteocytes, or bone cells that have ceased activity and become embedded in the bone matrix.

Recent advances in the understanding of bone growth and in the diagnosis and treatment of bone disease have brought about the discovery of messenger substances that can motivate these three cell types or, in worst case scenarios, demotivate them or cause them to dysfunction.

Bones are dynamic tissue

Bones are made up of dynamic tissue, which is subject to a continuous, coordinated restructuring process. This process is regulated by a balance between bone formation and resorption characteristic of a given age.

The spinal cord keeps changing until age 35

During bone formation, the osteoblasts are more active than the osteoclasts. A balance between osteoblasts and osteoclasts is reached when all the bone mass has been formed. But the formation of bone mass does not end with linear growth. For example, thigh bones are usually fully grown around the age of 25, but bone formation in the spinal cord continues until the age of 30 or 35. At this point, people reach their individual "peak bone mass."

The higher the peak bone mass, the fewer the problems

Every person has his or her own peak bone mass—the maximum mass of bones that is formed over the course of a lifetime. The larger the peak bone mass, the fewer problems there will be once osteoporosis sets in. Thus, the peak bone mass is an important factor when it comes to determining a person's risk level.

The Skeleton—An Eternal Construction Site

So, what determines whether a man has more or less bone mass? What can we do to stimulate bone formation?

After reaching its peak bone mass, the system remains stable for a time. Following a period that lasts several years (plateau phase), bone mass starts to decline as a result of the aging process. That decline is usually 0.5% to 1.5% of the original mass per year. Osteoporosis affects everyone, including people who feel perfectly healthy.

The reduction in bone mass is currently attributed to two phenomena:

1. A relatively incomplete formation of bone mass during adolescence and early adulthood, so that the bone density and mineral content of the bones are insufficient at the time the skeleton stops growing
2. A loss of bone mass that exceeds normal age-related attrition

The coordination of the rebuilding of bones is the result of systemic and local regulatory processes. Bone remodeling is a local and cyclic process that consists of the following phases:

1. activation
2. resorption
3. new formation
4. idle phase

The Interaction of Hormones

Bone metabolism is controlled by a network that includes the cellular effects of certain hormones, growth factors and cytokines.

The 'concrete'—calcium—is supplied by the vitamin D hormone (1,25-dihydroxy vitamin D3), the parathyroid hormone and calcitonin.

In addition to these, various other hormones affect the bone metabolism. These include the thyroid hormones as well as the male (testosterone) and female (estrogen/estradiol) sex hormones. Also important are cortisone and the growth hormone. Among the growth factors, interleukins/cytokines and prostaglandin bear mentioning.

Osteoporosis may be caused by impaired bone formation, by a permanent accelerated loss of bone mass, or by an accelerated loss of bone mass for a limited period of time.

Generally, there are two types of osteoporosis:
- Type 1 is almost exclusive to women; it affects the vertebral bodies of the thoracic and lumbar parts of the column.
- Type 2 affects women and men in a ratio of three to two; it affects the ver-

tebrae and the tubular bones, often in combination with femoral neck fractures or fractures of the lower arm.

Warning Signs of Osteoporosis in Men

Being underweight is bad for the skeleton

Unfortunately, there are no clear warning signs. The general risk factors include alcohol, poorly balanced diets, impaired absorption of calcium and vitamin D in the intestines, nicotine and insufficient body weight.

Recently, two very different, yet typical, male patients came to see us in our office. One of them, a 45-year-old manager in the cosmetics industry, had spent about $10,000 on dental implants. But only a few months later, the implants had fallen out. The man, who had not had any medical problems and who appeared in good health, could not explain it. So, he had them replaced at great expense. After a few weeks, the new implants had also started to come loose. He came to us for some advice. After taking his case history, gauging his risk factors and measuring his bone density, the case was clear. He had osteoporosis, at age 45.

The other patient, a 50-year-old manager in the automotive industry, complained of constant back pains. He believed that the pains were caused by his sedentary work—spending many hours in the car driving to see customers—and stress. He told us what happened when he was shopping in his usual men's clothing store. The salesperson joked with him and said that he appeared to be getting smaller, and that his arms suddenly seemed longer relative to his height.

After a short examination, X-rays of the entire spinal column and the pelvis as well as a bone density test afterward, the diagnosis was quite clear. A small partial fracture of the upper plate of a vertebra was the source of his pain, and the distance between several other vertebrae was diminished as a result of osteoporosis.

Diagnosis of osteoporosis in men is relatively easy

These two examples illustrate very well how simple the diagnosis of osteoporosis can be. First, the doctor talks with the patient to take his case history (genetic factors) and to learn more about his earlier diseases, lifestyle and exposure to the risk factors. Laboratory tests are then done on the blood, urine and hormones. The so-called bone metabolism parameters are also determined. In addition, X-ray and computer tomography tests are done. The bone density can be measured by means of an ultrasonic bone evaluation and DXA (dual X-ray absorptiometry), which can also be used with children.

It is recommended that women first have a basic bone density test around the age of 50. Men should do the same by the age of 55. There are many possible prophylaxes and treatments. Bones are very hormone-sensitive, and we can often detect hormone deficiencies by just looking at them. Hormone-replacement therapy is possible here.

Tip: after age 55, regular check of basic bone density

But it should be our goal to avoid having to undergo treatment (with or without drugs). Early detection must be the ultimate objective. There should be genetic screening and tests of peak bone mass, even in adolescents and young adults.

Individualized hormone-replacement therapy is helpful to men

On the basis of such early measurements, it is possible early on to identify those at risk of developing accelerated osteoporosis or complications later in life.

The public needs to be better informed of the risk factors. Men must realize that unhealthy bones are not just a "female thing." After all, men will one day soon be especially hard hit by osteoporosis. Educational materials to raise awareness of osteoporosis should be available through the media, insurance companies and doctors.

Proper Prevention

The following are essential to preventing osteoporosis:
- exercise
- an adequate supply of calcium (1,000 milligrams a day)
- sufficient levels of sex hormones

1,000mg of calcium per day can prevent osteoporosis

Physical exercise to maintain muscles and bones is important during the early years of bone formation, as well as between the ages of 20 and 60. The diminution of bone mass with age, according to international studies, is the consequence of muscular atrophy due to lack of exercise. You should exercise with weights up to the age of 40. Other effective prophylactic sports are jogging, walking, tennis, cycling, dancing, jumping rope, cross country skiing and weightlifting.

Light power training is important for the body

Here are some further measures for the prevention of osteoporosis:
- Cut down on coffee. You should not drink more than three cups a day.
- Avoid too much roughage in your diet, for it binds calcium in your intestines and can impair your calcium absorption.
- Avoid large quantities of protein in your diet.

Reduce coffee, roughage, protein and nicotine

● Cut down on alcohol and avoid nicotine. Do not go on drinking binges and stop smoking.

For treatment, there are a number of drugs, apart from sex-hormone replacement, that can be administered—so-called biophosphonates, calcitonin, calcium, vitamin D and fluorides. But their use must be closely monitored by a doctor. Medical research is constantly coming up with new kinds of treatment and better drug therapies for osteoporosis. Everything discussed here was state-of-the-art at the time of writing this book.

The Future: Genetic Risk Analysis

In the near future, it will be possible to identify high risk groups at birth by way of genetic testing. Preschools and schools will set up special exercise and dietary programs as osteoporosis prophylaxis, but there will also be special programs for society at large.

Special exercises in adolescence and early adulthood can work toward increasing the peak bone mass.

Around 2020: androlgists will fight osteoporosis

By about 2020, there should be specially trained andrologists, doctors for men, who will regularly measure bone density and check hormone levels for early preventive measures. May the human skeleton be as robust as the Eiffel Tower.

Heads Up

What You Can Do About Hair Loss and Baldness

Every man has 100,000 hairs, on average

It happens so slowly that you may not even notice it. But at some point, you are going to wake up to a receding hairline. It is a sign that the approximately 100,000 hairs on your head are disappearing, one at a time.

What happens next is every man's nightmare. The hair becomes thinner, bald spots appear at the back of your head and pouf, you are bald.

Baldness, or alopecia, is one of the worst signs of aging because it affects not only your hair, but also your ego.

A second type of male hair loss, which affects almost one in four men, is characterized by the hair at the top falling out, leaving a diffuse pattern. At the end, you are left with a circle of hair and a bit of hair on the temples.

Aromatherapy and Gene Therapy

For the longest time, there has been no remedy for baldness. It was only in 1999 that international headlines caught the attention of men: "Aromatherapy helps against circular hair loss." Hair loss, which is mostly hormone related, can be effectively treated with aromatherapy, using essential oils like thyme, rosemary, lavender or cedar. A controlled study in Scotland involving 84 patients confirmed this. After seven months of therapy, 44% of the treated patients showed a clear improvement against only 15% in the placebo group.

Aromatherapy helps in 44% of cases

Scientists at Columbia University created some headlines of their own. They managed to genetically transform normal skin cells of mice into hair cells. The key was in the genetic code for the protein beta carotine. This protein appears to be responsible for the "reprogramming" of the skin cells. But this process cannot be controlled yet. The mice used in the study ended up with uncontrolled cell growth.

What is hair loss? How does it happen? It is a dynamic process. Losing about 100 hairs a day is considered normal. The density of the hair not only depends on the amount of hair lost, but also on the hair that grows back. In general, everyone starts losing hair after the age of 25. For men, balding is part of the natural aging process.

Losing 100 hairs a day is normal

Hair loss seems to be caused by a number of factors, though there is still much research to be done. Genetic predisposition accounts for 90% of all cases. Other factors include the body's own immune system, psychological or nervous disorders, eating and metabolic disorders, the use of some drugs, high fever with severe diseases, hormonal imbalance, stress, shock, mechanical factors (some hairstyles, such as the ponytail, cause the roots to be pulled constantly, which may result in hair loss), iron deficiency as a result of anemia, and the treatment of cancer using drugs.

On average, our hair grows about one-third of a millimeter every day, which is 1.27 centimeters per month. Dark-haired people have about 100,000 hairs, red-haired people have about 80,000, and blonds have 120,000. If we take all the hairs and add them up, we can say that dark hair grows about 30 meters a day and blond hair about 36 meters a day, or 12 kilometers a year.

Our hair grows 30 meters every day

14% of our hair is dying off

Each hair has its own root, the so-called follicle, from which it grows. About 85% of all hairs are actively growing, which takes about three years. Roughly one per cent are in a transition period, meaning they grow more slowly and lose their connection with the root. The remaining 14% are dormant, and fall out when you comb, brush or wash your hair. Then, the cycle starts anew. With hereditary predisposition to excessive hair loss, hormones cause the follicles to shrink and the growth period is shortened. Finally, only a near-invisible fuzz is growing on the scalp.

The Fault Is in the Genes

90% of hair-loss cases are hereditary

About 90% to 95% of cases of excessive hair loss have genetic causes. Male hair loss is characterized initially by a receding hairline and a "tonsure" at the back of the head. By the end of the process, these two areas have merged into one, and only a circle of hair remains.

An article published in the British Medical Journal in 1998 summarized all the facts and information about hair loss known at the time. It states that premature male hair loss is due to a hereditary oversensitivity of the hair roots to male hormones. The article went on to point out that eunuchs were never bald.

By age 30, 30% of men experience hair loss

Every white male has this hereditary predisposition, with 96% losing their hair to a certain extent. By the age of 30, 30% of all white males suffer from male (androgenetic) hair loss. By 50, it is 50%. White males are four times as likely to go bald as black males.

Baldness takes 15 to 25 years

Hair loss does not usually set in before the end of puberty, but the rate can differ greatly. In some men, baldness takes less than five years. In most cases, it takes 15 to 25 years. The progressive loss of hair, in fact, is characterized by different phases with different rates. Such phases may last three to six months, followed by inter-phases of six to eighteen months.

The fact that hair loss only occurs in the presence of the male sex hormone testosterone shows very clearly how important hormones are to hair growth. Men produce testosterone in the testicles and the adrenal glands; women produce it in the ovaries. Not only testosterone, but its catabolite dihydrotestosterone (DHT), also plays a key role.

The question of whether hair loss is purely genetic can be answered by performing a trichogram—examining hair roots under a microscope. Dr. Angela

Christianof of Columbia University in New York City published an article on what she called the "nude gene" in the science magazine Nature in April 1999. The researchers believe that the nude gene works like a switch that can turn other genes on and off. The studies began with a bald patient who also suffered from a weakened immune system. In tests, the nude gene is to be transplanted to the scalp to see if it can trigger hair growth. Gene therapy is expected to provide a treatment for baldness.

Is the nude gene to blame?

I'm Bald—No Problem

Hair loss, for most men, is a major psychological blow, one that can seriously affect their self-esteem. Only 8% of men with normal hair growth say that baldness would be a problem for them. But this is in stark contrast to the results of a study that shows that 50% of men with light hair loss and 75% with medium to severe hair loss are, in fact, quite concerned. They said that they felt less attractive physically and sexually than men with a full head of hair.

75% of men have a problem with baldness

Androgenetic alopecia tends to occur when there is a high concentration of male hormones (androgens). A typical characteristic of androgenetic hair loss is a growth phase (anagen phase) that becomes shorter and shorter, while the dormant phase (telogen phase) becomes longer. Since the anagen phase is essential for hair growth, the hair itself becomes shorter. This progresses until the hair does not even reach the surface of the skin anymore. Another observation with androgenetic hair loss is that the entire follicle degenerates. The smaller the follicle, the thinner the hair and the fewer pigments it has.

It is the male sex hormones that, during puberty, enable very fine vellus hair on the face, in the armpits, on the chest and in the pubic area to be transformed into healthy terminal hair. On the head, however, these hormones have the opposite effect. Pigmented terminal hair degenerates into non-pigmented vellus hair. The exact causes are unknown. But it seems that the receptors for the male hormones in the area of the follicles are activated by the catabolite of testosterone, dihydrotestosterone.

Dihydrotestosterone activates hair loss in men

Stress and unhealthy diets are also often cited as reasons for hair loss. Experts suspect that the elevated cortisone level caused by anger could play a key role.

A high cortisol level influences baldness

If your diet is imbalanced, during fasting for example, your hair roots may suffer because your body lacks the trace elements zinc and iron, which are indispensable to healthy hair growth. Vitamin H (biotin, which is found in oranges) is also of great importance in this regard.

In ancient Egypt, there were some interesting remedies for hair loss. A mixture of dates, dog paws and donkey hooves was ground up and then cooked in oil. Once it cooled down, it would be massaged into the skin. The precise effect of this concoction has not been recorded. But desperate men will try even the strangest of brews if they think it might help: groundhog fat, honey, chicken droppings, garlic tinctures. They are all useless.

Strategies for Keeping Your Hair

There are four possible reactions to hair loss. You do not do anything and sport your bald head with pride; you put on a wig; you consult doctors; or you see a surgeon who will try to cover up your bald spots with hair from other parts of your body or artificial hair implants.

The first step: see your doctor

Have your hormone status checked

Before embarking on any form of therapy, you should always get the full story behind your hair loss. The first step is to see a dermatologist. Second, see your family doctor. The doctor will do a series of laboratory tests (blood count, blood sedimentation rate, serum iron, iron binding capacity, serum zinc, total IgE, thyroid status, vitamin status, blood sugar, antibodies against autoimmune disease, etc.) as well as a complete hormone analysis including male and female hormones. If he finds an underlying cause, he may decide on an appropriate treatment.

Third, you should see an andrologist or dermatologist in combination with a doctor specialized in this area to get more answers. They will analyze your hair roots and evaluate the test results. Fourth, the expert (andrologist/dermatologist) will prescribe the proper treatment.

Effective Remedies

1.5 million Austrian men suffer hair loss

About 1.5 million Austrian men and 500,000 Austrian women suffer from hair loss. Gynecologists usually prescribe estrogen pills, which can bring about an improvement in women within a few months. Unfortunately, men cannot be prescribed birth control pills for hair growth, because the female hormones would invariably lead to feminization.

● Minoxidil

Until the beginning of the 1980s, there had been no scientifically proven drug treatment for hair loss. The first effective remedy, Minoxidil, was discovered by accident. Originally, it had been used, in pill form, for treating high blood pressure. But women experienced an unpleasant side effect. Their body hair started growing at an accelerated rate. Needless to say, Minoxidil was taken off the market as a hypotensive drug.

The breakthrough came when a clever researcher at a pharmaceutical company had the idea of marketing Minoxidil as a solution, instead of as pills. The solution, he thought, could be rubbed onto bald spots. In large-scale double-blind studies it was shown that Minoxidil could stop hair loss 50% of the time. In some cases, new hair growth was even triggered. But, for it to work, Minoxidil must be taken permanently and you must have at least vellus hair on the scalp. Minoxidil must be applied everyday in the morning and again in the evening. Side effects include reddening of the skin, itching, and lower blood pressure. Effects on potency, if any, are still unknown. The substance is available under the name of Regaine® as a 2% or 5% solution. The 5% solution acts faster and the chances of growing new hair are higher.

Minoxidil stops hair-loss in 50% of all cases

● Aminexil

Aminexil is similar in structure to Minoxidil. But this substance has not been fully tested yet in terms of efficacy and safety.

A Pill Against Hair Loss—Miracle or Fraud?

So, what about the new miracle remedy, the "pill for men?"

With androgenetic hair loss, it appears that follicular androgen receptors are activated by DHT. Since 5-alpha reductase, an enzyme, triggers the transformation of testosterone into DHT, inhibitors of this enzyme may prove to be a good starting point. The active ingredient finasteride has been sold as a prostate drug (Proscar®) for some time now. This 5-alpha-reductase inhibitor, however, can do even more. By ingesting finasteride as a therapy for baldness (sold as Propecia®), the production of DHT can be reduced. Studies show that two-thirds of patients grow new hair after two years of finasteride therapy. In another third, hair loss can be stopped. Only 1% of patients continue to lose hair. But you have to be patient, since it takes at least four months before any results start to show. People whose hair growth has not yet fully ceased have the best chance. Once you are completely bald, Propecia will not help you.

5-alpha-reductase inhibitors: new kinds of therapy

Side effect: no sex drive

What are the side effects? Studies so far have shown side effects in about 2% to 5% of subjects. These effects were primarily reduced libido, erectile problems, decline in the quantity of ejaculate and a feminization of the chest, as well as an increased risk of cancer. There is no data yet on long-term consequences. But one thing is certain: women must never take this drug, for it could have disastrous effects on a male embryo if taken during pregnancy. This is why *Dangerous for pregnant women* the manufacturer recommends that men who take Propecia use a condom in order to lower that risk, as traces of finasteride end up in the sperm.

One scientifically proven alternative is the hormone derivative 17-alpha estradiol, which comes as a lotion and is rubbed into the scalp. Since not much of it gets into the bloodstream, there should not be any side effects.

Steroid solutions can stop hair loss as well

You will also find in the stores numerous other hair growth remedies, but they have not been tested clinically. These include alcohol solutions containing steroids, estrogen solutions (1% estradiol) that are massaged into the scalp three times a week, foltene, Priorin®, and others. You may also find tablets or capsules such as Gelacet (contains gelatin, vitamin A and L-cystine), Tamtogar (contains calcium-D panthotenate and L-cystine), biotin-H (contains vitamin H), siliceous earth, selenium, iron and zinc.

Hair Implants

Last but not least, there is always surgery. This involves the transplantation of artificial hair or hair from elsewhere on the body. For this purpose, real hair is woven together with the remaining hair. But this only lasts for about four to six weeks and the procedure has to be repeated. If you want something permanent, be careful. Experts warn of a relatively high rate of complications stemming from artificial hair implants. In more than 50% of cases, the implants fall out and leave scars on the scalp.

Half of artificial hair implants fall out again

In transplanting body hair, hair roots are taken from the neck and transplanted to the bald spots. If the hair is taken from a spot that is also affected by hair loss, it will fall out again after the transplant. The common methods are "punch-graft" and "slip-graft." In both cases, entire tufts of hair are taken from elsewhere and implanted in the bald spots. By the punch-graft method, the implants are punched in by means of a drill. By the slip-graft method, minuscule pieces of skin with one to three hairs are inserted into bald spots through a tiny incision, under a microscope. The whole procedure takes three sessions, six months apart.

> **TIPS FOR YOUR HAIR**
>
> ● Wash your hair as often as you like, but use mild shampoos.
> ● Avoid strong rubbing and massaging when washing your hair; also, when drying your hair with a towel, do not rub too hard.
> ● Do not blow dry oily hair for too long; just let it dry on its own.
> ● Do not wear tight hats, caps or scarves.
> ● Change your pillow more often than the rest of the bed linens.

Snoring as a Health Risk

How to Silence Those Nightly Disturbances

Has anyone ever told you that you snore? If so, did you react with disbelief and denial? But what if your partner is right? Or did she just dream it?

With increasing age, men are more likely to snore. A large-scale epidemiological study in the US has shown that about 30% of all men, nearly one in three, snore every night or every other night.

30% of men snore

Men are more likely to snore than women (only 15% of women snore), and older people are more likely to snore than younger ones. It is a proven fact that snoring increases significantly after the age of 35. About 60% of men between 40 and 65 are habitual snorers. Snoring is not only bothersome for the partner, it may also be the sign of a serious condition.

Snoring is caused by the vibration of the mucous-membrane muscles in the throat when you sleep. The muscles relax and the tongue falls back. People who snore often experience daytime fatigue, reduced performance and headaches in the morning. They gain more and more weigh, have high blood pressure and experience nocturnal arrhythmia. This may be the preliminary stage or symptom of a serious sleep-related condition, so-called obstructive sleep apnea. A number of scientific studies have shown that snoring may be a factor in cardiovascular disease, hypertension, angina pectoris and strokes. Snorers have considerably higher blood pressure even while sleeping than people who do not snore. This is important in terms of prognosis and treatment.

Relaxed mucous-membrane muscles vibrate

Snorers complain of daytime fatigue and reduced performance

The Triggers

Men's snoring: 70 to 90 decibels

Many men snore after consuming a lot of alcohol, with the snoring reaching levels of 70 to 90 decibels (about the same as a busy highway). If you are among those typical "party snorers," try spending a nice evening without alcohol.

Sleeping pills cause snoring

Certain drugs (sedatives, sleeping pills, allergy medication) can also trigger snoring.

Those who are 20% overweight snore

One of the main causes is obesity. It has been confirmed that men who are 20% to 30% overweight almost always snore. The extra weight results in the elevation of the diaphragm, reduces the lung volume and leads to more fat being deposited in the throat. Shallow respiration is another consequence.

Other causes include dry bedrooms that are not aired often enough and are overheated. If you snore, you should consider getting a humidifier, opening a window or, at least, airing the bedroom regularly. Optimal room temperature is about 18C (65F).

Breathing problems during sleep can be life threatening

Sleep-related respiratory problems may be life-threatening. During the day, you might doze off behind the steering wheel and cause an accident.

Are Hormones to Blame?

Other factors probably include the body's own hormones. Snoring and sleep disorders are often associated with hypothyroidism (diminished muscle strength). The hypothalamus hormones may also affect respiration.

Smokers more likely to snore than non-smokers

Another big risk factor is smoking. Smokers are more likely to snore than non-smokers. Even once they have quit, smokers are still more likely to snore. Scientists believe that nicotine makes the upper respiratory tract more sensitive. Genetic factors also come into play. You have a higher probability of snoring if there are, or have been, blood relatives who snore.

In children and adults, polyps of the nasal mucous membrane (benign growths) may trigger snoring or further aggravate it. Such polyps are relatively easy to remove. But often polyps are the result of allergies or a chronic inflammation of the sinuses. Tests are underway to see if polyps can be "washed out" using cortisone.

At times you will see athletes on TV using small strips of adhesive on the nose in order to stretch the nasal concha. These may also be used as a remedy for snoring.

How Do You Sleep?

Do you prefer to sleep on your side, back or belly? It is known that people who sleep on their backs are more likely to snore because the tongue pulls the lower jaw back, which constricts the throat. This is what causes those nasty noises. A harmless trick is to sew a tennis ball into the back of your pajama top. This way, you will wake up whenever you lie on your back and automatically turn over.

A tennis ball sewn into pajamas prevents snoring

First Aid Against Snoring

In the last twenty years, more than 300 different types of therapy or surgical intervention have been attempted. The variety of these experiments shows that snoring is not a uniform condition, but one that differs from person to person.

We believe that drug therapy involving treatments such as progesterone, protriptyline or other drugs is not really effective and even leads to side effects that clearly outweigh any benefits. Only patients with metabolic disorders, such as acromegaly or hypothyroidism, should undergo hormone therapy.

Progesterone is not a remedy for snoring

In serious or habitual cases of snoring, the first important step is to lose weight. Even a few pounds can improve the situation. If you are afflicted with this problem, stay away from alcohol before going to bed and do without sleeping pills and sedatives.

Interestingly, coffee and soft drinks that contain caffeine can actually bring some improvement when taken in the evening. The reason is that caffeine makes sleep easier and thus reduces snoring. However, this only works for people who do not suffer from sleep disorders.

Coffee can ease your snoring problem

If these simple measures do not help, you may want to consider surgery. Before you decide to undergo surgery, however, you should see an otorhinolaryngologist for an exam. The specialist will check whether the soft palate, the tonsils or the uvula are anatomically oversized. Depending on what is found, the situation may be correctible with a laser, by tightening the soft palate. The last resort for extreme snorers is to wear a facial mask during the night in order to create excess pressure, which keeps the respiratory tract open.

Otorhinolaryngologist checks the soft palate and tonsils

A SNORING SELF-TEST

	YES	NO
● Do you snore at night?	☐	☐
● Have you ever woken up because of snoring (or has your partner been woken up by it)?	☐	☐
● Have you (or your partner) ever noticed respiratory arrest?	☐	☐
● Do you sometimes have headaches in the morning?	☐	☐
● Do you often feel like you did not sleep well or enough?	☐	☐
● Do you tend to forget things?	☐	☐
● Do you often feel very tired during the day?	☐	☐
● Do you easily fall asleep over monotonous activities?	☐	☐
● Do you easily fall asleep watching TV or reading?	☐	☐

If you answered at least two questions with a yes, it is likely that there is a problem with your nocturnal respiration. Consult a specialist or a sleep clinic.

Obstructive Sleep Apnea

5% of men suffer from apnea

Five percent of men who snore suffer from obstructive sleep apnea. The relaxation of the throat muscles in your sleep that produces excessive snoring can close up your respiratory tract completely. This occlusion can be overcome initially by breathing harder and thus extending the muscles of the thorax. But often, even this effort is not enough to compensate.

Oxygen drops to a level comparable to being at an altitude of 6,000 meters

The result is an odd pattern of breathing. The thorax is lifted and the belly is lowered, but no breathing can be detected at the nose or mouth. Because of the occlusion, no air passes through the mouth when inhaling, which causes apnea, or respiratory arrest. Consequently, the blood oxygen drops to a level comparable to one that would be typical during a mountain tour in the Himalayas at 6,000 meters (20,000 feet).

Those drops in the oxygen level result in a "waking-up" response, which increases tension in the throat muscles. This is followed by heavy breathing and a triggering of the sympathetic nervous system which, in turn, may bring on tachycardia. In really serious cases, there may be as many as several hundred apneas a night.

Snoring is the most common symptom of this condition. If your partner observes such respiratory arrests, then it is the first sign that you have this condition. Someone who wakes up a hundred times a night cannot possibly be fully rested. Of course, the result will be daytime fatigue and a tendency to fall asleep the next day, especially when engaged in a boring or monotonous activity.

Daytime fatigue causes road accidents

In one of the classic causes of road accidents, the driver falls asleep behind the wheel. Other consequences may be headaches in the morning, mood swings, stupor and impotence.

If you are not sure if you suffer from this syndrome, go to a sleep clinic and have a polysomnography done. For this purpose, your brain activity, cardiovascular and pulmonary functions are measured while you sleep, with a series of sensors attached to your body and head. Also measured and evaluated are such things as oxygen saturation, heart rate, breathing movements of the thorax and abdomen, snoring sounds, respiration through the nose and mouth, and brain waves.

Sleep clinic: polysomnography sheds light on the situation

Treatment for minor cases of this condition may be the same as for snoring—special positioning (prone or lateral position) and abstinence from alcohol or sedatives. You may also want to try a drug that increases the oxygen saturation (theophyllin). Some people use a kind of "mouth prosthesis," similar to the gumshields used by boxers, but this is not very popular. In more severe cases, nasal masks are used to keep the respiratory tract open.

Theophyllin increases oxygen saturation

Darkness Envelops the Soul

Male Depression

"And men are flesh and blood, and apprehensive."
William Shakespeare, "Julius Caesar"

It is Sunday morning, shortly after 7 a.m.. The place—a nice house in Ketchum, Idaho. Ernest Hemingway, 62, Nobel laureate for literature, was sitting at his massive desk. The night had just passed, but the first rays of sunlight failed to light up the darkness that enveloped his soul. The gifted writer no longer noticed the luscious green of his garden. He took his gun and shot himself in the head. All the doctor, Scott Earl—called by Hemingway's wife, the journalist Mary Welsh—could do was to determine the time of death (7:40 a.m.).

Ernest Hemingway
shot himself
because of
depression

Hemingway, who wrote such powerful books as "The Old Man and The Sea" and "For Whom The Bell Tolls," suffered from depression all his life. When he killed himself on July 2, 1961, his wife tried to cover it up as "a tragic accident while cleaning a gun." In truth, he was running away for the last time. It was the last option left to him, a man whose expressiveness influenced the literature of his century.

Hemingway would often identify himself with the heroes in his stories, whom he always confronted with the same challenges—loss, love and death. The former war reporter, who had seen frontline action in the Spanish Civil War, enjoyed portraying himself as a boxer, an extreme athlete, a womanizer—he was married four times—and a "real man." This myth, which he created all by himself, was probably one of the many things that failed him.

The British prime minister, Sir Winston Churchill, resigned from office ten years before his death in 1965—for health reasons, it was said. But it had long been known that Churchill suffered from severe depression for years.

An Austrian
anchorman admits
to depression

Robert Hochner, one of Austria's leading TV news anchormen, who has suffered from depression since he was 21, says, "I think it is a real catastrophe that depression is still seen as a taboo you just don't talk about. When it comes to the diagnosis and treatment of depression, Austria is still a developing country."

More Than 150 Million Depressed People in the World

Dark clouds casting their shadows on your mind, sadness swallowing your soul, paralyzing fear robbing you of your will to live.

According to WHO, this diagnosis affects 150 to 200 million people around the globe. In recent years, the number of cases has increased rapidly. For example, 400,000 Austrians suffer from depression. But experts suspect the figure could be as high as 1.5 million (with some suffering only temporary bouts of depression).

"Sensitive, robust, old and young people, simple and brilliant minds and more and more often those that we would have never suspected—men. Successful managers, busy freelancers, glorious athletes. Behind such smooth façades often loom severe crises of the soul. The stronger sex succumbs to it like an epidemic," reported the German magazine Stern in February 1999. The afflicted person feels unimportant and worthless and withdraws from society more and more.

Depression among men is on the rise. In 1995, 9,932 depressed people committed suicide in Germany. Of that number, 7,081 were men. Moreover, the number of men suffering from severe depression has risen by 30% in the past 15 years. And this number includes only those who actually sought help.

According to German estimates, for every man diagnosed with depression, at least four others will continue to suffer by themselves. Recent studies show that the probability of becoming depressed at least once in your life is 10% to 12%. Depression mostly affects the age group between 35 and 50 (60 for men). Originally, depression was treated as a typically female problem. Only ten years ago, twice as many women as men suffered from depression.

10% probability of developing depression

Depression is a state of dejection, worry and deep sadness. Often connected to physical suffering, it can affect the entire body and all aspects of life. A person's physical well-being, emotions, and will to live and work are affected by this condition. Hippocrates even described the characteristic symptoms of depression, which he referred to as "melancholy." Another "affective disorder" is mania. It is a state of intensive activity for which there does not seem to be any reason. A manic person has a tremendous urge to talk, yet his or her thoughts are volatile. Mania rarely occurs by itself. Most patients alternate between phases of depression and mania.

Male Menopause and Depression

Depression is the most common problem associated with male menopause, and it is closely linked to impotence and sexual problems. Depression tends to occur intermittently—the episodes may be slow in coming or happen suddenly. About 40% of all men between the ages of 40 and 60 experience, in some way or another, a feeling of lethargy, depression, increased irritability, mood swings and erectile difficulty. The symptoms of male depression are often ignored, not least because they are different from the classic symptoms. Among the reasons for our failure to recognize male depression:

Depressed men often have erectile problems

- Men are programmed for success; they have to be tough and indestructible. So, they deny having a problem.
- Men refuse to admit to sexual problems and do not understand that depression and sexuality are linked.

● The different emotional and physical problems related to male depression have not been publicized enough; as a result, family members and even doctors or psychologists often fail to recognize those signs.

In his book, Male Menopause, Jed Diamond describes the catastrophic consequences of male depression:

80% of all those committing suicide are men

● In the US, 80% of all suicides are committed by men.
● The suicide rate among middle-aged men is three times higher than among women; for men over 65, it is seven times higher.
● According to a Swedish study, depression raises the risk of attempted suicide by 87%.
● Of depressed adults, 60% to 80% never get professional or medical help.
● Proof of an inadequate health care system: it often takes up to ten years and, on average, three different doctors before the patient is properly diagnosed. On the other hand, however, 80% to 90% of those seeking help see their situation improve after being diagnosed.
● The rate of suicide is very high: approximately 15% of all depressed patients commit suicide.

The fear of being ostracized is great

Today, it is important to be young, cool, dynamic and congenial at all times. You can be everything, but not sad. "Depression is a sickness and, thus, a taboo," says Carla Stanek, the founder of the "D&A" club (depression and anxiety). In Austria and Germany, for example, the fear of being shunned is still widespread. People in rural areas tend to go to a larger city to see a doctor about their depression, instead of going to a local doctor, because they are afraid of being an outcast in their community. They are terrified at the idea that people might gossip about them.

What Causes Depression?

Various factors are responsible for depression, but every patient has his own reasons for being depressed. The factors that trigger depression in some people may not affect others at all.

1. Genetic factors

If one parent is depressed, one in five children will be too

Scientific studies have shown that the immediate family members of patients suffering from depression are very likely to have the condition too. The probability of a child's developing depression is about 20% if one of the parents suffers from the condition. American studies have also shown that the child's probability of depression is 50% if both parents are afflicted.

American and British genetic researchers have now isolated the "happiness gene" in the chromosomes 18 and 21. This gene is thought to be responsible for depression. But the idea of simply "switching off" the gene and, thus, solving the problem of depression is for now still a dream.

2. Hormonal factors

Patients suffering from depression have dysfunctional hormone metabolism and problems with neurotransmitters, the chemical messenger substances that transmit nerve signals throughout the body. Clinical studies of depressed patients have clearly shown that they have a deficiency of serotonin and noradrenaline. Some also appear to have a surplus of the cortisol hormone. In depressed patients, the receptors that neurotransmitters react with are more sensitive. The brain shows changes in metabolic processes.

Depressed patients have a deficiency of serotonin and noradrenaline

3. Physical factors

Certain diseases, such as Parkinson's or cancer, can trigger depression and despair. Some drugs, such as cortisol, can do the same. Recently, researchers have reported that depression might be caused by a virus or, at least, that such a virus might be a concomitant factor of depression.

Diseases like Parkinson's can cause depression

4. Crises

Severe depression may also be a reaction to a crisis in a person's life. Depression would be more likely to occur at major turning points, such as puberty, male and female menopause, retirement, death of a spouse; or it might be triggered by ongoing conflicts in the person's private and professional life.

5. Seasonal depression

The key factor in so-called seasonal depression is light. Less daylight in the fall and winter may lead some people to become depressed. Almost a third of people experience such mood swings as a result of light deficiency. They perform less well, they develop a craving for chocolate and their sex drive is diminished.

Light therapy, which has become more and more popular in the last few years, has been able to help people by using special light sources instead of drugs. But there are different kinds of light. Sunlight, with its specific spectrum, is the only source of natural light. Nothing can fully replace it.

Light deficiency causes seasonal depression in winter

A visit to a solarium may help to ease seasonal depression. But be careful. Just like exposure to intensive sunlight with insufficient tanning lotion, going to a tanning studio may also result in skin cancer.

CAUSES OF DEPRESSION

1. Genetics. If one parent suffers from depression, the probability of the child's developing it too will be 20%. If both parents are afflicted with depression, the child will have a risk of 50%.
2. Hormonal imbalances. Depressed patients do not have enough serotonin and noradrenaline; often they have too much cortisol as well.
3. Diseases. Parkinson's, cancer and other diseases can trigger depression.
4. Life crises. Events such as the death of a spouse, retirement or job-related conflicts can cause depression.
5. Not enough sunlight. Light deficiency in the fall and winter can lead to seasonal depression.

Depression Is an Illness

Sigmund Freud: root of the problem in childhood

According to the famous psychologist Sigmund Freud, the roots of depression can probably be found in early childhood. If, during a formative phase (e.g., the oral phase), the needs of a small baby are not properly met (i.e., either too much or too little), the child will be likely to remain in this phase of development. Self-esteem in a young person strongly depends on their environment, and on parents and siblings.

Boys are taught to hide their feelings

If this child, now an adult, loses someone dear (loss is not automatically associated with death; it could also mean separation or rejection), he or she will identify with that person in order to compensate for the painful loss. Freud also said that we harbor negative feelings in our subconscious toward those we love. The child in our example would then direct those negative feelings at himself or herself. If the two people were very close, mourning and coping with the loss will be ineffective. The survivor will punish himself or herself, which leads to depression.

Other theories are based on the notion that depression is caused by behavioral patterns imposed on a person. Boys are taught to hide their emotions. Crying, or showing sadness and fear, is frowned upon. They have to be as "tough as Daddy." As a consequence, they respond by being stubborn and aggressive as well as by building a hard shell around themselves to hide the "softie" inside. Boys often distance themselves and learn to hide their real feelings. This creates the foundation of depression, which does not set in until they are adults.

Then, there are theories that base depression on negative experiences in childhood. They claim that children develop negative thinking and relate it back to these experiences. If these types of experience recur later in life, the negative thinking pattern will be reactivated. For example, if a waiter does not take the order of a depressed person because there are five other guests ahead of him, the depressive will believe the waiter is doing it because he does not like him.

Depression is an illness and not the sign of a flawed character. It can appear only once or recur periodically. The main symptoms are:
- feeling down
- listlessness
- lack of drive, sleep disorders

Other typical symptoms are:
- lack of concentration
- reduced self-esteem
- feelings of guilt
- inhibitions
- restlessness
- anxiety
- self-inflicted injury
- loss of appetite
- loss of energy (may lead to total exhaustion)
- diminished activity
- loss or gain of weight
- ignoring activities that used be considered fun (hobbies, sports)

Panic attacks may be caused by depression

Quite often, we also experience pain or tension that seem purely physical, such as headaches, tensing up of the chest, stomach or limbs. These symptoms have long been misdiagnosed. Panic attacks may sometimes be the result of depression. A panic attack is an exaggerated reaction of the body to fear. The main factor is probably the adrenaline hormone. If an excessive amount of adrenaline is produced and released, the person experiences highly unpleasant feelings, including even greater fear.

Such attacks may be rooted in depression, but they may also have emotional causes (anxiety and panic attacks brought on by exhaustion), psychological causes (despair, no future, fear of death) and physical causes (e.g., during and after weight-loss programs). Other possible physical triggers of panic attacks are low blood pressure, side effects of drugs, withdrawal of drugs, alcohol or nicotine, taking appetite suppressants and steroids to increase performance as well as stimulants such as cocaine, LSD or cannabis. People who were abused physically, emotionally or sexually as children often have panic attacks in adulthood.

SELF-TEST: AM I DEPRESSED?

- Do you find it harder nowadays to take pleasure in activities that you used to enjoy?
- Do you find it more difficult now to make decisions?
- Do you have difficulty concentrating?
- Have you lost your self-confidence?
- Have you lost your inner drive?
- Do you feel compelled to think about the same unpleasant things over and over again?
- Do you feel worthless and are you prone to self-reproach?
- Do you experience ups and downs during the day (morning low)?
- Has your sexual/erotic drive diminished?
- Do you suffer from sleep disorders?
- Do you often feel sad, down or hopeless?
- Has anyone in your immediate family suffered from depression, addiction, or attempted suicide?
- Have you ever thought about committing suicide?

If you have at least four affirmative answers, you should immediately consult a doctor (preferably a psychiatrist).

Depending on its degree of severity, the following forms of depression can be distinguished:

1. Depressive episodes
Symptoms: melancholy; slow, tortured thinking; inner restlessness leading to anxiety; problems sleeping. Depressive episodes include:

a. agitated depression (hectic, anxiety, restlessness)
b. inhibited depression (slow thinking, lack of drive)
c. psychotic depression (hallucinations, delusions)
d. masked depression (pains, physical problems)

2. Dysthymia
Symptoms: sleep disorders; fatigue; being unhappy with oneself; occurs in adulthood; is usually chronic. This includes:
a. exhaustion depression (permanent stress, no time for private life)
b. late depression (in men after the age of 50)
c. old-age depression (between the ages of 60 and 90).

Certain types like dysthymia are chronic

There is a special form found among women: postpartum depression (after giving birth).

3. Cyclothymia (manic depression)
Symptoms: mood swings between slight depression and euphoria. The change in mood occurs without any clear reason or motivation.

The Fine Difference

"With depression, there is a difference between men and women, based on very complex factors." This was the gist of a conference on "Depression in Men and Women—A Fine Difference?" at the university clinic for psychiatry in Vienna in the spring of 1999.

When medical scientists use the word "complex," they mean to say "not empirically confirmed." In other words, they assume something to be complex that, in fact, they do not know a lot about. Those attending the conference discussed women's greater dependence on interpersonal relationships and noted that women in conflict situations are more likely to develop feelings of guilt, which may lead to depression. Women were also said to experience more problems with relationships (separation, etc.), whereas men tend to get angry and suppress such problems.

The severity of the depression and the symptoms are similar in men and women. But women are more often affected by anxiety and eating disorders, while men, when depressed, show a strong tendency toward addiction to alcohol and other substances (pills, drugs, etc.).

Depressed men take to alcohol

For biological causes, researchers are now looking into hormones. Mood swings are often linked to hormonal changes that occur around the time of menstruation, shortly after giving birth (postpartum depression) or during menopause. Estrogen therapies have proven quite successful in treating postpartum depression.

Therefore, it will be the job of endocrinologists to consider depression in the treatment of the male climacteric and to find hormonal causes. They will have to find ways to neutralize these causes by way of hormone-replacement therapy.

One notable fact about depression is that two-thirds of patients and of psychotherapists are women. In order to flee from the feeling of inner emptiness and to rebuild their self-esteem, many men seek refuge in their work or in alcohol rather than by seeking professional counsel.

Men smoke when they are sad

A recent study on smoking habits, published by the Medical Tribune of the University of California at Irvine, clearly shows the difference between men and women in their reaction to depression. Men tend to smoke when they are tired or sad, while women also smoke when they are happy. Both like to light up when they are angry or when they have to concentrate, according to this study.

How to Defeat Depression

"Health is not everything, but without health, everything is useless."
Arthur Schopenhauer

Depression can be fought in many different ways. Start with easy steps that you can control yourself.

1. Share your feelings with others

Open up to a confidant

Talk to your friends, your spouse or family members. They can give you support and a new perspective on life. A study of the Carnegie-Mellon University in Pittsburgh, Pennsylvania, has found that people are more likely to develop physical problems when their social network is breaking down. That the mind and the physical condition are linked is nothing new. The authors of the study believe that being part of a larger social network also increases the motivation to stay healthy. They even suspect that there is a "feel good factor" that controls the hormones.

2. Spend more time with other people

Engage in activities that you used to really enjoy before you started neglecting them. Regular exercise can give your life more balance and improve your mood. Make sure that you have enough time to relax and that you maintain a balanced diet with a minimum of animal products.

Keep in touch with old friends whom you have neglected.

Do not try to do too much at once. When faced with bigger tasks, divide them into smaller units and set yourself realistic goals.

3. Antidepressants

Sometimes, drug therapy may be necessary in order to weather the depression. Make sure that your doctor does not simply follow the latest fads, such as "happy pills," but devises a treatment plan customized to your needs. Those happy pills include antidepressants from the group of serotonin reuptake inhibitors such as fluctine or seroxat. These are generally used in the treatment of depression, anxiety and panic disorders. In addition to nausea and restlessness, the side effects include sexual disinterest and other sexual disorders. These would be especially counterproductive for men going through andropause. By contributing to the symptoms of andropause, they would make matters even worse. Therefore, it is of the utmost importance to consult a doctor who is very experienced with these drugs and with depression.

Serotonin reuptake inhibitors often cause sexual dysfunction

The same is true of the recently approved antidepressant effectine, which, in combination with serotonin, inhibits the reuptake of noradrenaline. This antidepressant can also cause sleep- and sexual disorders as well as nausea. A new generation of antidepressants with the active ingredient NARI (Nor-Adrenaline Reuptake Inhibitor) is considered the new miracle weapon against depression. They are safe and they act quickly. After only ten days, the patient shows tremendous progress. And, as an added bonus, like Edronax® (reboxetine), these drugs are almost without side effects.

New antidepressants are veritable miracle cures

There is no "super pill" for treating male depression that will work for all ages and individuals. The best treatment is a customized therapy program. Compound medications exist as well, which have both antidepressant and sedative effects. Drug treatment is not usually for the short term. Rather, it is continued for several months beyond the point at which the symptoms have disappeared in order to avoid a relapse.

4. Psychotherapist or psychiatrist

One solution to depression is through professional client-based therapy or behavioral therapy. With interpersonal therapy and cognitive therapy, the goal is to correct the patient's negative attitude toward life and himself. Using examples from the life of the patient, his problems are analyzed and false expectations are exposed. In the process, the patient learns techniques for solving his

Interpersonal therapy: analysis of your problems

problems by himself. Check the credentials of your psychotherapist. The chemistry between you and your therapist must be right as well.

If you feel uncomfortable during the sessions, do not hesitate to change therapists. Do this until you have found one you can truly relax with and put your trust in. This is the key to successful therapy.

WAYS OUT OF DEPRESSION

Do not wait for the big collapse. Seek help before it all comes down on you.
Do not isolate yourself. Socialize.
Talk about your problems. Talk to your friends, spouse or family about everything that weighs heavily on your mind.
Think positively. Refer to the chapter on "Mental Fitness."
See a psychotherapist. Do not be embarrassed. In the USA, every Hollywood star has a personal psychotherapist and is proud of it.

Listen to Your Body

The Proper Prophylaxis for a Long Life

Health Is Not an Issue for Men

Male conversation topics: job, soccer, alcohol

When men are among themselves, they primarily talk about job-related topics, said a new study reported in Ärztewoche, a medical publication, in April 1999. The second most common topic of conversation among men (Europeans) is soccer, followed by alcohol—they not only like to drink the stuff, but they also talk about it enthusiastically. Then, they talk about vacations and politics. The arts and theater come in last, along with women, sex and health.

"It is outright shocking," says Prof. Ebert from Münster, Germany, the director of the psychological study that was reported in the magazine, "that many men go to bars to meet people whom they think they can use for favors at some later point in time." He also finds it shocking that alcohol should be such a hot topic. Men boast, joke, scream and drink. To talk about relationship problems is a big no-no. The same goes for sexual shortcomings. Personal defeats are never discussed among men, nor are topics like preventive examinations and checkups.

Austrians and Germans take no interest in their health unless they are seriously ill. As many as 32% of Austrians questioned for a survey by the organization Healthy Austria stated with conviction that their doctors were "responsible for their patients' health." Only 22% said that "everyone was responsible for their own health." Almost as many, 20%, felt that their health was the responsibility of the social security system. Only once they are afflicted with a serious illness do 90% feel that they are solely responsible for their own health.

Men think of their health only when they are sick

According to a Fessel survey in December 1998, 54% of Austrians think of themselves as athletic, but only 20% engage in regular, health-promoting, physical exercise. Only one in two overweight people think that their condition is due to a bad diet. "Small wonder that a quarter of Austrians are overweight to the extent that it is life-threatening, but only one in two of those affected blame it on their dietary mistakes," says Ärztewoche. With a complete lack of logic, Austrians are most afraid of cancer (62%), which is responsible for 23% of all deaths. But only 13% are afraid of cardiovascular disease, although this causes 50% of deaths. It might be concluded that health awareness among Austrians, as among Germans, is catastrophic.

Barely 20% of men exercise regularly

Only 13% are afraid of cardiovascular disease

Every Austrian in gainful employment has, on average, twelve sick days a year. Overall, the number of sick days has dropped to 35.5 million in recent years. The main health problems are diseases affecting the locomotor system (7.3 million sick days) and the respiratory tract (6.7 million), industrial accidents (3 million), non-industrial accidents (2.6 million) and one million working days lost because of headaches, sleep disorders and dizziness.

Austrians have 12 sick days a year

According to a survey by the Austrian newsmagazine NEWS, 62% of Austrians claim to exercise regularly, 60% say they watch their diet, 16% stay away from alcohol and nicotine, and 13% are actively concerned with prevention.

Many serious illnesses do not just appear out of the blue. They send out silent signals that need to be noticed and interpreted. The most important job of prevention and early detection is to recognize and decode these signals.

Many conditions send early warning signals

● Head
Headaches

If you suddenly get unusually pounding, splitting headaches, it is sign that something is seriously wrong. These may occur after physical exertion, e.g., sports. Go to see your doctor. The cause may be a vascular dilatation, or bleeding, in the brain.

Pounding headaches after sports: see your doctor

Speech problems, sensory problems or impaired motor functions

These symptoms point to circulatory problems and should be checked out at a hospital.

Swelling of lymph nodes in the neck near the head

Hard lymph nodes may be signs of cancer

The lymph nodes are located in the neck around the ears, below the lower jaw and in the cervical region. They can swell up as a result of infections (e.g., purulent tooth, tonsillitis). If the lymph nodes are hard and cannot be moved, are sensitive to pressure or extremely enlarged, you should immediately see a doctor to rule out cancer of the lymph nodes.

● Eyes
Yellow eyes

Yellow eyes may point to a disease of the liver or biliary tract

If you look at yourself in the mirror and see that the white of your eyes is yellow, you may have a condition known as icterus. It is a serious symptom that indicates a disease of the liver or the biliary tract. These diseases can be quickly diagnosed with a blood sample and an ultrasound exam.

Arch of the cornea

A pale-blue whitish ring that surrounds the eye on the inside can be a sign of aging or of a high cholesterol level. It is called the lipoid arch of the cornea. Sometimes, the skin in the area of the eyelids outside the eyes shows yellowish white nodes, so-called xanthelasmas. This is a sign of fat deposits that occur with abnormal serum-lipid levels.

Swelling of eyelids

Fatigue and pale skin point to liver problems

Swollen eyelids that are difficult to open in the morning may be the sign of an allergic reaction. But if there is also swelling of the legs, extreme fatigue or a pale or grayish skin color, then the liver may be affected as a result of hypothyroidism or kidney disease. Here, too, a blood test can provide quick answers.

Light flashes

Eye doctors call light flashes, stars or sparks before your eyes (like watching an old movie) muscae volitantes, or "small flies darting back and forth in front of the eyes." In most cases, this is quite normal, but it may be linked to nervousness and bad circulation. You should see a doctor if the condition becomes chronic.

● Lips
Chapped lips and corners of the mouth

Split corners of the mouth are a sure sign of vitamin deficiency, especially of vitamins B, C, and often of zinc, too. The problem can be controlled easily through a proper diet consisting of vitamins, trace elements and minerals, as well as by using lip lotions or creams.

Chapped lips speak of vitamin deficiency

● Throat
Problems with swallowing and sore throat

These problems usually occur together with mostly trivial bacterial infections, but they may also signal the enlargement of the thyroid gland (around the Adam's apple). In smokers, these symptoms may point to growths on the vocal cords and in the throat. If they last longer than seven days, you should see an otorhinolaryngologist.

● Respiratory organs
Coughing

White and clear sputum is normal for smokers. In the event of a viral or bacterial infection, the sputum usually has a yellow-green color. If there is fever and if the symptoms last for a longer period of time, you should have a chest X-ray and seek treatment. Red-colored or reddish-brown sputum may indicate that smaller vessels have ruptured. Again, you should see a doctor to rule out any dangerous or malignant conditions.

Reddish sputum: see a doctor immediately

● Heart
Irregular heartbeat or tachycardia

We all have extra heartbeats every minute. This is no reason for concern. But if there are more than ten irregular heartbeats per minute, combined with a very uncomfortable feeling (check your pulse), then you should see a doctor, just to be on the safe side. If your pulse is constantly over 90, it may be a sign of heart disease and needs to be looked into by a doctor.

● Intestines
Blood in the stool

In most cases, this is caused by small tears in the mucous membrane of the anus, or by hemorrhoids. But do not be too certain, because blood in the stools

Blood in stool: endoscopy required

may also be a symptom of tumors in the rectum or colon. Therefore, it is best to have a doctor perform an endoscopy to rule out any serious illness.

• Kidneys and urinary tract
Blood in urine

Reddish-colored urine may be due to your diet or to a certain drink. Apart from this harmless condition, it may also point to more serious problems affecting the kidneys and urethras or to tumors of the bladder. Quite often, blood vessels in the urethra rupture after sexual intercourse. This condition always needs to be checked out by a doctor.

• Skin
Melanoma

Changes to the skin: follow this rule

Suntanned skin is one of the fashion statements of the day. But because of an increasing rate of skin cancer (malignant melanoma), it is necessary to examine yourself regularly. For each mole or liver spot, the following factors can help you determine whether you have malignant melanoma: asymmetry, localization (irregular/ blurred), color (changing color within the center) and diameter (more than 5 mm).

Watch out for dark-brown, blue or blue-black moles that resurface within a few months, grow fast and change color, itch or even bleed.

• Muscles and joints
Nocturnal spasms of the calf muscles

The most common cause of muscular tremors or spasms of the calf muscles during the night is a deficiency of magnesium. Magnesium effervescent tablets can bring fast relief. Other causes include overexertion, sore muscles or too much strain on the joints. Cold toes and pains in the calf during and after a longer walk may also be a sign of circulatory problems.

WHEN AND HOW TO CHECK

- Cholesterol: the first time at age 20, then every five years; after age 45, once a year (in the case of a family history, have the level checked sooner and more frequently).

- Blood sugar: the first time at age 20, then every five years; after age 45, once a year (in the case of a family history, have the level checked sooner and more frequently).
- Blood pressure: once a year or, in the case of a family history, regular and more frequent checkups.
- Prostate: after age 45, once a year (urologist); in the case of a family history, sooner and more frequently. Make sure that the doctor checks your PSA level.
- Complete physical exam (family physician): in your twenties, twice a year; three times in your thirties, four times in your forties, five times in your fifties; after age 60, once a year.
- Colon-cancer prevention: after age 50, have your stools checked for blood once a year and have a coloscopy every three to five years (in the case of a family history, more frequently).
- Dental checkup: at least once a year.
- Eye exam: every four to five years.

The Patient Who Has Come of Age

One in three American women and one in four American men use the Internet as a source of medical information. In the age group 18 to 40, 35% of those surveyed routinely go on the Internet to get answers to their medical queries. Among those over 55, the figure is 20%. A recent study published in the British Medical Journal clearly demonstrates that patients want more information from their doctors than they actually get. This demonstrates the necessity of providing better information and developing an effective model for prevention.

One in four men gets medical information from the Internet

The Austrian publisher of this book has set up a website (www.ueberreuter.at) where you can go to get updated facts and information about "Men's Health and the Hormone Revolution." For now, this website is available only in German, but there are many more sites out there. Just browse with your favorite search engine.

Tons of medical information is available on the Internet

Regardless of these new sources of information, it should not be forgotten that everyone is responsible for looking after their own health. Prof. Fletcher of the Harvard Medical School put it quite succinctly, "Some people want to be told what to do. Others want information to be able to participate in decisions."

This means that patients and doctors share a huge responsibility. In a time of genetic engineering, molecular-biological diagnostics, gene therapy and cloning, comprehensive counseling is more important than ever before.

Your Medical Pedigree

Know your family's
case history

About 15% of people suffering from colon cancer have a family history. One in four children whose family has a history of alcoholism will become an alcoholic later in life. The same is true of high blood pressure, diabetes and many types of cancer.

Therefore, it would be a good idea to inquire about the case histories of your direct blood relatives—great grandparents, grandparents, uncles, aunts, etc., at your next family reunion. This way, you could find out if you are at risk of one or another condition. Then, consult your doctor to plan your individual prophylactic program.

A Healthy Attitude Toward Work Is Half the Battle

Many men spend ten to twelve hours a day engaged in sedentary activities. Your work is one of the key determinants in the state of your health.

Poor posture is a
health risk

Avoid bad posture. Sit upright. You should rest your thighs on the seat of the chair and refrain from crossing your legs. Put your hands on the desk or some other surface to prevent tenosynovitis. Your computer screen should not be too high.

Drink sufficient quantities of (mineral) water, at least two liters (almost half a gallon) per day, because the air in an office dries out your body. After thirty minutes in front of a computer screen, you should take at least a five-minute break. Get up whenever you can and talk to people while standing up. Avoid large meals—it is better to have several smaller meals.

Try to reduce stress and make sure you have time to relax. Listen to your own biorhythm. When are you most active? When do you get tired? Follow your internal clock and make up your schedule accordingly. Make sure you get enough sleep and that it is regular. Try to structure your working day.

Relaxing music and full body massages are perfect means of relaxation at the end of the day. Meditation and relaxation exercises, which are easy to learn and take only ten minutes a day, can truly work miracles for you.

TEN TIPS ABOUT YOUR MEDICATIONS

1. Read the instructions carefully and follow them.
2. Inform your doctor before you abruptly stop taking a certain medication.
3. Immediately inform your doctor if you experience any side effects.
4. Inform your doctor of any over-the-counter medications that you have taken.
5. Keep your drugs in a proper place, out of the sunlight. Some drugs need to be stored in the refrigerator.
6. Dispose of expired drugs.
7. Always keep your drugs in their original packaging.
8. Never take drugs in the dark.
9. Never take drugs and alcohol at the same time—it can have disastrous effects.
10. If you take several drugs at the same time, always keep a list of these drugs with the exact time that you took them.

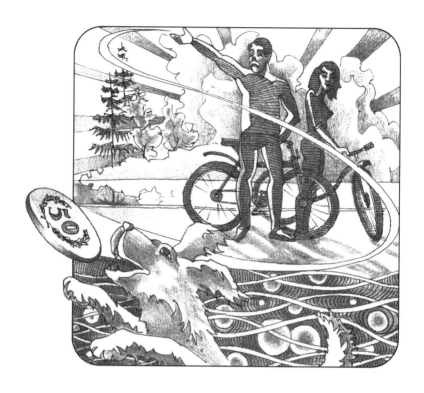

Defeating the Aging Process

The 50-Plus Generation

The Comeback of the Mature Man

He once chased after Dr. No, sent love from Russia, thwarted Goldfinger, and even lived twice. At the film festival of Cannes in 1999, he was celebrated as the actor of the century. Women go on about his sex appeal, men admire his impressive masculinity and that streak of Scottish audacity that is part of his charisma.

Sean Connery a sex symbol at 70   The American magazine People called the actor from Edinburgh the "sexiest man alive." It is hard to believe—the man is almost 70.

Sean Connery, the first and probably the best to ever play the role of James

Bond, is a textbook example of attractiveness and strength having nothing to do with age: "I feel good about myself, although I would have liked to grow old with a nice face, like Hitchcock or Picasso," says the actor, downplaying the effect he has on people. Connery's motto is to lead a healthy lifestyle and to exercise a lot. He does have a good deal of experience in that area. In real life, agent 007 used to be an athlete. He came in third in the 1953 Mister Universe competition.

The New Generation

Sociologically of no importance until a few years ago, the aging man has become a gigantic money making machine. Advertising that in the last decade only catered to a young audience with its beauty ideals and images of virility has now discovered the 50-plus generation, the "new generation." Hugo Boss, the fashion house, plays upon the charm of graying temples in its latest campaign. For the first time, men on the other side of 50 are depicted as down-to-earth, handsome and even sensuous, images that used to be reserved for youthful models.

The New Generation—the mature man as an engine of economic growth

Marco de Felice, executive creative director of the Vienna advertising agency Barci & Partner, wrote about the advantages of the protagonist of this latest trend in the Austrian daily, Kurier. "Visual stimuli suggest a certain degree of intelligence. A product advertised by someone over 30 has more credibility than a product plugged by a young model."

But this trend is extending its reach even farther. Companies are bringing back their retired top managers to train their young employees. The Austrian Broadcasting Company (ORF), for example, states in one of its advertising folders, "Age means new forms of work."

Betty Friedan, the American psychologist and social scientist who deconstructed the myths surrounding women's roles in society in her book, "The Feminine Mystique," published in the 1960s, has recently written a book on aging entitled, "The Fountain of Age." In it, Friedan argues that the cliché about aging, i.e., intellectual and physical degeneration, does not fit the reality of most older people, and that it is not scientifically proven. Convincingly, she shows, on the basis of the latest gerontological research, that cognitive and psychosocial skills increase in the course of a person's life and that the physical changes can, for the most part, be influenced.

Aging does not automatically mean decline

End to youth cult

This is a clear about-face when compared to the youth cult that has been dominant for decades. It is a definite rejection of the "deficit" model of aging. But this trend is not only about the advertising industry's discovery of the "Golden Oldies" and "senior models," or about the fact that business now views retirees as a potential new workforce. It is also about a reassessment of aging in our society, a new image of aging people.

Until recently, age, aging and death have been taboo subjects. A study done by the American MacArthur Foundation, the largest study of its kind in the world, has concluded that older people are more independent, productive and healthier than previously assumed. The fear of aging is unjustified because the gradual decline does not occur until the "bad years" set in, i.e., actual "old age."

How to Stay Young

Our society is getting older quickly. The life expectancy of an Austrian male, for example, was 74.3 years in 1997, according to the Austrian Statistical Office (women: 80.6).

In 2036, there will 82% more 60-year-olds than there are today

The number of people over 60 in Austria will be 2.07 million in 2015, which is an increase of 30% compared to 1997. The peak in the 60-plus group will be reached in 2036 with 2.9 million, an increase of 82% compared to 1997.

Life expectancy climbed by 25 years in a span of only 50 years

Anthropologists believe that the life expectancy of European men in the first millennium BC was about 20 years. By 1900 AD, this had risen to between 45 and 47 years. Yet in the following half century, that is, between 1900 and 1950, life expectancy rose to about 70 years. Is it really possible that it took nearly three thousand years to increase our life span by 25 years, but only fifty years to add another 25 years to the life expectancy of men in the West?

This doubling of life expectancy is impressive, but it is also subject to a statistical fallacy. A man who reached the age of 60 toward the end of the 19th century had a high probability of living for another nine years. On the other hand, a 60-year-old man in 1999 had a similarly high probability of enjoying another twelve years.

Quality or quantity: which is more important?

The true gain in the life span has thus only been three years. This raises the essential question: which is more important, quality or quantity?

The most substantial factor making for changes to the population pyramid was infectious disease. At the end of the 19th and at the beginning of the 20th century, infectious diseases were responsible for the premature death of many people, which minimized the statistical life expectancy.

But effective sociopolitical measures and medical progress have ensured that infectious diseases no longer have the same influence on our life span.

How to Grow Old Successfully

Today, we have a new concept of growing old successfully. The main risks nowadays are cardiovascular disease and cancer. According to recent statistical biological models, we will soon be able to vanquish all cardiovascular disease and cancer and, thus, extend our life expectancy by an additional six to nine years, but we will not be able to cross the biological limit of 120 years. As we live longer, it will become ever more important to ensure "quality aging." It really comes down to having fun in our later years, staying active and enjoying life.

Why do some people age faster than others? This is a question that has kept scientists busy for a very long time. In some families, everyone reaches the ripe old age of 100.

Some people age more slowly

We have a lot of questions, but only a few of them can be answered on the basis of what we know today. Some factors, however, are beginning to become clearer. For example, it is striking that our blood pressure rises with age (especially the systolic pressure), that serum-lipid levels increase, that body fat grows, that receptors become less sensitive to the insulin hormone that controls the blood-sugar metabolism, that our muscle mass and strength diminish, that our immune system becomes less effective and that our cardiovascular system becomes oxygen-deficient.

The blood vessels of young people, regardless of the influence of cardiovascular risk factors, show the signs of deposits typical of the early stages of arteriosclerosis. Arteriosclerosis thus seems, to a certain extent, to be a physiological phenomenon.

Blood pressure and serum lipids increase with age

But problems arise when that condition becomes more aggressive and accelerates, whether because of a genetic predisposition, or the exogenous risk factors that we can control. It is becoming clearer and clearer that the problem is

Polymorphisms of genes influence aging

not caused by a single gene, but by a constellation of polymorphisms of many different genes. The "inherited risk" does not exist unless various such polymorphisms collide. This phenomenon also explains why it is that different people react differently to the same drug, and it has an influence on the usefulness of therapy.

Genetic diagnostics will become routine

The routine use of new tools and techniques, such as genetic diagnostics (DNA chip), and our better understanding of human genes will, in the not too distant future, have a tremendous influence on medicine, on our lifestyles and on the recognition of risk factors, as well as on prophylaxis and specific treatment. But the genetic aspects aside, today it is hormones and lifestyle that determine the quality of the aging process.

THE THREE FACTORS IN GROWING OLD SUCCESSFULLY

Prophylaxis
With the right prophylaxis, it is possible to reduce the risk of disease. Have regular checkups and do not hesitate to see a doctor at the first sign of trouble.

Always learn new things
"Use it or lose it," says hormone expert Bruno Lunenfeld. "This is true of the brain as well as the muscles and the penis." You can only maintain your mental and physical functions by actively doing something with them.

Embrace life
Aging does not automatically mean that you are "over the hill." An active and positive attitude toward life is important to growing old in style.

A Doctor for Men

Comprehensive Preventive Care for Men

The time is right for andrologists

The hormone revolution, the discovery of andropause, and its scientific analysis will produce a new kind of doctor in the new millennium. The andrologist will be a doctor just for men.

In the last few decades, more attention has been given to researching female health concerns than male ones. It is high time that men also have a doctor of their own. Women have always been able to go to their gynecologist. But for this to work, it will be important to depart from the urogenital fixation and move toward a more complex view of men. Endocrinology will certainly play an important part in this. The complexity of the male body requires an equally complex therapeutic response.

Men must be viewed as complex, not only in urogenital terms

The reasons that the andrologist—a doctor who examines and treats men throughout the many stages of his life—still has not become reality are easy to explain.

- Women, because of pregnancy and childbirth, are usually more often confronted with medical care than men.
- Men have a different attitude toward aging. While women are abruptly made aware of the aging process (menstruation stops), men tend to ease into it. Men do not think it necessary to see a doctor who would guide them through this process. As a rule, men feel healthy all the time.

Men always feel healthy

- In early childhood, men learn certain behavioral patterns that shape their lives: "Real men don't feel pain," "Real men don't cry." Among friends, men never discuss their health or their sexuality. The openness that is so characteristic of friendship among women is completely non-existent among men. Male friendship may last longer, but it is never as deep as that of women, especially when it comes to health and sexuality.

Is the Typical Andrologist a Woman?

So, what should the andrologist of the future look like? It is self-evident that the urologist, with his expertise in genital and urologic matters, would be first choice. But the problems affecting the endocrine system and the influence of hormones on the body (the various extragenital organs and especially the prostate gland) have been largely ignored so far. Even the chairman of the first congress of urologists in Vienna, speaking on "Andropause—Myth or Reality?" acknowledged that urologists were about 10 to 15 years behind gynecologists as far as hormones were concerned.

Influence of hormones has been ignored so far

But there are also differences from country to country: iln Germany, internists have dealt with hormonal problems in men for a long time, whereas in Austria, hormones have been the specialty of gynecologists.

The ideal andrologist should combine the urogenital expertise of a urologist, the knowledge of general medicine of a family doctor, and the practical

Ideal: urologist-cum-family doctor-cum-endocrinologist

endocrinological competence of a gynecologist. Since there is no single person with all these skills, there will be institutes of urologists, general practitioners and gynecologists who combine their expertise to treat men. At such institutes, it will be easy to perform all the necessary tests, such as bone density scans, hormone status assessments, prostate screening, and memory tests. Extensive questionnaires will be used to assess the patient's anamnesis, and additional examinations and tests will rule out other diseases and the various types of cancer.

Diagnosis in terms of hormones

Once this analysis is complete, the doctor can draw up, say, a hormone chart. According to such a plan, one or several hormones might be supplemented or replaced. But the plan might also focus on the enzymes, i.e., those substances that produce hormones from other hormones. The andrologist should also discuss a "lifestyle plan" with the patient. By controlling the hormones, the general condition of the patient can be greatly improved, and the aging process can be effectively slowed down.

This leads to the next question. Why was all this not done 15 to 20 years ago? The answer is simple. Such examinations and tests were not practical or affordable back then, but now they are.

Hormone therapy costs about $1,500 per month in the USA

A few American centers already include the complete package in hormonal therapy, with analyses of everything from the growth hormone to testosterone. Such treatment can cost around $1,500 per month. But it can restore well-being, libido and potency in 60- or 70-year-olds.

An andrologist would basically do the same, but he would be more down-to-earth and objective about it. He would be more cautious in his approach, but work toward the same goal. Europe often copies US trends with a delay of ten years, e.g., jogging, nutritional awareness, functional food, etc. In this area, too, the gap is shrinking.

Women would make more empathetic andrologists

When looking for the ideal andrologist, we should also ask ourselves if "he" should be a woman. Many gynecologists are men. Members of the opposite sex can often analyze a situation better from the outside; women are usually more empathetic when dealing with men, yet they keep a distance.

The most successful sexologists and sex counselors are quite often women, and a particular type of woman at that—about 50 years old and motherly. This is the kind of woman that men confide in.

It should also be pointed out that it was women who started the discussion of the male climacteric. They consulted their gynecologists to find out if the symptoms in their spouses, which were quite similar to theirs, could be explained by some kind of male menopause.

Poor Medical Care

For the health of women, a lot has been done in the last few decades. Thanks to hormone-replacement therapy, it has been possible to increase average life expectancy by one-and-a-half years. What is more, this kind of therapy has also improved their quality of life.

For men, medical care is still anything but perfect. Some hospitals have outpatient departments for prostate problems, but there is no such thing for hormonal therapy or andropause. Also, the problems related to the aging process in men have always been reduced to erectile dysfunction. The treatment of more general problems was never even discussed.

Why is there no menopausal treatment for men?

While prostate cancer has about the same mortality rate as breast cancer in women, only 30% as much money that goes into breast-cancer prevention and research every year is put into prostate research.

Insurance does not even cover the costs of the annual routine check of the prostate-specific antigen (PSA), which is absolutely crucial to the diagnosis of cancer. Routine mammograms, however, are covered.

Insurance does not even cover PSA checkups

This attitude will have to change completely in the next few years. The first world congress "For the Aging Male" met in Geneva in 1998. The congress will convene every two years from now on and may have to be held every year, given the rapid development and explosion of information in this field. In any event, it has set new standards for dealing with male health issues.

World congress "For the Aging Male" to be held every two years

The authors of this book, Markus Metka and Siegfried Meryn, are involved in the organization of this world congress. They also organized the first Austrian andropause congress in May 1999.

Are Men Becoming Extinct?

The importance of having andrologists in the future is indicated by the most recent population statistics of the World Health Organization. For example, in

By 2010, 90% of 70-year-olds will be women

Russia, for 100 women over 60, there are only 60 men over 60. The WHO estimates that by 2010, the percentage of the Russian population made up of women over 70 will be 90%, while men will make up a paltry 10%. So, the question is, will men at some point become extinct?

Focus will be on prophylaxis

Clearly, it will be of the utmost importance to shift the medical treatment of men from purely curative to predominantly preventive care.

In 1998, an international association was founded in Vienna that takes a holistic and interdisciplinary approach to male health:

Institute ANDROX
The Society for the Aging Male
Rotenturmstr. 29
A-1010 Vienna, Austria
E-mail: androx@mmc.at

The Ten Golden Rules for Non-Aging

How to Grow Old Successfully

"Will you still need me, will you still feed me, when I am 64…"
The Beatles (visionaries of the 1960s)

It happened at the end of the 1920s during military maneuvers somewhere in the Mediterranean. A battleship had been out at sea for a week—the weather was bad and the seas heavy. Shortly after nightfall, the ship's mate reported to the bridge, "Light ahead."

"Is it stationary or is it moving?" asked the captain. The mate replied, "It is stationary, captain." In fact, they were on a dangerous collision course.

The captain said, "Signal to the other ship: 'We are on a collision course. Please change course by 20 degrees.'" A short time later, the other ship responded to the signal, "You should change your course by 20 degrees."

The captain got angry, "This is the captain speaking. Change your course by 20 degrees immediately." The reply: "I'm only a second-class seaman. You had better change your course." The captain was furious now and screamed, "Send the following message: 'This is a battleship. Change your course this instant.'" Then, the answer: "This is a lighthouse." The battleship changed course.

Principles are like lighthouses. They are as immutable as the laws of nature. But the principle of "Non-Aging—Anti-Aging—Successful Aging" is the responsibility of the individual. You are in charge of your own aging. It is up to you what you do with it.

Principles, like the laws of nature, are not to be broken

A study by the MacArthur Foundation published in 1998, "Successful Aging," lists three pillars of aging:
● Prevention of disease
● Maintenance of high level of cognitive functionality
● Active participation in everyday life

The three pillars of aging

Those three components fit into a clear hierarchy. The absence of disease and disability makes it possible to maintain the mental and physical functions. Mental and physical fitness, in turn, allow us to actively engage in life. The combination of all three, however, guarantees successful aging.

Of course, each of these pillars is a combination of other factors. Most of the "successful young geriatric crowd" surveyed by the MacArthur Foundation said, when asked about the secret of their success, responded that they "just keep on going."

The ideal attitude: "Just keep on going."

The three pillars of aging apply to every facet and every stage of a person's life. It is how they are dealt with that changes from person to person and with each new stage of life.

The Ten Golden Rules of Personal Responsibility

"The whole is greater than the sum of its parts."

Pythagoras

You are the only one who can redefine your life. It is you who decides the influence that aging has on your mental and physical well-being. Does aging control you or do you control aging? It is never too late to change course. The ten golden rules of non-aging will help you in achieving that goal.

1. "I"—the most important person in your life is YOU
● Eliminate "If only...," "I can't do it" and "I must..." from your vocabulary. Commit yourself to personal freedom and to making your own decisions. The greatest advantage of growing older is that you no longer have to strike

compromises. Approach your problems proactively by working on what you can control, and proceed to change your self-limiting behavior.

Set priorities
- Set priorities. Do only what you truly consider important. You wasted plenty of time on silly things in your youth. Growing older—when the path ahead of you is shorter than the one behind—gives you a new perspective on time.
- Be active—in a positive way.

Inner harmony is a prerequisite for happiness
- Start from the end: formulate your goal first, then decide how to get there.
- Listen to your body and try to achieve inner peace. Happiness is only possible through an inner balance or harmony.

2. The social "I"—socialize more.

Do not become socially isolated
- The darkest side of aging is loneliness and isolation. Try to avoid this. Look for synergies and creative cooperation in interpersonal contacts.
- Do not isolate yourself. Get out and meet new people.
- Try to understand others first so that they can understand you.
- Always think positively and be generous in problem situations, i.e., think about what you can do to ensure that both sides gain.

3. Joy, happiness, laughter—never do without them

"Most people are about as happy as they make up their minds to be."

Abraham Lincoln, U.S. president

- Happiness mostly comes from within; it has little to do with outside influences. You alone are responsible for your personal happiness.

Do not forget how to laugh
- If you are not satisfied with yourself, you will have a hard time dealing with other people when you are older.
- Do not forget how to laugh.

4. A healthy diet—essential to a long life
- Make sure to reduce your calorie intake as you grow older. Also, your diet should be balanced, and rich in fiber, vitamins and minerals.
- Do not forget about water. Drink at least two liters of water everyday.

Eat right
- Eat a lot of fruit and vegetables.
- Eat low-fat foods.
- Cut down on meat and protein. It is also better to have several small meals spread over the day than one or two large meals.

Take vitamins C and E regularly
- Make sure you get enough vitamins, especially vitamins C, D, E, B and folic acid. Vitamins C and E act as antioxidants.
- In some cases, aspirin can be taken as a prophylaxis against arteriosclerosis. Consult your physician.

5. Body and mind—always exercise both

- Any kind of exercise will make you feel better and strengthen your body.
- Climbing stairs, going for long walks or slow running—every step you take has a positive effect on your health.
- Feed your brain. It also needs daily exercise.
- Memorize telephone numbers, names, or anything to exercise and improve your memory.
- Read a lot and try to summarize the content afterward. If you find this difficult, repeat the exercise until you notice an improvement.

Exercise your brain daily

6. The proper prophylaxis and early detection of diseases

- Have your colon, rectum, prostate, lungs and skin checked by a doctor regularly.
- Heart attack and stroke prophylaxes must include an EKG and other diagnostic procedures such as ergometry.
- Watch your blood pressure, blood sugar, homocystein and serum lipids.
- Beginning with middle age, you should periodically (annually) be vaccinated for hepatitis A and B, tetanus, polio, influenza and pneumococci. Before going traveling, consult a doctor about inoculation against tropical and other diseases.

7. Normal weight—try to keep those extra pounds off

- Calculate your body mass index (BMI) and the fat distribution in your body ("apple-shaped," "pear-shaped").
- Watch your weight. Being overweight puts a strain on your heart and the cardiovascular system, even more so when you grow older. By losing weight, you can gain years on your life.

Watch your weight

8. Osteoporosis—do not underestimate the risk to men

- Increase your bone density and bone mass by exercising (the sooner you start, the better).
- Keep exercising and have your bone density checked regularly.

Sports can improve bone density

9. Alcohol and nicotine—try to avoid or cut down on both

- Stay away from smoking, and even secondhand smoke; either can shorten your life span.
- Reduce your consumption of alcohol. One eighth of a liter of red wine may actually have a positive effect on your body, but excessive consumption will counter any benefits.

Stay away from smoking and from secondhand smoke

10. Hormones—therapy can give you new strength

Hormone-replacement therapy gives you new strength

- A decline in hormone levels is what makes you grow older. You can counter this with hormone-replacement therapy.
- Consult an endocrinologist, who will explain the benefits and disadvantages to you.

Good Luck!

By following these rules, you will grow old a happy man. Life is one dimensional, with only one way to go—FORWARD!

The future is in your hands.